Intensive Coronary Care: A Manual for Nurses, 4th Edition

Library of Congress Cataloging in Publication Data

Meltzer, Lawrence E.
    Intensive coronary care.

    Includes index.
    1. Coronary heart disease—Nursing. 2. Arrhythmia—
Nursing. 3. Coronary care units. I. Pinneo, Rose.
II. Kitchell, J. Roderick. III. Title. [DNLM:
1. Arrhythmia—Nursing texts. 2. Coronary care
units—Nursing texts. 3. Coronary disease—Therapy—
Nursing texts. 4. Myocardial infarction—Therapy—
Nursing texts. WY 152.5 M528i]
RC685.C6M44   1983   616.1′2   83-2748

ISBN 0-89303-247-6

Prentice-Hall International, Inc., London
Prentice-Hall Canada, Inc., Scarborough, Ontario
Prentice-Hall of Australia, Pty., Ltd., Sydney
Prentice-Hall of India Private Limited, New Delhi
Prentice-Hall of Japan, Inc., Tokyo
Prentice-Hall of Southeast Asia Pte. Ltd., Singapore
Whitehall Books, Limited, Petone, New Zealand
Editora Prentice-Hall Do Brasil LTDA., Rio de Janeiro

Printed in the United States of America

92 93   10 9 8

Contents

TO THE STUDENT

A self-instructional workbook for this text is available through your college bookstore under the title, *Workbook to Accompany Intensive Coronary Care, Fourth Edition*, by Jacquelyn Deal, RN, (title code D2484-6). If not in stock, ask the bookstore manager to order a copy for you. If your course is being offered off-campus, ask your instructor where to obtain a copy. The workbook can help you with course material by acting as a tutorial review and study aid.

To the best of our knowledge, recommended measures and dosages herein are accurate and conform to prevalent standards at time of publication. Please check the manufacturer's product information sheet for any changes in the dosage schedule or contraindications.

Preface

The system of intensive coronary care proposed in the original edition of this book (1965) is now a well established, standard method of hospital care throughout the world; indeed, very few medical advances have been accepted as readily or with as much enthusiasm. It has been our premise from the outset that intensive coronary care is primarily and above all a system of specialized nursing care. The effectiveness of the plan in saving lives of patients with acute myocardial infarction depends finally on the ability of nurses to function as decision-making members of the coronary care team, capable of acting on their observations and judgment, particularly in emergency situations or whenever therapeutic decisions cannot be delayed. By demonstrating remarkable competence in this demanding role (and accepting the responsibilities that accompany it), coronary care nurses have broadened the horizons of clinical nursing, and have earned the sincere respect of their colleagues and patients.

We are extremely grateful for the extraordinary reception accorded the three previous editions of this book. *Intensive Coronary Care—A Manual for Nurses* has served as the standard textbook of coronary care nursing for the past 18 years; it has been translated into four languages, and more than 1 million copies are in print.

In preparing this fourth edition, we have attempted to increase the scope and depth of the presentation, while preserving its simplicity and clarity. In effect, the style of the book remains unchanged, but the text has been revised and expanded considerably. The revisions and additions are designed not only to update current principles and practices of intensive coronary care (and the management of acute myocardial infarction) but, equally important, to keep pace with the growing sophistication and quality of nursing education and nursing practice. To this end, we have provided substantially more information about all aspects of the pathophysiology and treatment of acute myocardial infarction and its complications. Also included in this new edition are:

- a brand new chapter on electrocardiographic diagnosis of acute myocardial infarction, injury and ischemia
- updated diagnostic procedures
- more anatomy and physiology
- more emphasis on ECG arrhythmia interpretation
- information on new antiarrhythmic drugs including calcium antagonists

We are grateful to Elizabeth Meholick for her indispensable help in preparing the typescript.

Lawrence E. Meltzer, M.D.
Rose Pinneo, R.N., M.S.
J. Roderick Kitchell, M.D.

Philadelphia, Pennsylvania
May, 1983

1

Coronary Heart Disease

When the incredible complexity of the human system is considered along with the vast number of possible sources of illness and death, it seems incongruous that the life of so many depends finally on the health of two small arteries; but the fact is undeniable. Disease of the coronary arteries has become the single greatest threat to life in industrialized countries throughout the world. In the United States, for example, more than 650,000 deaths a year—or one-third of *all* deaths—are directly attributable to this one disease.

As the sole blood supply to the heart musculature (myocardium), the coronary arteries assume extreme importance. Any significant interference with blood flow through these vessels can impair the entire function of the myocardium, with dire consequences including sudden death. Before describing the clinical aspects of coronary disease it is pertinent first to consider the coronary arteries and the basic disease process that affects them.

THE CORONARY ARTERIES

The two coronary arteries, the left and right, arise from the aorta just above the aortic valve. The left coronary artery then divides into two large branches: the left anterior descending artery and the left circumflex artery. The relationship of these three arteries is shown in Figure 1.1.

Each artery supplies a different area of the heart. Briefly, the left anterior descending artery supplies most of the anterior wall of the left ventricle, the anterior portion of the interventricular septum, as well as the anterior wall of the right ventricle. The left circumflex artery supplies the lateral aspect of the left ventricle and the left atrium. The right coronary artery supplies the right atrium and the right ventricle, along with the posterior portions of the left ventricle and interventricular septum. The arteries lie on the outer surface of the ventricles and give off numerous branches that penetrate all parts of the heart (Figure 1.2). The terminal branches of the arteries have many interconnections, forming an extensive vascular network throughout the myocardium.

The function of the coronary arteries is to bring oxygen-carrying blood to the myocardium, oxygen

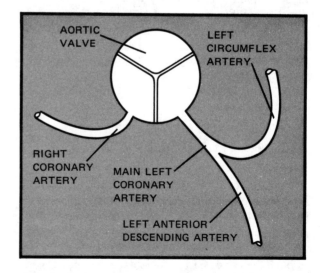

Figure 1.1. The coronary arteries as viewed from above (looking down at the aortic valve).

1

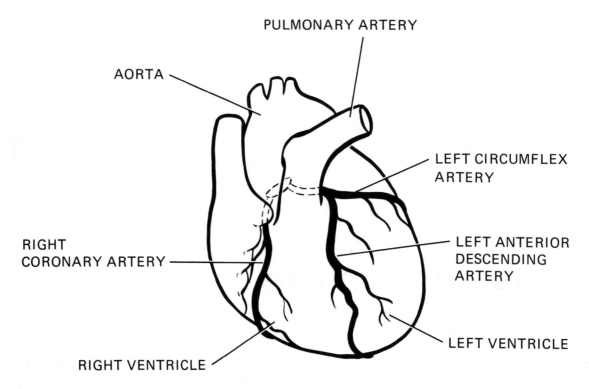

Figure 1.2. Coronary circulation.

being an essential ingredient in producing the energy the heart requires to contract. As a pump that works incessantly (contracting more than 100,000 times a day), the myocardium has very great oxygen needs. This constant demand can be met only by an adequate coronary blood flow. Indeed, 250 cc of blood per minute—or 36,000 liters per day—pass through the coronary arteries to oxygenate the myocardium under normal conditions. The oxygen demands of the myocardium increase greatly with exercise or emotional stress. Since the heart utilizes nearly all of its available oxygen supply even with normal activity and has a very limited oxygen reserve, these additional needs can only be satisfied by an increase in coronary blood flow.

CORONARY ATHEROSCLEROSIS

The primary disease affecting the coronary arteries is atherosclerosis, a process in which fatty substances (particularly cholesterol) deposit as plaques along the inner lining of the vessels and narrow the passages. If the narrowing reaches a stage where the blood flow through the arteries is insufficient to meet the oxygen demands of the myocardium, then coronary heart disease (CHD) is said to exist.

Coronary atherosclerosis usually develops gradually over a period of years. However, the process begins at an early age so that by adulthood most men (and women, to a lesser degree) have some evidence of atherosclerosis in the coronary arteries. Autopsy studies have shown, for example, that among young American soldiers (average age of 22 years) killed in action during the Korean war nearly 80% had definite signs of coronary atherosclerosis. It is essential to realize, however, that the critical determinant of coronary heart disease is not the mere presence of atherosclerosis but rather the extent of arterial narrowing and the reduction in blood flow the lesions produce. Atherosclerosis can be categorized into four grades according to the degree of arterial obstruction. Grade 1 atherosclerosis indicates that the diameter (lumen) of the artery is reduced by no more than 25%; grade 2 represents a 50% reduction, grade 3 a 75% reduction, and grade 4 complete (100%) obstruction of the vessel (Figure 1.3). An obstruction of at least 75% is necessary to produce a significant reduction in coronary blood flow; lesser degrees of narrowing can usually be tolerated without affecting myocardial function. Obstruction may occur in any (or all) of the coronary arteries, but involvement of the left anterior descending artery is particularly dangerous. This vessel supplies a much larger portion of the total myocardial mass than the right coronary and left circumflex arteries and therefore has the greatest blood flow. Even more serious is obstruction of the left main coronary artery. Significant narrowing of this short (2 cm) vessel causes a reduction in blood flow through *both* the left anterior descending and left circumflex

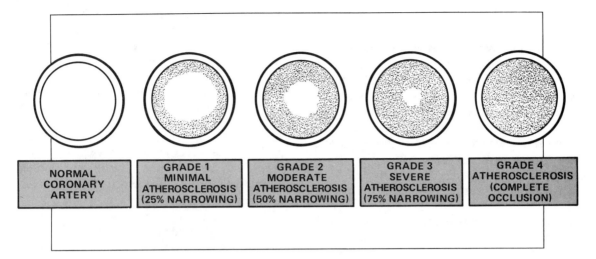

Figure 1.3. Criteria for the four grades of atherosclerosis.

arteries and therefore compromises the blood supply to nearly all of the left ventricle. Fortunately, obstruction of the left main coronary artery is the least common lesion of the coronary circulation, occurring in only 5-10% of patients with symptoms of CHD.

The site and extent of arterial narrowing can be determined by means of *coronary arteriography,* a technique that permits the arteries to be visualized by x-rays. The procedure involves the insertion of a catheter into the root of the aorta (by way of a peripheral artery) and the injection of a radiopaque dye through the openings (ostia) of the two coronary arteries. As the dye is being injected a rapid series of x-ray films or photographs (cineangiograms) are taken to outline the entire arterial tree; significant lesions can readily be detected in this way. Figure 1.4 compares a normal coronary artery with one that has a 90% obstruction.

CAUSES OF CORONARY HEART DISEASE

An unrelenting search has been in progress for more than 50 years attempting to ascertain why and how the coronary arteries are affected by atherosclerosis. The question has never been answered, and the cause of coronary atherosclerosis remains unknown. However, one fundamental fact has emerged: a combination of several factors is undoubtedly involved in the development of CHD; no single mechanism can be held responsible in its own right. According to this concept, all of the following factors (called risk factors) may contribute to the formation and progression of coronary atherosclerosis.

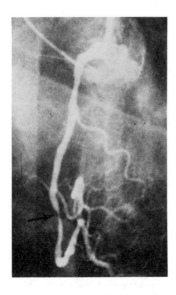 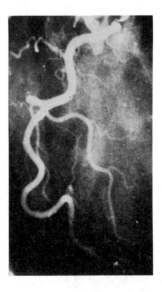

Figure 1.4. Arteriograms comparing a normal right coronary artery (right) with one that has a 90% obstruction (left).

Sex and Age

CHD is distinctly more prevalent in men than in women. Indeed, during the child-bearing years women are seemingly protected from CHD unless they have many other risk factors (e.g., hypertension and diabetes). After the menopause, however, the incidence of CHD in females rises rapidly and equals the male rate thereafter. In contrast, symptomatic CHD may occur in men as young as 30 years (or even younger). This sex-age discrepancy suggests that hormonal influences may be important in the disease process.

The incidence of CHD increases greatly with age in both sexes. For example, a man in his fifties has four times the risk of a heart attack as a man in his thirties. The fact, however, that young persons may develop CHD makes it clear that coronary atherosclerosis is not simply a disease of aging.

Diet, Cholesterol, and Lipoproteins

Several epidemiologic studies have demonstrated that the incidence of premature CHD (i.e., coronary disease occurring before the age of 60) can be correlated with the different dietary patterns of various societies. Specifically, in affluent countries (as the United States), where animal fats constitute a large percentage of the total diet, the frequency of CHD is very high; and in poorer countries, where animal fat intake is much less, the incidence of the disease is low. The gross disparity in the amount of animal fat eaten (e.g., eggs, butter, cream, milk, and fatty meats) in different parts of the world is believed to account for the fact that "normal" serum cholesterol levels in the United States may be 200-240 mg%, whereas in those countries in which CHD is uncommon the comparable levels are only 100-120 mg%. Further evidence in support of the danger of high-fat diets is the reported decrease in the number of deaths from CHD during World War II in those countries where animal fats became scarce, followed by a prompt increase in the death rate after the war ended, when the economy improved and fats again became available. From data of this type many researchers have concluded that overeating of animal fats (also called saturated fats) is a prime factor in the etiology of CHD.

More specific information about the danger of high serum cholesterol levels has been obtained from the Framingham Heart Study. In this study more than 5000 men and women in the town of Framingham, Massachusetts, have been examined at regular intervals for more than 25 years to determine which factors contribute to the development of CHD. The results indicate that the risk of a heart attack is at least three times greater in men with serum cholesterol levels of more than 240 mg% than it is in those with levels of less than 200 mg%.

Although serum cholesterol has received the most attention, other serum lipids (e.g., triglycerides) and substances that transport lipids in the blood (lipoproteins) are also recognized as important risk factors for CHD in their own right. It has been shown, for example, that elevated serum triglyceride levels (above 200 mg%) are associated with an increased incidence of CHD even though serum cholesterol levels may be normal or only slightly elevated. In other words, cholesterol and triglyceride levels are not necessarily related and a high concentration of either lipid may indicate an increased risk of CHD. Elevated triglyceride levels, unlike elevated cholesterol levels, are usually induced by the ingestion of carbohydrates (rather than saturated fats) and are commonly associated with diabetes or abnormal glucose tolerance.

Cholesterol and triglycerides, as lipids, are insoluble in plasma and are carried in the blood in combination with a group of proteins, called *lipoproteins,* that are soluble. Lipoproteins can be separated into three main classes: low-density lipoproteins (LDLs), very low-density lipoproteins (VLDLs), and high-density lipoproteins (HDLs). About two-thirds of the cholesterol in the blood is carried by LDLs while HDLs carry less than one-third. (VLDLs are involved primarily in the transport of triglycerides and carry only small amounts of cholesterol.) Epidemiologic studies have revealed that the higher the concentration of LDH cholesterol, the greater the risk of CHD. On the other hand, there is an inverse association between HDL cholesterol and the incidence of CHD. This means that the higher the percentage of HDL cholesterol (of the total serum cholesterol), the lower the risk of CHD. In fact this latter relationship appears so definite that HDL cholesterol actually seems to *protect* against CHD.*
Consequently, prediction of risk of CHD can be enhanced substantially by measuring HDL and LDL cholesterol in conjunction with the total serum cholesterol levels.

Hypertension

High blood pressure is thought to predispose to CHD by accelerating the rate of atherosclerosis and

---

*That a high level of HDL is associated with a low incidence of CHD, and affords protection against the disease, may be difficult to perceive since this type of inverse association is certainly an anomaly in medicine. Also curious is the apparently beneficial effect of alcohol on HDL cholesterol levels. Several studies have confirmed that HDL cholesterol levels are higher among those who consume moderate amounts of alcohol than among non-drinkers. The mechanism and significance of this latter relationship are unknown.

by increasing the oxygen demands of the myocardium. In the Framingham Heart Study it was observed that blood pressures in excess of 160/95 were associated with a fivefold increase in the incidence of CHD compared with normal pressures. Thus from a statistical standpoint hypertension appears to be one of the most serious risk factors.

Cigarette Smoking

There is firm statistical evidence to indicate that heavy cigarette smokers have a higher incidence of CHD than nonsmokers. In the Framingham Study the risk of a heart attack was nearly twice as great in cigarette smokers. However, the risk was associated primarily with middle-aged men and was less impressive in older men and in women. Curiously, cigar and pipe smokers are at no greater risk than nonsmokers, presumably because they do not inhale. The manner in which cigarette smoking affects the coronary arteries is not understood. The suggestion that nicotine may cause sufficient constriction of the arteries to reduce coronary blood flow has not been confirmed. On the other hand, nicotine increases the work of the heart (by increasing the heart rate and blood pressure) and could produce a relative oxygen deficiency. Moreover, cigarette smoking is associated with elevated carbon monoxide levels in the blood, which may also interfere with myocardial oxygenation. Regardless of its mechanism of action, cigarette smoking is generally considered among the most serious risk factors for premature CHD.

Heredity

A familial pattern of CHD has long been recognized, but the degree of risk is still uncertain (because family histories are unreliable in many instances). However, our own experience suggests that heredity ranks among the highest risk factors, particularly when CHD occurs during the fourth or fifth decade of life. In these latter cases it is commonly found that a man's father, grandfather, and brothers often developed CHD at about the same age. It has been postulated (but not proven) that the physical structure of the coronary arteries and the rate of atherosclerosis may be genetically determined.

Diabetes

CHD develops more frequently and at an earlier age among diabetic patients than among nondiabetics. Even when diabetes is mild or well controlled the risk of CHD remains substantially greater. These facts along with data indicating that other metabolic diseases (e.g., gout) are associated with a high incidence of CHD suggest that a biochemical disturbance may be central to the underlying disease process.

Sedentary Life

Lack of physical activity has been incriminated as a risk factor in CHD, but the evidence for this belief is still inconclusive. Several studies have revealed, for example, that CHD occurs more frequently in sedentary workers (e.g., postal clerks) than in those whose occupations demand substantial physical activity (e.g., mail carriers); yet many observers have questioned the significance of these findings, noting that there were so many other variables between the two groups that physical inactivity should not be singled out as a risk factor in its own right. Although there is good reason to believe that exercise may benefit the myocardium, it remains to be seen if physical activity (or inactivity) affects coronary arteries and influences atherosclerosis.

Obesity

Insurance company statistics suggest that obesity predisposes to fatal CHD, but (as with physical inactivity) the issue is by no means settled. In fact in the Framingham Study moderate obesity by itself was not associated with an increased incidence of CHD. However, overweight persons are especially prone to hypertension, diabetes, and elevated lipid levels, and it may be that the risk of obesity lies with these secondary effects. In any case obesity is classified as a risk factor even though its mechanism of action is uncertain.

Emotional Stress

Epidemiologic studies have consistently shown a markedly higher increase of CHD in industrialized (civilized) countries than in primitive, less-demanding societies. Many believe that this gross disparity is a reflection or a direct result of emotional stress imposed by modern, fast-paced styles of life. For this reason CHD is considered by some to be a disease of "overcivilization." According to this theory, civilized man has developed chronic anxiety in attempting to cope with rapidly changing socioeconomic and sociocultural forces, and this tension in some way promotes atherosclerosis. In principle, this is an attractive concept since it has been demonstrated that anxiety is often accompanied by a distinct rise in serum cholesterol, which could favor the development of atherosclerotic plaques. Moreover, stress is known to accelerate blood coagulation, allowing small clots to form within the coronary arteries. Nevertheless, the relationship between emotional stress and CHD has been difficult to prove, particularly since there are no available methods to actually measure degrees of stress. Some research studies in fact have cast doubt on the importance of stress as a risk factor. For example, one large investigation involving telephone company employees showed that the incidence of CHD was actually less common among high-level executives (who presumably function under great stress) than it was among workers who installed or repaired equipment. Further study will be needed to determine the significance of emotional stress as a risk factor.

Behavioral Patterns

Attempts have been made to correlate CHD with certain personality traits and behavioral patterns. The coronary-prone person—called a type A personality—is said to be one who is aggressive, ambitious, highly competitive, and, most of all, possessed with a profound sense of the urgency of time. Those with this type behavioral pattern reportedly have significantly higher cholesterol levels and an increased incidence of CHD than their counterparts (type B personalities), in whom these particular characteristics are not as apparent. This interesting observation requires confirmation, but many now accept type A behavior as a distinct risk factor.

Summary of Risk Factors

It is essential to point out that there is no definite evidence that any of the risk factors just described actually *cause* CHD. All that can be said is that individuals with multiple risk factors are high-risk candidates for CHD; conversely, the absence of these factors predicts little likelihood of developing the disease. For example, a man with hypertension and a high serum cholesterol level who is a heavy cigarette smoker may have ten times the risk of sustaining a heart attack than a person with none of these factors. In other terms, there is a statistical association between risk factors and CHD but, on the other hand, no proof that these risk factors in themselves are the direct cause of coronary atherosclerosis.

THE CLINICAL SPECTRUM OF CORONARY ATHEROSCLEROSIS

Asymptomatic Coronary Atherosclerosis

If the degree of arterial obstruction is moderate and does not significantly reduce the blood supply to the myocardium, the disease may never be suspected by the patient or the physician. Results of autopsy studies among persons dying of other causes indicate that this is a common situation. In fact, practically all men in the United States have evidence of coronary atherosclerosis by age 50; it is only the degree of involvement that varies.

Even if the coronary arteries are grossly narrowed by intimal plaques, it still does not follow that the disease will be clinically evident or produce symptoms. This paradox can be explained partly by the fact that as the coronary arteries gradually narrow small branches of these vessels may enlarge or new branches may form in order to bring more blood to the myocardium. This additional blood supply, called *collateral circulation,* is of great importance in determining the clinical effects of coronary atherosclerosis since this network of vessels is often substantial enough to maintain an adequate blood supply to portions of the myocardium despite the presence of advanced atherosclerosis in a major vessel. It is the *total* blood supply to the myocardium rather than the state of the main coronary arteries that determines whether the disease will be symptomatic.

It is important to realize there is no definite correlation between the extent of coronary artery disease and symptoms. In fact, about 30% of patients who die of CHD experience no symptoms of the disease before the fatal event.

Symptomatic Coronary Disease

Coronary heart disease, by definition, implies that the myocardium is affected by inadequate coronary blood flow. The symptoms of CHD are due to myocardial oxygen deprivation and are manifested in progressive order of severity by three main clinical patterns: angina pectoris, intermediate coronary syndrome (unstable angina), and acute myocardial infarction. Each of these syndromes is described separately in the following pages.

Angina Pectoris

The classic indication of impaired circulation to the myocardium is a distinctive type of chest pain called *angina pectoris.* The pain signifies insufficient oxygenation *(ischemia)* of the myocardium; it occurs when the oxygen demands of the myocardium exceed the capacity of the coronary circulation to supply oxygen. In other words, angina represents a signal from the heart, indicating that the myocardium is not receiving sufficient oxygen to meet its needs at the moment. Because angina pectoris is usually the key to the diagnosis of CHD, it is essential to understand its clinical features.

Site of Pain. The pain of myocardial ischemia is located most often directly under the center of the breastbone. It may radiate from this substernal location to both sides of the chest, the left or right arm, the neck, the jaws, or the shoulders and upper back. In some instances the pain occurs only at these latter sites without a substernal component; this pattern, however, is much less common than central chest pain.

Quality of Pain. The discomfort is usually described as pressure, tightness, or constriction within the chest. Some patients place a clenched fist against the sternum in attempting to characterize the tight, constricting nature of the sensation. Although angina generally lasts for only a few minutes (as described below), the pain is steady and is not influenced by breathing, breath-holding, or change in body position. This constancy of the pain is a characteristic aspect of angina and is often more significant than other descriptive qualities (e.g., burning, pressure, or "indigestion").

Occurrence of Pain. Any situation that increases the myocardial demand for oxygen is capable of producing angina. In general, oxygen demand is determined by the amount of work the heart performs. As would be anticipated on this basis, the pain is usually brought on by physical effort which increases the heart rate and work and, in turn, myocardial oxygen requirements. Certain activities are especially prone to precipitate angina: walking uphill or against the wind, hurrying after meals, unaccustomed exercise. Conversely, angina is relieved by rest. As soon as physical activity stops the oxygen demand falls promptly and as a consequence the pain subsides. This relationship (activity → pain, rest → disappearance of pain) is typical of transient myocardial ischemia and distinguishes angina of effort from other nonischemic causes of chest pain in which this pattern does not occur. In addition to physical exertion, sudden emotional stress (e.g., anger, fear, or even the excitement of watching a football game) may induce an anginal episode. The mechanism is the same as with angina of effort: the workload of the heart is transiently increased beyond the ability of coronary circulation to satisfy the additional demands. In all, any physical or emotional stress that produces a sudden increase in the heart rate or elevation in blood pressure may induce angina.

Duration of Pain. Angina is characteristically of *brief* duration, lasting usually from 1-5 minutes before abating with rest. Occasionally the pain may last for more than 5 minutes, particularly if the stimulus for the attack persists. The cessation of pain indicates that the myocardial demand for oxygen has been met and that the oxygen deficit was only transient and not destructive to the myocardium. If the pain does not subside within minutes after rest, myocardial damage may be suspected.

Relief of Pain. Another distinctive feature of angina is the prompt relief of pain that follows the use of nitroglycerin. Failure of nitroglycerin, administered sublingually, to terminate ischemic pain is unusual and is cause for suspicion that the attack is not due to angina of effort. Nitroglycerin (and other nitrates) acts by dilating the coronary vessels, thus increasing the blood flow and oxygen supply to the myocardium. At the same time, nitrates lower the blood pressure and thereby reduce the workload of the heart by diminishing pumping resistance.

Diagnosis of Angina Pectoris

The most important diagnostic evidence of angina pectoris is the patient's history. If the chest pain is central in location, brief in duration, oppressive in quality and related to effort, the diagnosis of angina pectoris is virtually assured; no other confirmation is necessary. Physical examination and electrocardiograms at rest are normal in the majority of patients and seldom contribute directly to the diagnosis. When the chest pain pattern is suspicious but not entirely characteristic of angina, several diagnostic tests may be performed to determine if the pain is ischemic in origin.

Exercise (Stress) Testing. The simplest and most widely used diagnostic method is the exercise, or stress, test. It consists of recording an electrocardiogram during progressively strenuous exercise when the oxygen demands of the myocardium increase greatly and electrocardiographic signs of myocardial ischemia are most likely to appear. The exercise is performed by riding a stationary bicycle or walking on a treadmill while the heart rate, blood pressure and electrocardiogram are monitored continuously. The test starts with low level exercise and builds up in stages until a target heart rate (based on the patient's age) is achieved. In patients with significant obstructive disease of the coronary arteries a point is soon reached where myocardial oxygen demand exceeds oxygen supply and, as a consequence, electrocardiographic signs of myocardial ischemia appear. Although chest pain may develop during exercise, a positive stress test is defined only on the basis of characteristic electrocardiographic changes of ischemia (as described in Chapter 15), not the presence or absence of angina. One of the main limitations of stress testing is that many elderly or sedentary patients are unable to exercise sufficiently to achieve the target heart rate; the test must often be terminated prematurely in this group because of fatigue, leg weakness or shortness of breath.

Radionuclide Studies. In recent years various nuclear scanning techniques have assumed an increasingly useful role in the diagnosis and assessment of CHD. One of these methods, known as *radionuclide angiography,* provides indirect information about myocardial blood flow and is used in combination with exercise testing to confirm the diagnosis of angina pectoris. The test is based on the fact that myocardial ischemia, in addition to producing typical electrocardiographic signs, also causes abnormalities in contraction of segments (regions) of the left ventricle. These transient abnormalities in regional ventricular wall motion with exercise can be detected by nuclear scanning of the heart. The procedure involves the intravenous injection of a radioactive isotope at the peak exercise period and then sequentially recording ventricular wall motion with a nuclear camera. With significant coronary artery disease blood flow to the region supplied by the involved vessel is reduced, as reflected by the abnormal contractile pattern of that portion of the ventricle. Radionuclide angiography has greater diagnostic accuracy than customary stress testing alone, but it is much more costly. (Radionuclide scanning is described additionally in Chapter 2.)

Coronary Arteriography. The most definitive method for the diagnosis of coronary obstructive disease is *coronary arteriography.* In fact it serves as the standard of accuracy for the comparison of all other tests used in the diagnosis of CHD. As mentioned previously, coronary arteriography permits visualization of the coronary arteries (with a radiopaque dye) and thereby defines the precise number of arteries involved, the extent of narrowing in each vessel, and the degree of collateral circulation. This anatomic description of the disease process is particularly important in evaluating patients for coronary bypass surgery.

In addition to coronary arteriography, cardiac catherization and ventriculography are also performed as part of a complete study. *Cardiac catheterization* involves the introduction of catheters into the cardiac chambers and great vessels in order to measure pressures and oxygen concentrations in each of these sites. These data are essential for patients in whom coronary surgery is contemplated. *Ventriculography* is used to assess ventricular pumping function and to detect regional wall abnormalities. The technique consists of injecting a radiopaque dye through a catheter placed in the left ventricle and recording motion pictures of ventricular motion. This latter information is similar, but more precise, than that obtained by radionuclide studies. The main disadvantage of coronary arteriography (and the other components of the test) is that heart catheterization is an invasive procedure not entirely without risk, and requires expensive hospitalization.

Stable and Variant Angina Pectoris

Classic angina pectoris, as described above, behaves in a predictable and reproducible manner: it is brought on by physical activity or emotional stress, which increases myocardial oxygen demands, and is relieved promptly by rest, which decreases oxygen requirements. This established pain pattern is called *stable* angina pectoris. It is associated with fixed narrowing of the coronary arteries, resulting from advanced atherosclerosis. Coronary arteriograms usually show at least 75% narrowing of one or more of the arteries; most often, two or three vessels are involved.

Angina pectoris may also result from coronary artery spasm. The arterial spasm reduces coronary blood flow sufficiently to produce ischemic artery disease. Coronary artery spasm may be manifested clinically in several ways, but its most typical form is described as *variant* angina, or Prinzmetal's angina. The pain pattern of variant angina differs greatly from stable angina; indeed, it is almost the opposite in many of its characteristics. The main feature of variant angina is that the pain occurs with *rest* and not with activity. In fact, patients with variant angina do not develop chest pain or characteristic electrocardiographic signs of ischemia even during exercise testing. Also, the pain has an unusual cyclic pattern, often awakening the patient each night at about the same time. Furthermore, the electrocardiographic changes that accompany variant angina are entirely different than those associated with stable angina (see Chapter 15). The cause of coronary artery spasm is still unknown, but it is related somehow to abnormal contraction of the smooth muscles in the walls of arteries.

Although variant angina is very uncommon compared to stable angina, it has commanded increasing attention in recent years. Part of this interest can be attributed to a new class of drugs, called *calcium antagonists* or calcium blocking agents, that have proved very effective in inhibiting or releasing coronary spasm and relieving variant angina. Much more important is that these drugs also seem to benefit certain patients with fixed coronary artery obstruction. This implies that coronary spasm may contribute to the classic anginal syndrome even when the dominant cause of ischemia is advanced coronary atherosclerosis. However, the mechanism of action of these drugs in controlling stable angina is not known with certainty, but the very fact that calcium antagonists are effective for this purpose has caused a reevaluation of the causes and treatment of ischemic heart disease. Clinical research now in progress is likely to produce many new concepts about an old disease.

Intermediate Coronary Syndrome (Unstable Angina)

The term *intermediate coronary syndrome* has been used to characterize a clinical state that lies between stable angina pectoris and acute myocardial infarction. The syndrome has several different patterns, which accounts for the variety of names given to this condition in the past. Among the older (but still used) terms are: impending myocardial infarction, preinfarction angina, crescendo angina, accelerated angina, and acute coronary insufficiency. At present the preferred term is *unstable angina,* connoting that the common feature of the syndrome is its clinical instability.

Unstable angina may occur as the initial symptom of CHD or, more often, as a sudden worsening of stable angina. The chest pain, instead of lasting briefly as with stable angina, usually persists for 10-20 minutes or longer. It develops with increasing frequency and is provoked by less effort, often occurring at rest. Nitroglycerin provides incomplete or no relief in most cases of unstable angina. Electrocardiographic signs of ischemia are common but without definite evidence of acute myocardial infarction.

The mechanism of unstable angina is not entirely clear but progressive narrowing of the coronary arteries probably plays a major role, especially in patients with stable angina previously. In any case,

unstable angina is more serious than stable angina since frequently it is an immediate forerunner of acute myocardial infarction.

The diagnosis of unstable angina implies, theoretically, that despite prolonged ischemia adequate oxygenation was restored before actual myocardial destruction occurred. However from a clinical standpoint it is often difficult to rule out the possibility that small areas of the myocardium were in fact injured or destroyed during the ischemic episodes. For this reason and because of the changing and unpredictable course of the condition, patients with unstable angina are admitted to a coronary care unit, at least until the diagnosis of acute myocardial infarction has been excluded.

Acute Myocardial Infarction

When there is profound and sustained ischemia to a portion of the myocardium the cells deprived of oxygen cannot survive, and local death of tissue (necrosis) develops in the involved area. This destructive process is termed *acute myocardial infarction.* The event that produces this irreversible tissue damage (infarction) is often called a coronary thrombosis, a coronary occlusion, a coronary, or a heart attack. These latter terms are used synonymously in clinical practice to describe what properly should be designated acute myocardial infarction.

With few exceptions acute myocardial infarction results from advanced atherosclerosis of the coronary arteries. The final insult of progressive coronary atherosclerosis usually occurs when one of the main coronary arteries or its branches becomes occluded (Figure 1.5). Although the narrowing process is gradual, the obstruction takes place suddenly in most

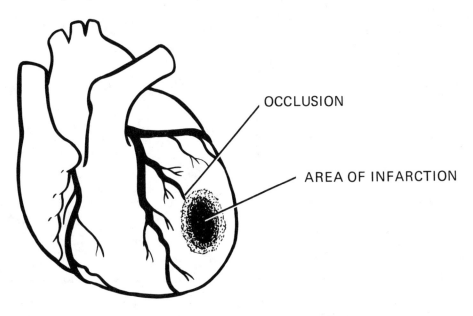

Figure 1.5. Anterior myocardial infarction.

instances. The exact reason that a coronary artery blocks off at a certain moment is not fully understood, but three main causes have been incriminated: 1) a clot may develop on the roughened surface of an atherosclerotic plaque and occlude the lumen of the artery; 2) the atherosclerotic lesions may irritate the underlying arterial wall, causing bleeding beneath the plaque (subintimal hemorrhage), which dislodges the plaque and obstructs the artery; 3) a piece of a large plaque may break off and block a small distal artery. Although all of these mechanisms offer a logical explanation for the suddenness of the event, it is now clear that none of them can account for *all* myocardial infarctions. Autopsy studies have shown, for instance, that acute myocardial infarction can occur even though the coronary arteries have no clots and are not completely obstructed. In these latter instances, it is presumed that at a particular moment the heart is faced with an enormous oxygen demand (e.g., during intense physical activity, such as shoveling snow) which cannot be met by the available blood supply through partially narrowed arteries. In effect, even though the coronary arteries are not completely obstructed, the persistent myocardial demand for oxygen simply overwhelms the limited supply and tissue necrosis develops because of this relative oxygen deprivation. Another possibility is that coronary artery spasm may be superimposed on existing coronary artery disease, causing a partially narrowed vessel to close completely during the transient spasm. (Although this is an attractive concept, the role of coronary artery spasm in acute myocardial infarction has not been determined as yet.)

The site of an infarction depends fundamentally on which coronary artery (or arteries) is blocked. When the left coronary artery or its branches are occluded, the infarction involves primarily the anterior wall of the left ventricle and is called an *anterior infarction*. Occlusion of the right coronary artery results in infarction of the inferior (diaphragmatic) wall of the left ventricle—an *inferior infarction* (Figure 1.6). Very often more than one area of the left ventricle is damaged by the ischemic process; in these cases more specific terms are used to describe the location of the infarct. For example, if the infarction involves both the anterior and lateral walls of the left ventricle, it is termed an *anterolateral infarction*. Similarly, damage to the anterior wall of the left ventricle and to the interventricular septum is called an *anteroseptal infarction*.

Myocardial infarction involving the *right* ventricle alone is very rare because this chamber receives a relatively greater proportion of blood for its (smaller) muscle mass than the left ventricle, and also has less oxygen requirements. However, right ventricular infarction is not uncommon in conjunction with inferior myocardial infarction. This relationship is understandable since the right ventricle and the inferior wall of the left ventricle share a common blood supply through the right coronary artery. Nevertheless, the frequency of these combined infarctions was not appreciated until the recent introduction of radionuclide methods for the diagnosis of acute myocardial infarction (as described in the next chapter). With these (and other) means it has been shown that at least 25% of patients with acute inferior myocardial infarction also have some evidence of right ventricular damage.

The extent of an infarction is determined first by the size of the vessel obstructed and second by the

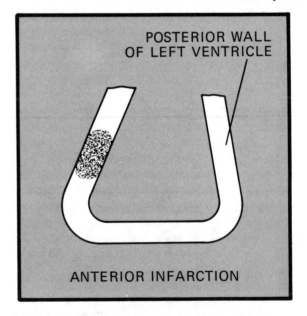

Figure 1.6. Side view of the left ventricle showing the respective locations of an inferior and and anterior infarction. Because the inferior surface of the left ventricle faces the diaphragm, inferior infarctions are also called *diaphragmatic infarctions.*

capacity of the collateral circulation to bring additional blood to the oxygen-deprived areas. If there is widespread myocardial necrosis extending through and through the entire ventricular wall (from the endocardium to the pericardium), the infarction is termed *transmural* (Figure 1.7A). Lesser degrees of damage which do not involve the full thickness of the ventricular wall are categorized as *nontransmural* infarctions (Figure 1.7B). Other descriptive terms for nontransmural infarctions are intramural and subendocardial infarctions.

In the early stages of acute myocardial infarction there are, at least in concept, three zones of tissue damage (Figure 1.8). The first zone consists of necrotic myocardial tissue that has been irreversibly destroyed by prolonged deprivation of oxygen. Surrounding this dead tissue is a second zone (zone of injury) in which the myocardial cells, although injured and jeopardized, may still survive if adequate circulation to the area is restored. Zone 3, called the zone of ischemia, represents cells that have not received

adequate oxygen but can be expected to recover unless the ischemic process worsens. In effect, the ultimate size of an infarction may depend on the fate of the zones of injury and ischemia. (These latter zones are not actually distinct or separate areas as the foregoing description suggests. Instead, they appear histologically as a combined outer zone surrounding the central zone of necrosis. This outer zone is diffuse and consists of patchy areas of necrotic, injured and ischemic tissues, merging with normal myocardium. Because of its in-between location and status, this peripheral zone is usually described as the *border* zone or twilight zone.)

Once the coronary circulation is interrupted and a myocardial infarction occurs, a series of events follows which places life and death in balance. This book is concerned with these events and describes a concept of specialized care, known as *intensive coronary care,* designed to lower the death rate from acute myocardial infarction.

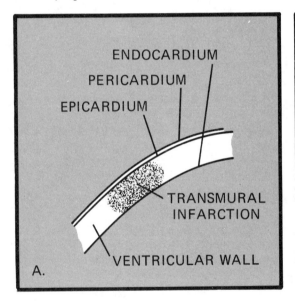
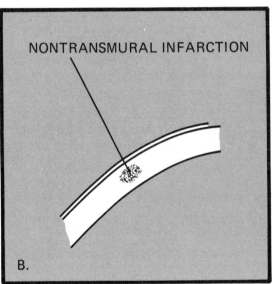

Figure 1.7(A). Transmural myocardial infarction. Note that the necrotic area extends all the way through the ventricular wall from the endocardium to the pericardium. **(B).** With a nontransmural infarction the damage is less extensive, involving only a portion of the ventricular wall.

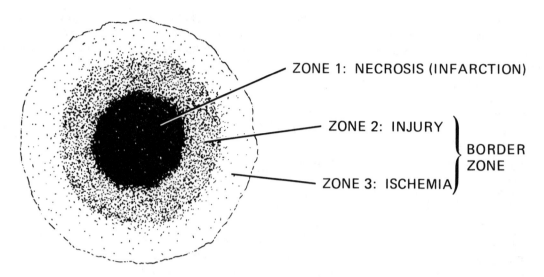

Figure 1.8. Three zones of tissue damage associated with acute myocardial infarction. Zone 1 is irreversibly damaged, but zones 2 and 3 may recover if adequate circulation to these areas is restored by collateral circulation.

2

Acute Myocardial Infarction

THE ONSET OF THE ATTACK

Most patients with acute myocardial infarction seek medical assistance because of *chest pain*. The pain is usually quite distinctive; it occurs suddenly and is of severe, crushing quality. It is more intense than the pain of angina or the intermediate coronary syndrome and may be unlike any sensation the patient has experienced previously. Typically, the pain is concentrated directly beneath the sternum, but it frequently radiates across the chest or to the arms and neck. Patients commonly describe the pain as a heavy weight or pressure or a knot in the chest. Unlike angina, the pain does not necessarily occur with exertion; in fact, it frequently begins during sleep. Its occurrence after eating explains why many patients interpret the pain as indigestion. The chest pain is continuous and is not relieved by change in body position, breath-holding, or by home remedies (e.g., bicarbonate) the patient may try. It usually persists for 30 minutes or more and may not subside until morphine is administered. Nitroglycerin seldom influences the duration or severity of the pain. Shortly after the onset of the substernal pain drenching perspiration usually begins, and nausea and vomiting often occur at the same time. Fear and apprehension are usual, and most patients sense that a catastrophe has happened. Within minutes, many patients are aware of dyspnea and marked weakness. This symptom complex of substernal pain, sweating, nausea, and vomiting along with dyspnea and sudden weakness can be considered the typical history of acute myocardial infarction.

Not all patients, of course, present such typical histories and there are many variations of the story. Sometimes the pain is centered not in the chest but, as with angina, may be located in the arms, neck, or shoulders. Sweating, nausea, vomiting, and dyspnea are not constant features of the attack and may not appear at all. The severity and duration of chest pain can vary greatly and it is often difficult to distinguish angina pectoris, the intermediate coronary syndrome, and acute myocardial infarction on the basis of the quality of pain alone.

Some patients experience acute myocardial infarction apparently without any chest pain or other clear-cut symptoms. The diagnosis becomes evident when signs of an old infarction are found on a routine electrocardiogram and yet the patient denies any previous symptoms; these are called *silent* infarctions. It is estimated that at least 20% of all infarctions are in this category.

At the other end of the spectrum are patients who develop serious or fatal complications of acute myocardial infarction immediately after the onset of the attack. In these cases it is the complication itself (e.g., pulmonary edema or a death-producing arrhythmia) that suggests an acute myocardial infarction has occurred.

THE CLINICAL COURSE IMMEDIATELY AFTER INFARCTION

It is apparent from the foregoing description of the onset of the attack that the heart may respond in several different ways to the interruption of its blood supply. Some patients develop serious or lethal complications almost instantly while others never experience any difficulties at all. It is not known with certainty which factors actually influence the heart's behavior in the immediate post-infarction period. There is good reason to believe however, that the size of the infarction is the most critical determinant of the clinical course. In general, if a main coronary artery is occluded and produces extensive myocardial damage (transmural infarction), the course and prognosis are much poorer than when a branch artery is blocked and the resultant injury is small (nontransmural infarction). This relationship, however, is not always constant and patients with modest areas of tissue destruction can indeed develop serious complications. Because of this disparity it is evident that other factors contribute to the initial and subsequent outcome of the attack. One important factor is the extent of the collateral blood supply. If sufficient blood can be diverted immediately to the border zone surrounding the necrotic area the jeopardized tissues may be preserved, thus limiting the size of the infarction. Conversely, if the collateral supply is poor, widespread myocardial destruction may result since tissue oxygenization cannot be enhanced. Along this same line, the extent of an infarction is probably influenced by the particular oxygen demands of the myocardium immediately after the attack. If, for example, the heart rate is rapid and the blood pressure high, the oxygen requirements are increased greatly; consequently, the jeopardized zone of ischemic tissue cannot survive, causing the infarction to enlarge. (As explained in Chapter 3, attempts are now being made to limit the size of infarctions with various techniques carried out in the first few hours after the attack.) Regardless of the mechanism accounting for the different responses to obstruction of coronary blood flow, the immediate clinical course can be categorized generally in the following order of severity:

1. If the infarcted area is limited in size and enough blood is diverted to the site by collateral channels, the myocardium may continue to function quite normally. The heart's pumping action may not be affected, and the rate and rhythm of the heart are not necessarily disturbed. The pain gradually subsides in these instances, and the patient appears in no distress at the time of admission.

2. When the involved area is larger and if there is only trivial collateral assistance, the myocar-

dium may become sufficiently embarrassed and its function impaired. This may be manifested by signs of decreased pumping action of the heart (heart failure) or by disturbances in the rate and rhythm of the heartbeat (arrhythmias). The degree of impairment may vary greatly; some patients have only mild shortness of breath and minor arrhythmias while others are critically ill with marked dyspnea, pulmonary edema, and life-threatening arrhythmias.

3. If the pumping action of the heart is grossly reduced as a result of extensive structural damage to the myocardium, the left ventricle is simply unable to pump sufficient blood throughout the body to sustain circulation to the vital organs. Accordingly, the blood pressure falls, the heart rate increases, the urinary output decreases, and the skin becomes cold and clammy. This state is called *cardiogenic shock;* most patients with this complication die within hours.

4. For some patients death occurs almost instantly after interruption of coronary blood flow. These *sudden* deaths are almost always due to lethal arrhythmias resulting from extraordinary changes in the electrical activity of the heart, probably induced by myocardial ischemia. By far the most common arrhythmic mechanism of sudden death is *ventricular fibrillation,* a condition in which the ventricles are stimulated incessantly so that they merely quiver without propelling blood. There is no clear relationship between the size of an infarction and the occurrence of sudden arrhythmic deaths. It is estimated that probably 50% of *all* deaths from acute myocardial infarction occur within the first few hours after the attack as a result of arrhythmic disorders.

Because of these different possibilities it can be appreciated that some patients admitted to the hospital with acute myocardial infarction have no pain by the time they arrive and are not in distress, whereas others are near death from cardiogenic shock or acute heart failure when first seen. The ultimate clinical course is related to a large degree, but certainly not entirely, to the clinical picture on admission. However, *complications can develop at any time in any patient!*

THE COMPLICATIONS OF ACUTE MYOCARDIAL INFARCTION

There are five major complications that threaten life after acute myocardial infarction. Each of these complications is considered in detail in subsequent chapters. They are mentioned here to provide an overview of the clinical course of the illness.

1. Arrhythmias

Disturbances in the cardiac rate or rhythm (arrhythmias) are the most common complication of acute myocardial infarction. At least 90% of patients with acute infarction develop some form of arrhythmia during the acute phase of the illness. Arrhythmias pose two serious threats: they may reduce the pumping efficiency of the heart, precipitating acute heart failure; and, above all, they may produce *sudden death*. Alhough not all disorders of rate and rhythm are life-threatening, the critical fact is that *death-producing arrhythmias, particularly ventricular fibrillation, can occur at any time.*

2. Acute Left Ventricular Failure

The contractile ability of the myocardium is inevitably reduced after infarction, often causing the heart to fail as a pumping system. Such failure can occur suddenly, resulting in acute pulmonary edema, or gradually (if the ventricle recovers from the original ischemia but falters subsequently). Clinical signs of heart failure are observed in about 60% of patients, but the degree of this pumping deficit varies considerably.

3. Cardiogenic Shock

The most advanced form of left ventricular pumping failure is described as cardiogenic shock. It results when the heart is unable to sustain the circulation and provide adequate oxygen to the vital organs and tissues. Cardiogenic shock is an extremely serious complication: despite all present forms of treatment the mortality is at least 80%. Although cardiogenic shock develops most often during the first 12 hours after the attack, it can occur several days later.

4. Thromboembolism

There is a propensity for blood to clot on the inner wall of the injured left ventricle. These clots may break loose and leave the heart (as emboli) to block the arterial supply to the brain, abdomen, or extremities. Emboli may also rise from the deep veins of the legs (presumably due to stasis of blood) and eventually find their way to the lungs and produce pulmonary infarction. Embolic phenomena, from either the left ventricle or the leg veins, can produce sudden death, but this complication is not common and accounts for a relatively small percentage of deaths after infarction.

5. Rupture of the Left Ventricle

When there is extensive damage to the ventricular wall the necrotic area may weaken, leading to rupture of the left ventricle. When this catastrophe occurs blood from the ventricle instantly fills the surrounding pericardial sac and causes compression of the heart (cardiac tamponade). Death occurs usually within minutes. Ventricular rupture may develop at any time during hospitalization, but the highest incidence is within the first 7-10 days. Less than 5% of the total mortality from acute myocardial infarction is due to ventricular rupture.

THE DIAGNOSIS OF ACUTE MYOCARDIAL INFARCTION

The diagnosis of acute myocardial infarction is made essentially in three steps: the patient's history, the electrocardiogram, and enzyme studies. In the event a definite conclusion cannot be reached on this basis, radionuclide imaging studies may be needed to confirm the patient's diagnosis.

The Patient's History

In many ways the patient's story of his illness is the prime factor in reaching the diagnosis of acute myocardial infarction. It is because of the history that the physician *suspects* the diagnosis and admits the patient to the hospital. The development of severe, substernal pain associated with nausea, sweating, and the other features already mentioned is often so distinctive the physician can safely anticipate subsequent confirmation of his diagnosis by the electrocardiogram and enzyme studies. However, the history, regardless of how typical it may be, is not diagnostic in its own right and other steps must be taken to prove that acute infarction has actually occurred.

The Electrocardiogram

The diagnosis of acute myocardial infarction can be made *definitively* only by electrocardiographic means. When injury and local death (infarction) of myocardial tissue occurs, characteristic findings reflecting these changes are found in the electrocardiographic tracing. On many occasions the initial diagnostic (12-lead) electrocardiogram fails to show specific evidence of an infarction, and additional (serial) tracings must be obtained over the next several days until definite electrocardiographic proof has evolved. The diagnosis of acute infarction cannot and should not be made unless characteristic electrocardiographic changes are finally demonstrated. It is important to realize that the electrocardiogram does not show the actual extent of damage and by itself is not a true index of the seriousness of the attack. (The electrocardiographic signs of acute myocardial infarction are described in Chapter 15.)

Enzyme Studies

Patients may give an impressive history suggesting acute myocardial infarction, but the electrocardiograms show equivocal (rather than definite) changes. In these cases other studies are necessary to verify the diagnosis. The most important of these laboratory determinations involves the measurement of certain enzymes in the blood. The basis of these tests is as follows: several enzymes are normally present within the cells comprising the myocardium. When the myocardium is injured, these enzymes escape into the bloodstream where they can be detected and mea-

sured. Thus, a characteristic elevation of these enzymes in the serum is to be expected after acute myocardial infarction. The three enzyme studies most frequently used to confirm the diagnosis of acute myocardial infarction are creatine phosphokinase (CPK), serum glutamic oxaloacetic transaminase (SGOT), and lactic dehydrogenase (LDH).

Creatine Phosphokinase (CPK)

CPK is the first enzyme to increase after myocardial infarction, and elevated levels can be detected within 2-6 hours after the attack. The peak level usually is reached during the first 24 hours. After 2-3 days the CPK levels generally return to normal (Figure 2.1). Accordingly, CPK levels should be measured at the time of admission, 24 hours later, and then at the end of the second and third days. Unfortunately, creatine phosphokinase is not only a myocardial enzyme but is produced also by the brain and the skeletal muscles. Therefore, elevated CPK levels may be noted after brain damage (e.g., strokes) or with various muscle diseases or injuries. Even an intramuscular injection may cause a significant rise in serum CPK. (For this reason it is wise, when possible, to draw a blood sample for CPK determination

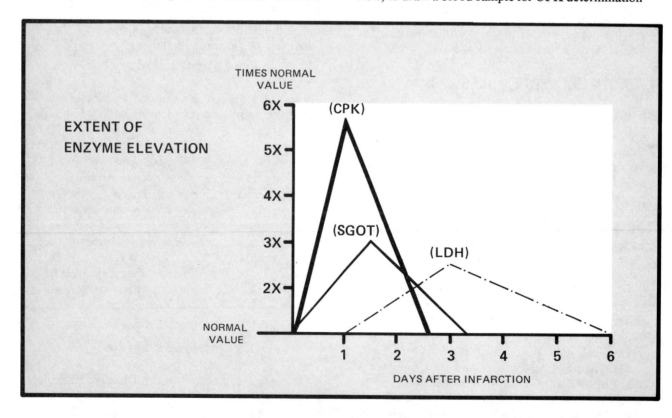

Figure 2.1. Typical enzyme elevation patterns after acute myocardial infarction. Note that the peak levels occur on different days; also that the extent of increase (i.e., two times, three times, or four times the normal value) is not the same for each enzyme. The normal values for the enzymes depend on the particular laboratory method used and therefore may vary from hospital to hospital. (It is important to ascertain the normal values at your own hospital in order to interpret the results of enzyme studies.)

before any intramuscular injections are administered.)

To exclude the possibility that elevated CPK levels are due to causes other than acute myocardial infarction most laboratories also measure *CPK-MB,* one of three components (isoenzymes) of CPK. This particular isoenzyme is found only in the myocardium and is therefore a very sensitive index of myocardial necrosis. CPK-MB levels become abnormal 2-3 hours after an attack and peak at 12 hours; they then decrease rapidly and may return to normal in 24 hours. If CPK-MB is greater than 5% of the total CPK level, the diagnosis of acute myocardial infarction is nearly certain. Because the separation and assay of CPK-MB is time-consuming and costly, this test is usually reserved for cases in which the diagnosis is in question on the basis of total CPK levels. On the other hand, little purpose is served in measuring CPK-MB if the patient's history is typical and the total CPK level is, for example, 20 times the normal value.

Serum Glutamic Oxaloacetic Transaminase (SGOT)*

SGOT levels rise less rapidly than CPK after myocardial infarction. Although minor increases in SGOT may be detected after 8 hours, the peak level does not occur until 24-48 hours have elapsed. The levels usually return to normal after 3-4 days. Therefore the concentration of this enzyme should be measured at 24, 48, and 72 hours after the attack. While SGOT levels are generally reliable in confirming myocardial damage, other diseases may also produce elevations of this enzyme. High SGOT levels are especially common in liver disease (hepatocellular damage) and, to a lesser degree, in congestive heart failure and after muscle injury.

Lactic Dehydrogenase (LDH)

Serum levels of LDH increase after infarction at a slower rate than CPK or SGOT. Peak concentrations do not occur usually until the second or third day, after which the levels return to normal on about the

*Although SGOT has been one of the standard enzymatic tests for acute myocardial infarction for many years, its value as a diagnostic procedure is now in question. It is argued that since the introduction of CPK-MB determinations, SGOT studies are much less important because they do not increase the specificity of the diagnosis. For this reason, the World Health Organization and the American Heart Association have recommended that SGOT tests be abandoned in the diagnosis of acute myocardial infarction. Nevertheless, SGOT studies have served a valuable purpose over the years and will probably remain one of the basic diagnostic tests, at least until all hospitals are prepared to measure CPK-MB routinely.

fifth or sixth day. This laboratory determination should therefore be performed on days 3, 4, and 5, but only if CPK and SGOT levels have not already confirmed the diagnosis. As with CPK and SGOT, LDH levels may increase from causes other than acute myocardial infarction. Elevations of LDH are known to occur with pulmonary, renal, and skeletal muscle diseases. These latter causes can be excluded by measuring the isoenzymes of LDH. It has been shown that the ratio of two LDH isoenzymes, LDH_1/LDH_2, is a far more specific indicator of acute myocardial infarction than the total LDH level.

Significance of Enzyme Studies

Although the degree of serum enzyme elevation cannot be correlated precisely with the size or severity of myocardial infarction, the levels do provide a general indication of the extent of tissue destruction. Markedly increased serum enzyme levels, especially CPK-MB, appearing promptly after infarction and remaining elevated longer than anticipated usually suggest an extensive myocardial infarction.

Despite the sensitivity of isoenzyme determinations, the diagnosis of acute myocardial infarction should not be made solely on the basis of elevated enzyme levels; the value of these tests is only supplemental. Conversely, negative results of enzyme studies should not be grounds to abandon the diagnosis of acute myocardial findings.

Radionuclide Imaging

Occasionally the diagnosis of acute myocardial infarction cannot be definitely confirmed by either electrocardiograms or enzyme studies. For example, characteristic electrocardiographic signs of an acute infarction may be obscured by preexisting abnormalities, such as an old infarction. Even CPK-MB, the most sensitive enzyme study, can be misleading at times. If, for instance, the test is delayed more than 12 hours after a small infarction, the diagnosis may be missed because the peak level has passed and CPK-MB may be returning toward normal. A more common diagnostic problem is acute myocardial infarction occurring during or after open heart surgery. In this circumstance there is no way to tell if the elevated postoperative enzyme levels are due to a heart attack or to myocardial injury from the surgical procedure itself. It has been proposed that these (and other) diagnostic dilemmas can be resolved in many instances by means of a new technique called *radionuclide imaging.*

Radionuclide imaging to diagnose acute myocardial infarction can be performed in two basic ways: "hot spot" imaging and "cold spot" imaging.

"Hot spot" imaging involves the intravenous injection of a radionuclide substance, most often technetium 99ᵐ pyrophosphate, which selectively accumulates in areas of myocardial necrosis. The uptake of the radionuclide in the infarcted area can be visualized in the form of emission images with a specialized nuclear camera. Acute myocardial infarction appears on the images as an area of increased uptake (greater radioactivity), called a "hot spot." By contrast, normal myocardial tissue demonstrates no visible uptake of the radioactive agent. Therefore the zone of necrosis and normal myocardium are demarcated, which in effect defines the size and location of an acute infarction. An example of acute myocardial infarction as determined by "hot spot" imaging is shown in Figure 2.2. Images reflecting acute myocardial infarction become evident about 10-12 hours after the attack and peak at 24-72 hours; they may remain positive for 7-10 days. Although this diagnostic concept is very attractive and has been received enthusiastically, there are several pitfalls associated with "hot spot" imaging, including varying results with different types of infarction, and the timing of the test. At present it is estimated that the sensitivity of technetium 99ᵐ pyrophosphate in the diagnosis of acute myocardial infarction is about 80-90% for transmural infarctions and 50% for small, nontransmural infarctions. Many believe, however, that the reliability of the test will increase as technology improves.

"Cold spot" imaging is based on a different principle. It has been demonstrated that certain radionuclides, especially thallium-201, are taken up by the myocardium in direct relation to coronary blood flow (myocardial perfusion). If myocardial perfusion is normal, radionuclide imaging following the intravenous injection of thallium-201 reveals an even, homogenous distribution of radioactivity throughout the myocardium, mostly the left ventricle. The images show a horseshoe or doughnut appearance, reflecting the configuration of the left ventricle (Figure 2.3). On the other hand, if an area of the myocardium is infarcted there is no uptake in this nonperfused segment and a void or "cold spot" is seen on the myocardial images. In other words, myocardial infarction is revealed by a "cold spot" with thallium perfusion and by a "hot spot" with technetium pyrophosphate. The relative accuracy of these two tests is still undetermined, but one drawback of the thallium-201 study is that an area of old infarction will also produce a "cold spot" and, therefore, an acute infarction cannot be distinguished from an old one.

As noted in the previous chapter, thallium-201 studies are also used to confirm the diagnosis of angina pectoris and the intermediate coronary syndrome; in fact the greatest usefulness of the test is for this latter purpose. Since the thallium study reflects myocardial perfusion, ischemia of the myocardium is manifested by abnormalities in the perfusion pattern, particularly the development of transient "cold spots." The thallium technique is especially useful in conjunction with exercise testing designed to induce temporary ischemia. In normal myocardium there is a brisk uptake of thallium after exercise, but the ischemic area shows scant or no uptake. However as the ischemia subsides the "cold spot" gradually assumes a normal appearance because of redistribution of the isotope. A positive thallium exercise test is considered strong evidence for CHD and is probably more reliable than exercise testing alone (as described in Chapter 1).

PHYSICAL EXAMINATION

In examining a patient with acute myocardial infarction the fundamental objective is to ascertain

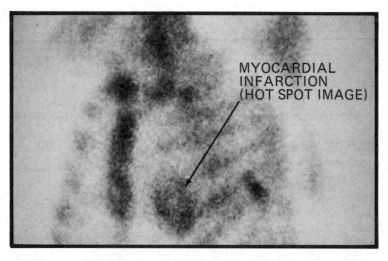

Figure 2.2. Technetium scan showing a large myocardial infarction (arrow). A smaller old infarction is also apparent.

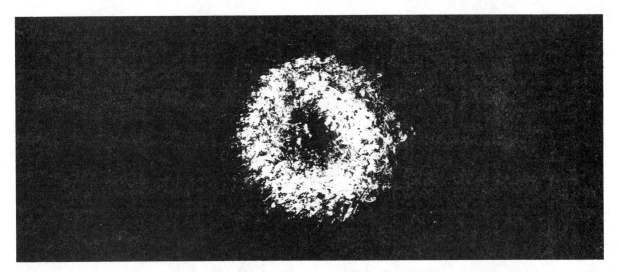

Figure 2.3. Normal thallium scan showing homogenous uptake of radioactive isotope by the left ventricle.

whether complications of the infarction have developed. Myocardial infarction in its own right does not produce abnormal physical findings; it is only the complications that can be detected by clinical examination.

As described in later chapters, each complication is associated with characteristic physical signs. For example, left ventricular failure is manifested by rales at the bases of the lungs and a gallop rhythm (among other findings). Hypotension, a rapid pulse rate, decreased urinary output, mental confusion, and cold clammy skin are found with cardiogenic shock. Arrhythmic disturbances are characterized by changes in the rate and rhythm of the heart.

It is understandable that the physical examination may be normal in patients who have not developed complications. Furthermore, it should be realized that acute myocardial infarction cannot be distinguished from other forms of heart disease solely on the basis of physical examination since circulatory failure and arrhythmias also occur with many different cardiac disorders.

THE ACUTE PHASE OF MYOCARDIAL INFARCTION

In general, the clinical course after infarction can be considered in two phases: the *acute* phase, which usually involves the first 4-5 days following the attack, and the *subacute* phase, which concerns the remaining period of hospitalization. During the acute phase patients are treated in a coronary care unit.

Clinical Course

The most characteristic aspect of the acute phase of myocardial infarction is its uncertainty; there is no typical course. The variation in the clinical picture is quite remarkable, but three broad patterns can be described.

There are some patients whose clinical course is truly uncomplicated. They show no evidence of cardiogenic shock, acute left ventricular failure, arrhythmias, or other major problems during this critical period of the illness. Most of these patients make uneventful recoveries regardless of the type of treatment employed.

In other patients the illness appears benign at the time of admission, but suddenly major complications develop. These complications account for nearly all deaths, and it is the unpredictability of these catastrophes that makes myocardial infarction such a lethal disease. The concept of intensive coronary care is based on the prevention or the immediate detection and treatment of life-threatening complications. By its ability to prevent sudden unexpected death in this group of patients, the system of intensive coronary care has made its greatest contribution.

When serious complications already exist at the time of admission, the clinical course is usually hectic and the prognosis becomes extremely poor. For example, if shock is present when the patient is admitted, there is more than a 90% likelihood that the patient will die within the next 48 hours. If acute heart failure is evident on admission, the mortality rate may be as high as 50%. Therefore the original clinical picture is very important in determining the ultimate course of the attack; but an uncomplicated picture on admission should not lead to a false sense of security for reasons stated in the preceding paragraphs.

That acute myocardial infarction may have such widely divergent courses explains why the death rate may be 90% at one extreme and 0%-5% at the other. Probably no other disease behaves in this unpredictable fashion.

The treatment program during the acute phase is described in detail in later chapters.

Other Aspects of the Acute Phase

In addition to major complications, many other problems may develop during the acute phase. Some of these effects represent natural responses to tissue damage, whereas others can be considered actual complications.

Fever

Most patients with acute myocardial infarction develop temperature elevations during the acute phase of the illness. Typically, the body temperature rises after the first 24 hours of the attack to levels of 100°-101° F (or more) and remains elevated for 2-3 days before declining gradually. By the fifth day the temperature has usually returned to normal (Figure 2.4). It is thought that this febrile pattern reflects local death of myocardial tissue. (The white blood cell count and the erythrocyte sedimentation rate also increase during this period for the same reason.) Thus the presence of fever is an anticipated finding and ordinarily does not indicate an infectious process in patients with acute infarction. However, if the fever is prolonged, excessively high, or develops after the first few days, the possibility of pneumonia, thrombophlebitis, or other systemic infection must be considered.

Pericarditis

Myocardial infarctions frequently extend to the epicardial surface of the heart and produce inflammation of the overlying pericardium. In most cases the pericardial reaction (pericarditis) is confined to the area over the infarction, but occasionally diffuse pericardial irritation may develop, probably from inflammation at the surface of the infarction site. Patients with pericarditis secondary to acute myocardial infarction usually experience chest pain, which is often increased by deep breathing or changes in body position. The characteristic physical finding of pericarditis is a pericardial friction rub—a grating sound occurring each time the heart beats. A transient friction rub can be detected in nearly 50% of patients with acute myocardial infarction. Pericarditis usually disappears spontaneously within a few days and seldom causes serious problems.

Recurrent Chest Pain

Some patients develop additional episodes of ischemic chest pain during the acute phase of myocardial infarction. This pain may represent angina pectoris or, worse, an extension of the original infarction. (The possibility that the pain is caused by pericarditis must also be considered.) Recurrent ischemic pain generally indicates that the acute process has not stabilized and that further damage may occur. Serial electrocardiograms and enzyme studies should be performed after any significant chest pain episode.

Emotional Disturbances

Profound emotional reactions are frequent among patients with acute myocardial infarction during the period of intensive coronary care. The basis of this response can be readily appreciated: the abrupt interruption of normal life, the fear of death, and the possibility of permanent invalidism are powerful psychological threats. Because the patient's response to this stress is influenced by numerous factors inherent in his personality, the spectrum of reactions is very wide. The most common emotional problems associated with acute myocardial infarction are discussed in Chapter 5.

THE SUBACUTE PHASE OF MYOCARDIAL INFARCTION

The overall incidence of complications lessens greatly after the first 5 days and for this reason patients are usually transferred from the coronary care unit (CCU) at that time, assuming of course that their clinical condition is stable.

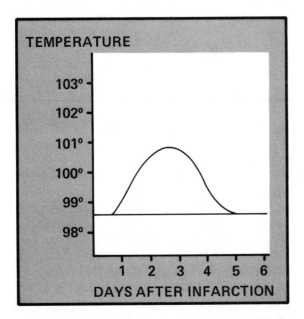

Figure 2.4. Characteristic temperature pattern after acute myocardial infarction.

During the subacute phase, while the infarction is healing, the main objective is to observe the clinical course carefully, focusing on the prevention of new complications. At the same time it is important to prepare the patient for hospital discharge and resumption of normal life by instructing and counseling him about his illness and by starting a planned program of physical rehabilitation.

In general, physical activity is restricted during the subacute phase in order to limit the work of the heart as its heals. However, complete bed rest is not necessary and it is customary to allow patients to sit in arm chairs and to walk to the bathroom. (The use of chair rest rather than bed rest is beneficial not only for the emotional support derived from being out of bed, but also because the sitting position is more effective in terms of circulatory efficiency.) In recent years, increasing emphasis has been placed on *early ambulation,* particularly for patients with uncomplicated or minimally complicated courses during the acute phase. The objective of early ambulation is to prevent the deleterious physiologic and psychologic effects of prolonged bed rest, especially cardiovascular deconditioning, skeletal muscle wasting, and anxiety or depression. This is accomplished by a program of progressive physical activity starting with low intensity exercise and building up gradually to a level that will enable the patient to return home not as an invalid.

The hospital course of patients who develop complications during the acute phase varies with the nature of the problem and the response to treatment. Understandably, the basic program of care just described must be adapted according to the clinical picture.

Although the subacute phase is undoubtedly less hazardous than the acute phase, there is substantial evidence indicating that the period after transfer from the CCU is by no means without danger. *Indeed, complications, especially sudden death from arrhythmias, may develop at any time during the hospital stay.*

In an effort to reduce mortality during the subacute phase, some institutions have established special care facilities for the postcoronary care unit period. These units, designated variously as intermediate coronary care units (ICCU), step-down units, or after-care wards, allow careful observation to be continued for a week or two after transfer from the CCU in a less-intensive but nonetheless prepared setting. The actual value of this intermediate care concept is still a subject of debate, particularly from the standpoint of the number of lives saved compared to the cost and effort involved. (In some centers, telemetry is used as an alternative method of monitoring patients who have experienced serious arrhythmias during the CCU period.)

HOSPITAL DISCHARGE

The usual hospital stay for most patients with acute myocardial infarction is about three weeks in duration, including the period in the CCU. However, patients who experience no significant complications are sometimes discharged after two weeks (or even sooner with nontransmural infarctions). Although early discharge of selected patients has been reported to be safe and not associated with a higher mortality subsequently, many physicians still prefer the more conservative approach.

In keeping with the trend toward early mobilization, some cardiologists now perform a *treadmill exercise test* before hospital discharge. Unlike a maximal (or submaximal) stress test used for the diagnosis of angina pectoris, the exercise level is of low-intensity, designed to increase the heart rate only moderately. The primary purpose of the procedure is to assess the patient's clinical and electrocardiographic response to exercise as a means of determining the type and amount of activity that can be safely tolerated at home and then at work. In addition, there is some indication that exercise testing soon after acute myocardial infarction may provide prognostic information about the future course of the patient's illness. According to a few recent studies, the risk of developing angina pectoris, recurrent myocardial infarction, and sudden death in the first year or two after infarction may be predicted on the basis of the results of low level exercise testing. Predischarge exercise testing is reserved only for patients whose hospital course is uncomplicated; it is not performed in those with arrhythmias, heart failure, or angina. Nevertheless, the procedure is not without potential risk and there is always the possibility of provoking serious myocardial ischemia or dangerous arrhythmias. Since the value of the test compared to its risks is still uncertain, predischarge exercise testing is not a standard procedure in most hospitals as yet.

CONVALESCENCE AFTER ACUTE MYOCARDIAL INFARCTION

After discharge from the hospital, it is customary for patients to remain at home on a limited activity program until the infarction has healed. As a general rule, necrotic areas of the myocardium heal within 6-8 weeks after the attack. Thus if a patient was hospitalized for 3 weeks, the period of convalescence at home would be an additional 3-5 weeks. The duration of convalescence depends on several factors, the most important of which are the functional capacity of the heart and the patient's age.

Physical activity is increased gradually during the convalescent phase. Excessive rest is unnecessary, but stair-climbing or household chores should be minimized (unless the patient has already progressed to this stage with an early ambulation program or if predischarge exercise testing indicates that these activities can be tolerated safely). Toward the end of the healing phase a deliberate program of progressive physical activity is started in order to promote cardiac reconditioning and the development of collateral circulation to the myocardium. Although it is difficult to prove that the growth of collateral blood vessels is directly related to physical activity, the consensus is that regulated exercise is distinctly beneficial for this purpose. In concept, regular exercise may help to create what is in effect an additional blood supply to the myocardium, taking over the role of the previously occluded artery. Walking is considered to be the most sensible and effective exercise to achieve this goal and should be encouraged, with the distance (and then pace) being increased daily. In addition to its helpful effect on the heart and circulation, physical activity at this stage of the illness is of great value in combating the weakness and fatigue that are so common after myocardial infarction. These symptoms, resulting mostly from disuse of the skeletal muscles during the period of hospitalization, are usually alleviated soon after a regular walking program is instituted.

Most patients, especially those without serious complications, are able to resume their customary lives and return to work about 2-3 months after the original attack. This time schedule must be flexible and adjusted according to the patient's age, general health, and cardiac status. It has become increasingly clear that the resumption of normal activity is highly desirable and every effort should be made to fulfill this objective. There is no reason to believe that deliberate inactivity or retirement from work after a myocardial infarction is conducive to longevity; in fact, the evidence is strictly to the contrary.

The resumption of a normal, useful life after a heart attack depends not only on physical recovery but also on emotional recovery. Some patients, despite excellent physical recoveries, develop such profound psychological reactions to their illness that they in fact become invalids. Emotionally-induced cardiac inva-

lidism is a common problem and produces no less functional impairment than true physical invalidism. The clinical features of this distressing problem are inability to tolerate physical activity, weakness and fatigue (which are often overwhelming), and an intense awareness and concern about any discomfort or pain occurring anywhere above the waist.

PROGNOSIS OF ACUTE MYOCARDIAL INFARCTION

The outcome of acute myocardial infarction during the period of hospitalization depends on several factors, including the size and location of the infarction, the extent of coronary artery disease and, of course, the occurrence of complications. However, the key determinant of prognosis is the pumping ability (ventricular function) after the attack. If ventricular function is not affected significantly and there are no signs of left ventricular failure, the prognosis is usually very good; but if ventricular function is reduced substantially, the outcome is generally poor. The relationship between the degree of left ventricular failure (LVF) and hospital mortality is shown in Figure 2.5. Note that among patients with no evidence of heart failure (categorized as Class I) the hospital mortality averages about 7%, while among those with cardiogenic shock (Class IV) the mortality is 85%. The overall hospital mortality from acute myocardial infarction with the present system of intensive coronary care in most institutions is 15-18%.

Of those who survive the period of hospitalization, another 10-15% die within the next 12 months. Thus approximately 30% of all patients hospitalized with acute myocardial infarction are dead within one year after the attack. After the first year the mortality decreases substantially to about 5% each year, and remains at this level thereafter. This means that after 5 years the total mortality is approximately 50% (i.e., 30% the first year and 20% during the next 4 years). It must be emphasized that these are *average* mortality rates and, therefore, do not define the prognosis for an individual patient. Indeed, some patients survive 15-20 years or more, especially those who are young and those with normal ventricular function.

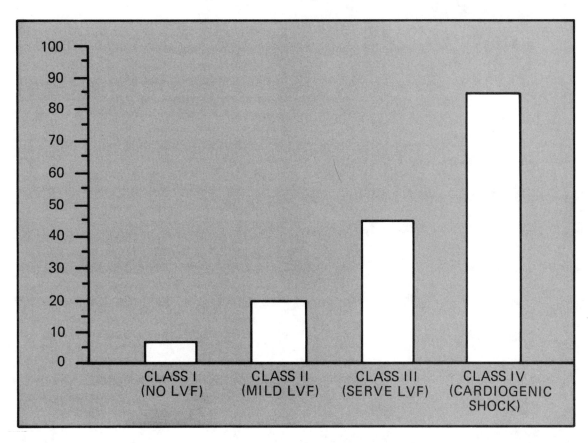

Figure 2.5. Hospital mortality from acute myocardial infarction according to degree of left ventricular failure (LVF).

3

The System Of Intensive Coronary Care

THE PROBLEM OF CORONARY HEART DISEASE

A means to halt the awesome death toll from coronary heart disease (CHD) is desperately needed. Consider the magnitude of the problem in the United States alone: nearly 2000 persons a day—more than 650,000 a year—die from this one disease. The enormity of this mortality is brought into perspective by noting that all forms of cancer together—the second leading cause of death—take less than half this number of lives per year. Understandably, CHD has been described as the greatest epidemic modern man has ever faced. It is not only its extraordinary death rate that makes CHD such an overwhelming problem, but also the fact that the disease disables millions of other people, many of whom are in the most productive years of life. Current estimates indicate that at least 5 million Americans now suffer from CHD, with 1 million new cases being added annually.

What can possibly be done about such a devastating disease? Certainly the main attack should be directed toward the prevention of coronary atherosclerosis. Indeed, for more than a half century a relentless search has been in progress attempting to identify the cause of atherosclerosis with the underlying hope that once the mechanism was uncovered, it would prove to be preventable or at least reversible. Unfortunately, this search has not been fruitful thus far, and it is clear that a practical way of inhibiting or preventing coronary atherosclerosis will not be forth-

coming in the near future. Although certain risk factors associated with CHD have been identified (e.g., high serum cholesterol levels, smoking, and hypertension, among many others), there is still no proof that any of these factors specifically *cause* coronary atherosclerosis, or, even more significantly, that by reducing these risks CHD can in fact be prevented. Present indications are that it will take many more years to unravel this complex, multifactorial process and reach a point where coronary atherosclerosis can possibly be averted. (Those who believe that CHD is an effect of "overcivilization" or the emotional stresses of our times might have an even more pessimistic outlook, since the likelihood of slowing the pace of present-day life is difficult to envision.) On the positive side it should be pointed out that there is still hope that CHD may ultimately yield to *primary* prevention. This means that deliberate efforts will have to be made to control risk factors beginning in childhood and continuing throughout life. Specifically, forthcoming generations would have to recognize the danger of overeating, smoking, emotional stress, and other potential risk factors, and avoid these threats from an early age. This approach differs from the current plan of *secondary* prevention, which attempts to correct these habits (risk factors) after they have already become established. It remains to be seen if future generations will heed this advice or if primary prevention is in fact more effective than secondary prevention.

If we must accept the conclusion that there is no definite means at present to prevent or reverse coronary atherosclerosis, what other measures can be used to reduce the death rate from CHD?

Surgical Treatment

One possibility for lowering mortality from CHD involves the use of surgical techniques to increase the blood supply to the myocardium after the coronary arteries have become critically narrowed. Many surgical methods have been attempted during the past 30 years in an effort to provide the heart with additional blood flow, but it was not until 1970, with the introduction of a new operation called the *coronary artery bypass graft* (CABG), that the surgical approach to CHD achieved widespread popularity. The procedure consists of suturing a segment of a vein (taken from the saphenous vein of the patient's leg) to a small opening made in the aorta at one end and to a coronary artery at the other. This vein graft bypasses the obstructed portion of a diseased artery and permits blood to pass from the aorta to the myocardium (Figure 3.1). For the operation to succeed in its purpose, the distal end of the vein graft must be attached to a portion of the coronary artery that is relatively free of advanced atherosclerotic disease (as determined preoperatively by coronary arteriography). If the disease process is diffuse and extends throughout the entire length of the artery, the bypass will not be effective. Fortunately, atherosclerotic narrowing is most likely to occur near the point of origin of the artery, thus permitting vein grafts to be applied in most patients with CHD. Because more than one coronary artery is involved in the majority of patients with symptomatic CHD, usually two or three (or more) grafts are placed during the procedure. The operation can be accomplished with a low surgical mortality; indeed, many large medical centers report an operative mortality of only 1%.

Bypass surgery was conceived originally as a means of treating severe disabling angina that could not be controlled by medical management; but now it is also being used as a therapeutic as well as prophylactic measure in many other situations, including stable angina pectoris, unstable angina, and acute myocardial infarction. In principle, the revascularization procedure produces an immediate increase in coronary blood flow (and myocardial oxygen supply) and in this way controls angina and possibly prevents serious complications of myocardial ischemia.

Extensive clinical experience during the past decade has clearly demonstrated that CABG surgery is extremely effective in relieving angina pectoris. About 85% of patients describe symptomatic improvement after a bypass procedure and 65% show increased exercise tolerance. Much less certain is the value of the operation for other purposes. In fact there has been no evidence thus far to even suggest that CABG surgery can inhibit progression of the disease, avert impending myocardial infarction (in patients with unstable angina), or prevent complications of CHD

(e.g., heart failure or arrhythmias). Above all, it is not known if bypass surgery prolongs life. In other words, it is clear that the operation produces marked improvement in symptoms and the quality of life—certainly very important benefits—but it is still uncertain whether patients undergoing surgery actually live longer than those who are treated by medical means.* (One exception to this uncertainty is a small subset of patients with obstructive lesions of the all-important left main coronary artery. Research studies have shown that survival in this group is distinctly better with surgical than medical treatment.)

If coronary bypass surgery ultimately proves effective in prolonging life, it will certainly represent a major advance in the treatment of CHD in selected patients. However, it should be recognized that this (or any other) surgical method can have only limited application in terms of the overall problem of CHD throughout the world. It is not only that relatively few hospitals have facilities for open-heart surgery, but also that the cost of this surgery is so high that economic considerations preclude this approach on a wide-scale basis. For example, the overall cost of CABG surgery in the United States at present (about 100,000 operations per year) already exceeds $1 billion a year! Few societies can afford an expense of this magnitude to treat only a small percentage of the population.

Prevention of Clots

Another possibility for combating CHD concerns the prevention of clot formation within the coronary arteries. Recognizing that extensive atherosclerosis may be present for years without ever producing CHD (and its lethal complications), it can be postulated that unless a clot developed an atherosclerotic plaque, acute myocardial infarction might never occur in many instances. The basic question is what causes a clot (thrombosis) to form in the coronary arteries, and why does it develop on one particular day rather than a month earlier or a year later.

---

*In an effort to answer this critically important question, a large cooperative study was conducted in the early 1970s by 13 Veterans Administration hospitals. About 600 patients with angina and (arteriographic) documented evidence of advanced obstruction of at least one artery were randomly assigned to either surgical or medical treatment. The results after 4 years revealed that survival was essentially the same in both groups: surgery was no better than medical treatment in prolonging life. However, the methods and conclusions of the study have been challenged, and the issue of survival remains controversial. Fortunately, other major trials are now in progress, and perhaps the question will be settled or clarified within the next few years.

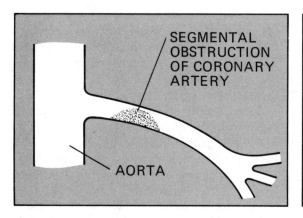
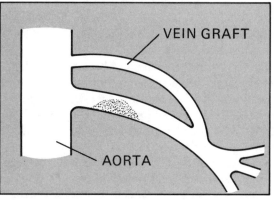

Figure 3.1. Coronary artery bypass graft. The saphenous vein graft extends from the aorta to a point distal to the obstructed segment of the coronary artery.

Research studies have revealed that clot formation within arteries (in contrast to clots within veins) is the result of increased adhesiveness of blood platelets. Because of this unusual "stickiness," platelets tend to clump together and form the framework for a larger clot. Also, it has been suggested that blood platelets may somehow be involved in the development of atherosclerotic plaque formation as well. If this general concept is correct it might be possible not only to prevent clot formation in arteries, but, conceivably, to impede atherosclerosis by administering drugs that inhibit platelet aggregation. Several drugs are known to have this ability, including aspirin, Persantine, and Anturane. These latter antiplatelet agents have been carefully studied in large clinical trials to determine their effectiveness in reducing mortality from CHD (among patients with previous myocardial infarction). The results, in general, have been encouraging but, unfortunately, are not entirely conclusive. All of the studies showed that patients treated with aspirin, Persantine, or Anturane had a somewhat lower mortality in ensuing years than those receiving a placebo; but the differences in mortality were too small to be considered statistically significant. (This means that the lower mortality may have occurred simply by chance, not because of drug therapy.) However, one striking finding that emerged from the Anturane trial has created a new wave of enthusiasm about the potential value of this (and perhaps other) antiplatelet agents in the management of CHD: the drug seemed to reduce the incidence of sudden cardiac death by nearly 75% during the high risk period 2–7 months after acute myocardial infarction (but not beyond this time). The mechanism of this unusual protective action against arrhythmic deaths, and why it persists for only 7 months, is not known. At any rate, on the basis of present evidence it appears that antiplatelet drugs may be beneficial in lowering mortality in post-infarction patients, particularly if treatment is started early after an attack, but, clearly, further research is needed to answer this question.

Medical Treatment

Several important advances in the medical treatment of symptomatic CHD in recent years have brought hope that drug treatment may in one way or other inhibit serious complications of myocardial ischemia and promote long-term survival.

The first advance was the introduction of a group of drugs called *beta-blocking agents.* These drugs represented a breakthrough in the treatment of angina pectoris as they provided the first effective means of *preventing* anginal attacks rather than relieving them (with sublingual nitroglycerin) after they occurred. By blocking the sympathetic nervous system's effects on the heart, beta-blockers reduce the heart rate and blood pressure, thus diminishing the work of the heart and its oxygen demands. Beta-blocking agents are generally used in combination with long-acting nitrates such as isosorbide dinitrate; together, these drugs are highly efficacious in managing angina pectoris or the intermediate coronary syndrome. Despite the proven ability of beta-blockers to inhibit myocardial ischemia and improve exercise tolerance in patients with angina, there is no documentation that these agents can prevent progression of the atherosclerotic disease process. However, there is impressive evidence to indicate that beta-blocking drugs may prolong life in patients who have recovered from an acute myocardial infarction. For example, a large cooperative study conducted throughout Norway showed that patients treated with a beta-blocking agent following myocardial infarction had a 40% lower mortality than a control group during the next two years. Moreover, the incidence of sudden death and recurrent myocardial infarction were reduced markedly in the drug-treated patients. These encouraging results have been confirmed in subsequent trials in the United States (and elsewhere) and it now appears that treatment with beta-blockers after myocardial infarction has considerable value in improving long-term survival. Unfortunately, this form of treatment has many contraindications (especially heart failure and obstructive lung disease) that precludes its use on a routine basis.

Another medical advance has been the development of a new class of drugs categorized as calcium antagonists or *calcium-blocking agents.* These drugs have several different actions, foremost of which is their ability to increase coronary blood flow and improve myocardial oxygenation. The exact mechanism of this beneficial effect is still uncertain, but it is believed that these agents reduce coronary vascular resistance by relaxing the smooth muscles within the arterial walls. In other words, the drugs inhibit smooth muscle contraction, which in effect allows the arteries to dilate fully. (Smooth muscle contraction depends on calcium ions; by blocking the entry of calcium through cell membranes these agents prevent contraction.) Because of this antispasmodic action, calcium-blocking agents were used initially to treat coronary artery spasm (variant angina), and the results of several studies indicate that these drugs are extremely effective for this purpose. Calcium antagonists have also been employed in the treatment of stable angina, again with considerable success. (Present evidence suggests that calcium antagonists have about the same efficacy as beta-blockers in controlling stable angina, although the mechanism of action of the two drugs is entirely different.) In addition to preventing myocardial ischemia, calcium-blocking agents are reported to be effective in the treatment of resistant arrhythmias, heart failure, and hypertension. In all, it seems clear that this class of drugs has great potential and will provide a new avenue of medical treatment for CHD; however, the role and ultimate value of this therapy remains to be determined.

Balloon Dilatation of Coronary Arteries

The newest approach to the treatment of symptomatic CHD involves dilatation of narrowed segments of coronary arteries by means of a small balloon catheter inserted into the obstructed vessel by way of a peripheral artery. The technique is described as *percutaneous transluminal coronary angioplasty (PTCA).* It is primarily used to treat patients with disabling angina who might otherwise be candidates for bypass surgery.

The procedure is performed as follows: a relatively large catheter, called a guiding catheter, is introduced percutaneously through either a femoral or brachial artery and positioned at the ostium of the involved vessel. Coronary angiography is performed through the guiding catheter to visualize the exact location of the lesion. A second catheter—the coronary dilatation catheter—is then inserted through the guiding catheter to the site of obstruction. The dilatation catheter, which has a short, flexible wire guide at its tip, is advanced until the guide wire passes through the obstruction and the deflated balloon segment of the catheter straddles the stenotic area (Figure 3.2). The balloon is then inflated for 3-5 seconds with a pressure sufficient to dilate the obstructed segment. If the first response is not satisfactory, the inflation cycle may be repeated several times. After the procedure, patients are monitored for 6-8 hours and may be discharged after 1-2 days.

The main advantage of PTCA, at least in principle, is that it unblocks obstructed arteries and produces an immediate increase in coronary blood flow without the need for surgery. Moreover, the procedure involves a minimal hospital stay with rapid convalescence and is much less expensive than bypass surgery. Also, PTCA can be repeated, if necessary, in the event the vessel becomes obstructed again. In practice, however, the technique seems to have limited application at present. Clinical experience suggests that PTCA is useful primarily in patients with one vessel disease, and should be restricted to this particular group. Accordingly, only 5%-10% of patients who might otherwise undergo coronary bypass surgery are considered suitable candidates for PTCA. Furthermore, this catheterization procedure is not without risk: it may cause sudden occlusion or deterioration in flow in the obstructed artery, resulting in acute myocardial infarction or worsening of symptoms. Further evaluation of the benefits, risks, and long-term effects of PTCA will be necessary to define the eventual role of this innovative method of treatment.

THE CONCEPT OF INTENSIVE CORONARY CARE

Of the various methods proposed to reduce the overwhelming death rate from CHD, only one thus far has proved to be feasible, practical, and of definite benefit: the plan is called *intensive coronary care.* It is based on the premise that unless acute myocardial infarction can be prevented the best hope for reducing mortality is to provide specialized care soon after the attack has occurred, when the death rate is highest, and to salvage lives in this way. Admittedly, this after-the-fact approach to the overall problem of CHD is less meaningful than attempting to avert acute myocardial infarction, but the value of this concept is clearly evident. Before the introduction of intensive coronary care in 1962, *at least 30%* of all patients admitted to hospitals with acute myocardial infarc-

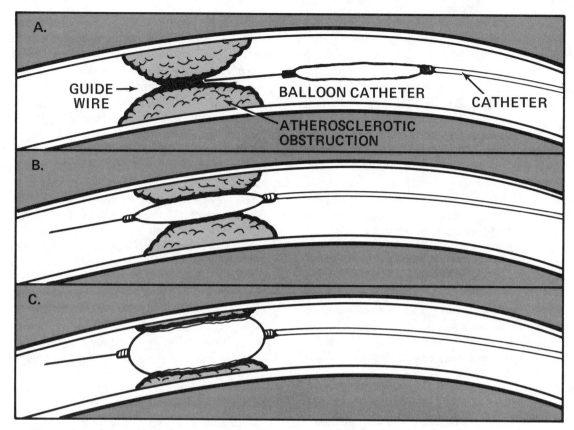

Figure 3.2. A) Guide wire of dilatation catheter (with balloon deflated) being inserted into obstructed segment. B) Balloon inflated within stenotic area, thereby enlarging lumen of artery.

tion died during the period of hospitalization. This means that about one out of every three patients with acute myocardial infarction who was fortunate enough to even reach a hospital did not survive. Since that time, as a direct result of the coronary care system, the hospital death rate from acute myocardial infarction has fallen to about 15%-17%, or to about one-half of the previous mortality. The total number of lives saved each year by intensive coronary care is difficult to estimate, but it is noteworthy that in the United States the mortality from CHD, after rising steadily for many decades, fell for the first time (by about 23%) during the years 1968 through 1977, when all but the smallest hospitals had established coronary care units.* In any case, intensive coronary care is now a standard method of care in hospitals throughout the world. It is the strongest and most dependable method presently available for combating the overall problem of CHD, and it promises to remain so in the foreseeable future.

---

*It would not be fair to assume that this very significant reduction in mortality was due entirely to intensive coronary care; many other factors undoubtedly contributed to the decline. Not only did medical and surgical treatment of CHD improve greatly during this same period, but smoking decreased substantially and hypertension was treated more vigorously.

THE DEVELOPMENT OF INTENSIVE CORONARY CARE

The concept of intensive coronary care was conceived in 1962 when two parallel avenues of research were finally brought together as a functional system of care. One area of research concerned the manner and mechanisms by which acute myocardial infarction causes death; the other involved new techniques of cardiac resuscitation.

It had been known for many years that death from acute myocardial infarction was always the result of *complications* of the attack, not occlusion of a coronary artery itself. However, the relative frequency in which the five main complications of acute myocardial infarction (as described in Chapter 2) produce death was uncertain. In 1961 Meltzer and Kitchell answered this question by studying the mechanisms of death in 171 patients who died of acute myocardial infarction. On the basis of their investigation they concluded that death was attributable to the following causes:

Arrhythmias	47%	
Left ventricular failure	28%	} 43%
Cardiogenic shock	15%	
Emboli	8%	
Rupture of ventricle	2%	

These findings were extremely important in pointing out a way toward improving the survival rate after acute myocardial infarction. It was evident that rupture of the ventricle and embolism, the two complications that rarely can be treated successfully, were not common causes of death, comprising only 2% and 8%, respectively, of the total mortality. Left ventricular failure and cardiogenic shock, representing failure of the heart to pump effectively, collectively produced 43% of the deaths. *By far the most important observation was the unusually high percentage (47%) of deaths due to arrhythmias.* Although sudden and unanticipated deaths resulting from electrical disturbances in the heart were not unfamiliar events, the actual incidence of this lethal complication had been grossly underestimated in the past. (Indeed before this study the impression existed that arrhythmic deaths were relatively uncommon.) The fact that nearly one-half of all deaths from acute myocardial infarction resulted from arrhythmias became the cornerstone for the concept of intensive coronary care since it was known that *arrhythmic deaths were preventable!*

In fact, it was known for more than 50 years that *ventricular fibrillation,* the arrhythmia responsible for at least 90% of all sudden deaths, could be terminated and the life saved if a powerful electric shock was delivered to the heart immediately after the onset of the arrhythmia. At first it was believed that the electrodes (which delivered the electric shock) had to be applied directly to the surface of the ventricles. Because this procedure required the chest to be opened (thoracotomy) to expose the heart, application of this livesaving measure was confined primarily to the prepared setting of operating rooms. For this reason the technique of open-chest cardiac resuscitation never became a practical method for preventing death from acute myocardial infarction.

In 1956 this particular problem was solved when Dr. Paul Zoll and his colleagues demonstrated that ventricular fibrillation could be terminated by means of an electric shock delivered *externally* through the intact chest wall, thus eliminating the need for thoracotomy. Even this major medical advance had limited practical application until the development of the coronary care concept because of the extraordinarily short interval between the onset of ventricular fibrillation and irreversible death. *Usually only 1-2 minutes are available to stop ventricular fibrillation and restore an effective heartbeat.* Understandably, the chance of accomplishing this maneuver (defibrillation) within this very brief period is remote under ordinary hospital circumstances. Specifically, successful defibrillation in the precoronary care era required that a physician be in attendance when the death-producing arrhythmia began, that an electro-cardiographic (ECG) machine (to identify the arrhythmia) and a defibrillator be brought to the bedside, and that an electric shock be delivered to the heart— *all within two precious minutes or less!* From the results of the study previously described in which nearly half of all deaths from acute myocardial infarction were due to arrhythmias, it is clearly apparent that these fortuitous circumstances rarely prevailed even though the hospitals involved had highly trained personnel and the necessary equipment to perform defibrillation.

Results of resuscitation from *ventricular stand-still*—the second of the arrhythmias that cause sudden death—were equally poor. There was good evidence that if the heartbeat stopped (asystole) it could be reactivated under certain conditions by rhythmic electric stimuli delivered to the myocardium by a device called a pacemaker. However, again, although pacing techniques had been known for more than a dozen years, very few lives were ever saved with this ingenious method because of the same time limitation; restoration of the heartbeat after ventricular standstill can be accomplished only if pacing is started within seconds after the onset of the arrhythmia.

Thus as late as 1960, despite the availability of methods and equipment to prevent arrhythmic deaths, little headway had actually been made in decreasing mortality from acute myocardial infarction. The fault was readily apparent: insufficient time to permit corrective action to be taken once a lethal arrhythmia developed. Attacking this critical problem, Kouwenhoven and co-workers at Johns Hopkins Hospital in 1960 devised a simple procedure to sustain the circulation until defibrillation or cardiac pacing could be performed. The method, now known as cardiopulmonary resuscitation (CPR), involves rhythmic compression of the lower sternum (to compress the heart) and mouth-to-mouth ventilation (to supply oxygen). With this technique the circulation can be adequately supported for many minutes (or longer), thus providing additional time to terminate the arrhythmia. Although CPR was instrumental in saving the lives of many patients who would have died otherwise, it soon became evident that this resuscitative method could not be expected to reduce substantially the total number of arrhythmic deaths. The reason was that most patients who died of lethal arrhythmias were unattended at the moment of the catastrophe, and by the time the event was recognized it was too late to initiate CPR because death was already irreversible.

Finally, in 1962, Day, at Bethany Hospital in Kansas City, Kansas, and Meltzer and Kitchell, at the Presbyterian-University of Pennsylvania Medical Center in Philadelphia, independently conceived a plan by which sudden arrhythmic deaths among patients hospitalized with acute myocardial infarction might be prevented in nearly all instances. Both research teams reasoned that, if patients were kept under constant surveillance in a special unit where the cardiac rhythm could be observed continuously and where resuscitative equipment was always ready for immediate use, it would be possible to detect and terminate lethal arrhythmias the instant they occurred. In this way, sudden, unexpected death from arrhythmias could be avoided. *Were this scheme successful, the in-hospital mortality rate from acute myocardial infarction might be reduced by nearly 50%.*

The development of monitoring equipment which permitted the cardiac rate and rhythm to be viewed constantly brought the plan closer to reality. One last step had to be accomplished before intensive coronary care could be implemented: to train personnel to assess the patient's clinical course, to identify and interpret arrhythmias, and, above all, to act on their own if necessary in terminating lethal arrhythmias. But who would assume this demanding role? At that time it seemed that only physicians could possibly undertake the responsibility, but then research studies at the Presbyterian-University of Pennsylvania Medical Center revealed that specially trained nurses were fully capable of serving in this critical position. It was with this background that the original system of intensive care was finally designed and tested.

THE BASIC SYSTEM OF INTENSIVE CORONARY CARE

Intensive coronary care is a *system* of care designed primarily to prevent death from the complications of acute myocardial infarction. As with any effective system, optimal function depends on the interrelationship of its various components; individually the components are not self-sufficient and cannot achieve the desired result. The interrelationship of the components of the system of coronary care is shown in the following diagram.

The patient (A) with suspected or confirmed acute myocardial infarction is admitted directly to the coronary care unit (CCU), a fully equipped facility within which all materials necessary for the detection and treatment of the complications of acute myocardial infarction are centralized. (The design of the unit and its equipment are described in Chapter 4.)

Monitoring equipment (B), attached to the patient, provides a continuous display of the electrocardiogram on an oscilloscopic screen. In this way the rate and rhythm of the heart is apparent at all times, and the onset of any arrhythmia can be detected immediately. Cardiac monitors also include rate meters which indicate the minute-to-minute heart rate as well

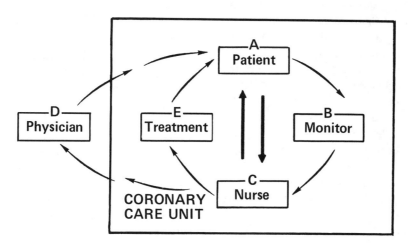

as alarm systems which alert personnel to significant changes in the heart rate. Thus if the rate of the heart exceeds or falls below preset limits, an alarm is triggered. (The details of cardiac monitoring are described in Chapter 6.) In addition to electrocardiographic monitors, other monitoring equipment to assess circulatory (hemodynamic) function is also available for diagnostic purposes.

The nurse (C), who has been specifically trained for this specialized role, remains in constant attendance within the unit. Of the multiple nursing duties and responsibilities, one of the most essential is to interpret the electrocardiographic findings displayed on the oscilloscope and to recognize the significance of changes in cardiac rate or rhythm. In addition the nurse must repeatedly assess the clinical condition of the patient at the bedside by planned careful observation and physical examination in order to detect signs of other complications of myocardial infarction. In the event of any change in the patient's status, either clinically or electrocardiographically, the nurse must decide upon a course of action which may involve either further observation, notifying a physician, or acting immediately on her own in emergency situations. (The nursing role is described in detail in Chapter 5.)

The physician (D), unlike the nurse, is not in constant attendance. He relies fundamentally on the observations made by the nurse members of the team who advise him of their assessments, particularly when there is a change in the clinical course. That the physician delegates unusual authority to the nurse members of the physician-nurse team is one of the most distinguishing characteristics of the system of intensive coronary care.

The treatment program (E) is designed to prevent lethal complications. The plan of therapy is directed by the physician but carried out, for the most part, by the nurse. In emergency situations—especially when lethal arrhythmias develop—the nurse must perform lifesaving measures (e.g., defibrillation) in the absence of the physician.

From the foregoing description of the coronary care system it is readily apparent that *the nurse is the key to the success of the entire system of coronary care.* This is not to say that nursing practice alone determines the effectiveness of intensive coronary care, but it does indeed mean that without specially trained, highly skilled nurses the system can never achieve full effectiveness. In fact, without specialized nursing practice intensive coronary care is no more than a token gesture. This concept of nursing care implies much more than simply having a nurse stationed in a CCU to observe the cardiac monitor and to call a physician when an alarm sounds or another problem arises. For the intensive care program to fullfill its objectives the nurse must be able to anticipate complications, assess each problem as it arises, and, above all, assume a *decision-making* role. Unless nurses are delegated authority to make and carry out therapeutic decisions based on their own observations and judgment, the coronary care system is weakened seriously. This point was demonstrated decisively by the initial experience with intensive coronary care at New York Hospital-Cornell Medical Center. When the coronary care unit began operation, the nursing staff was *not* empowered to act on its own in emergency situations and had to call a house officer to defibrillate patients. With this restrictive policy the mortality at the end of the first year among patients treated in the CCU was the same (31%) as that noted on the general medical wards. As soon as nurses were granted authority to defibrillate patients in the absence of a physician, the mortality in the unit fell promptly.

It should also be emphasized that monitoring equipment alone, regardless of its sophistication or elegance, must not be construed as intensive coronary care. Monitoring is only one component of the total system and can never be self-sufficient. In the absence of a skilled nursing staff monitoring equipment by itself does not even warrant its expense.

AGGRESSIVE MANAGEMENT OF ARRHYTHMIAS

As would be anticipated from its background, the original concept of intensive coronary care focused primarily on resuscitation from lethal arrhythmias. The fundamental objective was to identify ventricular fibrillation and ventricular standstill the moment they occurred, and to terminate them instantly.

When this plan of coronary care was first tested at the Bethany Hospital and the Presbyterian-University of Pennsylvania Medical Center it proved effective immediately. The mortality among patients treated in the coronary care units of both hospitals fell to 20% (in constrast to the previous death rate of 30%-35% with customary hospital care). In other words, intensive coronary care was successful in decreasing the hospital mortality from acute myocardial infarction by about one-third (33%). This reduction in mortality was achieved almost entirely by successful defibrillation and (to a much lesser extent) by emergency cardiac pacing.*

---

*In the first coronary care units cardiac pacing was performed by means of a pacing electrode attached to the chest wall that delivered electrical stimuli to the heart after ventricular standstill had occurred. This external method of pacing was seldom successful in resuscitation; and it was not until the introduction of intracardiac pacing, a few years later, that any significant inroad could be made against death from ventricular standstill.

It soon became evident that ventricular fibrillation and ventricular standstill seldom occurred spontaneously; in most instances the catastrophes were preceded by lesser (warning) arrhythmias. When it was demonstrated that warning arrhythmias could be controlled by antiarrhythmic drugs or by transvenous pacing, the theme and emphasis of coronary care switched abruptly from resuscitation to the *prevention* of lethal arrhythmias. This step marked the beginning of the second stage of development of the coronary care system—the aggressive management of warning arrhythmias.

According to the concept, vigorous treatment of warning arrhythmias would prevent ventricular fibrillation and ventricular standstill in most cases, relegating resuscitation to a role of lesser importance (at least in principle). The value of this plan was confirmed promptly. For example, Lown, at the Peter Bent Brigham Hospital in Boston, reported a zero incidence of ventricular fibrillation among 130 consecutive patients in whom this preventative approach was used. He concluded that "resuscitation even when successful represents a failure—a failure of anticipation and a failure of prophylactic therapy." Aggressive management became, and remains, the byword of coronary care.

THE ATTACK AGAINST DEATH FROM PUMP FAILURE

With the ability to prevent arrhythmic deaths an accomplished fact, coronary care entered its third stage of development: an attempt to reduce the death rate from left ventricular failure and cardiogenic shock (pump failure).

By 1970 (when many major medical centers had reported their experience with intensive coronary care) it was clear that the reduction in hospital mortality had already reached a plateau (at about 18-20%, as noted in Table 3.1), and that no further decrease in the death rate could be anticipated with the existing program of care. The reason for this limitation was readily apparent: the system of care was capable of preventing nearly all sudden arrhyth-

mic deaths, but it was not effective in saving lives from the other complications of acute myocardial infarction. In particular, the mortality from pump failure showed no improvement compared to the results obtained without coronary care. The inability to combat death from cardiogenic shock and advanced left ventricular failure made pump failure the most common cause of death among patients treated in CCUs. In fact more than 90% of the total mortality from acute myocardial infarction is now due to pump failure. The change in the relative incidence of death-producing complications before and (8 years) after the introduction of the coronary care system at the Presbyterian-University of Pennsylvania Medical Center is shown in Table 3.2.

Little headway was made in the battle against left ventricular failure and cardiogenic shock until the introduction of the Swan-Ganz balloon catheter in 1970. This simple, ingenious device permitted the heart's pumping performance to be measured safely and effectively at the bedside during the acute phase of myocardial infarction. With these pressure measurements treatment could be structured in a rational, deliberate way according to the particular hemodynamic disturbance. Moreover, it became possible to evaluate the actual effectiveness of various forms of drug therapy, which had been used indiscriminately in the past.

Of the several different approaches now being used to control pump failure, four methods seem to hold the greatest promise: 1) detecting heart failure at its earliest stages so that prompt treatment can be initiated in an attempt to prevent progression, 2) improving pumping efficiency by reducing the workload of the heart with drug therapy, 3) increasing left ventricular function (particularly in cardiogenic shock) by means of mechanical circulatory assist devices (e.g., intraaortic balloon pumping or external counterpulsation), and 4) performing emergency bypass surgery if other methods are unsuccessful. (All of these methods are described in Chapter 7.) Although the effectiveness of this multipronged approach must still be determined, it is fair to say that the possibility of reducing mortality from advanced left ventricular failure and cardiogenic shock is brighter than before, at least in selected patients.

Table 3.1. Mortality from Acute Myocardial Infarction at Major Medical Centers (1970)

Series	Place	No. of Patients	Hospital Mortality (%)
Day and Averill	Kansas City	280	20.0
Meltzer and Kitchell	Philadelphia	500	18.0
Lown et al.	Boston	300	17.7
Julian and Oliver	Scotland	552	19.2
Killip and Kimball	New York	300+	21.0
Sloman et al.	Australia	350	18.0

Table 3.2. Incidence of Death-Producing Complications Before and
After Introduction of Coronary Care

Complication	Complication Rate (%)	
	Before CCU	*After CCU*
Arrhythmias	47	2
Pump failure (left ventricular failure and cardiogenic shock)	43	91
Emboli	8	4
Ventricular rupture	2	3

REDUCTION OF MYOCARDIAL INFARCT SIZE

Despite the progress just described, the fact remains that no significant reduction in the overall mortality from pump failure has been achieved since the advent of intensive coronary care. Many believe that an entirely different approach to the problem will be necessary before the death rate can be lowered substantially. It has been proposed recently that the treatment program should be redirected toward *preventing* left ventricular failure and cardiogenic shock, rather than attempting to control these complications after they have occurred. This new approach is based on evidence that most patients who die of pump failure have extensive myocardial infarction, involving at least 40% of the left ventricle. Thus, were it possible to *limit the size of the infarct* the chances of developing serious pump failure would be reduced. Not only would this intervention decrease mortality during the acute phase of myocardial infarction, but it might also improve long-term survival since it is known that the size of the infarct and the degree of left ventricular function it produces are critical factors in determining the ultimate prognosis of CHD.

The concept of attempting to reduce the size of an infarct is based on the premise that in the early hours after acute coronary occlusion there are two general zones of myocardial damage: a central zone of severe ischemia and a border zone of lesser ischemia. The central zone undergoes necrosis and is irreversibly destroyed. The border zone, however, although injured and jeopardized, may survive and recover if the ischemic process can be controlled within 3 hours. Thus the ultimate size of an infarction depends, theoretically, on the fate of the border zone (as described in Chapter 1). The goal of treatment is to salvage the border zone and in this way to reduce (or limit) the size of the infarct. Among the drugs currently being tested for this purpose are beta-blockers (e.g., propranolol and metoprolol), intravenous nitroglycerin, glucose-potassium-insulin infusions, hyaluronidase, and calcium-blocking agents (e.g., nifedipine). Results of clinical trials with these drugs have been generally encouraging but it has been very difficult to prove that any of these agents can in fact reduce the size of the infarct. Ongoing research may provide an answer to this all-important question.

The newest (and perhaps most exciting) method of preserving ischemic myocardium involves reopening acutely occluded coronary arteries with the use of drugs that dissolve clots; this technique is called *intracoronary thrombolysis.* Since clot (thrombus) formation is the major cause of acute coronary artery occlusion it was reasoned that dissolution of thrombi by thrombolytic agents might restore blood flow immediately, thus reversing the ischemic process and reducing the area of tissue destruction. (In fact, animal experiments have shown that restoration of blood flow can completely prevent necrosis if reperfusion is accomplished within 20 minutes after coronary artery occlusion.) The technique consists of introducing a special catheter into the occluded vessel (by way of a peripheral artery) and infusing a thrombolytic substance (e.g., streptokinase or thrombolysin) for approximately one hour. The effect is very prompt and reopening of obstructed vessels has been demonstrated within 20-30 minutes. For thrombolytic therapy to be successful patients must be treated within 3 hours (and probably no later than 6 hours) after the onset of myocardial infarction. Clinical experience with intracoronary thrombolysis has been limited to date, and its potential risks have not been defined; however this method is now being utilized on a research basis in centers throughout the world. If effective, it will be important to the future treatment of acute myocardial infarction.

PREHOSPITAL CORONARY CARE

One of the inherent weaknesses of the basic coronary system is its inability to prevent death before hospitalization. Ordinarily intensive coronary care begins when the patient finally reaches a CCU, which often involves a delay of many hours after the onset of symptoms. This delay in initiating care is a very serious handicap since it is estimated that 50%-60% of deaths from acute myocardial infarction occur before hospital admission, usually in the first few hours after the attack, as a result of lethal arrhythmias.

In an effort to reduce *prehospital* mortality many communities now utilize mobile coronary care units. The primary purpose of these units is to prevent arrhythmic deaths at home or in transit to the hospital by initiating coronary care as soon as possible. The mobile units are large vehicles (or ambulances) specially designed and equipped for handling acute cardiac emergencies; they are usually staffed by allied health personnel (Emergency Medical Technicians) who have been carefully trained to defibrillate patients, administer intravenous drugs, and perform other lifesaving measures. This system of prehospital care has been of inestimable help in preventing early deaths from myocardial infarction. It promises to become even more effective as the public becomes better aware of the need for immediate medical attention after the onset of symptoms.

A related problem interfering with the prompt initiation of intensive coronary care is the prolonged period of time patients most often wait in busy emergency wards of hospitals before being examined and finally admitted to the CCU. There are two basic ways of removing this weak link in the chain of hospital care. One is to bypass the emergency facility and admit patients directly to the CCU. This plan functions in the following way: as soon as a patient whose history suggests acute myocardial infarction enters the receiving ward he is placed on a litter equipped with a battery-powered monitor and defibrillator, and cardiac monitoring is started immediately. The patient is then transported to the CCU accompanied by a nurse or physician. No attempt is made to confirm the diagnosis of acute myocardial infarction or to obtain customary hospital admission data in the emergency ward. An alternative approach is to equip and staff part of the emergency ward as a separate CCU, where intensive care can be started instantly. Unfortunately, only a few hospitals can afford to maintain and staff two CCUs; therefore this scheme is less feasible than rapid transfer to the CCU. *In any case, the sooner intensive coronary care can be initiated, the better the survival rate.*

BASIC PRACTICES OF INTENSIVE CORONARY CARE
Selection of Patients

The criteria for admission to a CCU are distinctly different from those used to determine the need for other forms of intensive care. Usually admission to an intensive care unit is based primarily on the level of patient care required rather than on a specific clinical disorder, but this is not the case with acute myocardial infarction and intensive coronary care. Every patient with acute myocardial infarction, regardless of the severity of the attack, should be admitted directly to a CCU. Admittedly, patients who show evidence of complications on arrival at the hospital have a far greater chance of developing additional problems than those who are free of complications initially; therefore it might be argued that intensive coronary care (being as comprehensive and expensive as it is) should be reserved for patients who are acutely ill when first seen. This reasoning is fallacious however because the clinical course during the acute phase of myocardial infarction is by no means predictable. *Many patients who appear perfectly stable on admission may be candidates for sudden death.* The fact is that arrhythmias and other complications can develop at any time. For example, in studying the clinical course of 100 patients *without* complications at the time of admission to the CCU at the Presbyterian-University of Pennsylvania Medical Center, we found that 38% of the group subsequently developed serious arrhythmias, 22% left ventricular failure, and 4% cardiogenic shock. The mortality among these so-called "good risk" patients was 9%. In other words, it is foolhardy to attempt to predict the outcome of acute myocardial infarction according to the clinical picture on admission: good risk patients can be identified only *in retrospect,* and therefore all patients with acute myocardial infarction should be treated in a CCU for at least the first few days.

This cautious policy also involves the admission of patients with *suspected* myocardial infarction. Very often patients arrive at a hospital with chest pain or other symptoms suspicious of acute myocardial infarction, but a positive diagnosis cannot be established at the time because the ECG fails to reveal characteristic findings of an acute infarction. Should these patients be admitted to a CCU to "rule out acute myocardial infarction" or should they be observed elsewhere in the hospital until a definitive diagnosis is made? The answer is clear: any patient whose *history* suggests the possibility of acute myocardial infarction should be admitted to a CCU and treated as if an infarction had in fact occurred. That the initial ECG does not show evidence of myocardial ischemia, injury, or necrosis is unimportant since these findings may take many hours or days to develop. If this practice is followed, the diagnosis of acute myocardial infarction will not be confirmed in approximately one of every three patients admitted to the unit (usually because the problem is finally diagnosed as angina or the intermediate coronary syndrome rather than acute infarction). Although this conservative approach may seem wasteful in terms of personnel, bed usage, and cost, it is nevertheless a sound principle to adopt, particularly since lethal arrhythmias may develop with bewildering speed in the presence of myocardial ischemia. Any compromise with this admission policy is a flirtation with danger.

Along this same line, all patients with *unstable angina* should be admitted directly to a CCU. The clinical course of this condition, as explained previously, is unpredictable and may progress abruptly to acute myocardial infarction. Constant observation of these patients is essential until the pain pattern can be controlled.

The Duration of Intensive Coronary Care

Under ordinary circumstances patients with acute transmural myocardial infarction usually remain in the CCU for 5 days. The reason for this particular duration of stay is that the majority of complications and hospital deaths from acute myocardial infarction occur within this period. As shown in Figure 3.3, approximately 40% of all deaths take place during the first day of hospitalization, and by the end of the fifth day 65% of the total mortality has already occurred. This is not to say, however, that a rigid discharge policy should be followed for all patients. For example, patients with *nontransmural* infarction who experience no complications can usually be transferred from the CCU after only 48 hours. Even those

with transmural infarction may not require 5 days of intensive coronary care, particularly if no significant complications have developed within the first 2 or 3 days. On the other hand, the occurrence of dangerous arrhythmias or even modest heart failure at any time during the period of intensive coronary care dictates a stay of 5 days (or longer).

Although (in the study shown in Figure 3.3) 65% of hospital deaths from acute myocardial infarction occurred in the first 5 days, 35% of the patients died after discharge from the CCU. (Some reports indicate that post-CCU mortality may be as high as 50%). On this basis it might seem logical to extend the period of intensive coronary care for one or two weeks or, indeed, for the entire hospital stay. This approach to the problem is not feasible for several reasons. First, the CCU would require an inordinately large number of beds to accommodate all patients with acute myocardial infarction for more than 5 days. (Surveys have shown that about 8% of the census of a general hospital on any given day consists of patients with acute myocardial infarction; thus a 300-bed institution would require a coronary care unit of neary 25 beds.) Second, intensive coronary care is prohibitively expensive and the total cost for prolonged sojourns in the unit would create an enormous economic burden for the patient and society. A final deterrent to extended coronary care is the adverse psychological effects it produces in most patients; depression, anxiety, and abnormal behavior occur frequently in this circumstance.

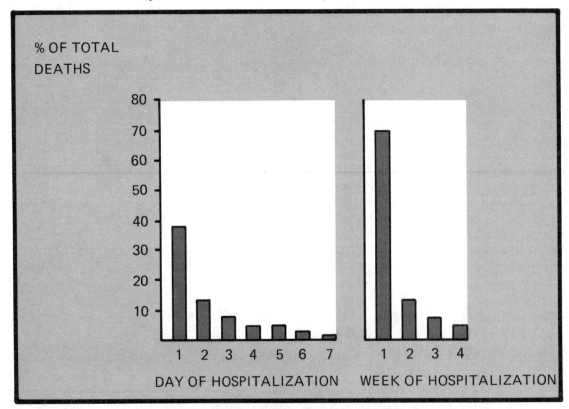

Figure 3.3. Mortality from acute myocardial infarction during hospitalization: an analysis of 350 deaths at the Presbyterian-University of Pennsylvania Medical Center.

In an effort to prevent death after transfer from the CCU, some hospitals have established intermediate coronary care units. The plan for this subacute care involves a separate facility (often contiguous with the CCU) to which patients are transferred after the period of intensive care. The subacute care unit permits additional surveillance of patients with myocardial infarction in a setting that is intermediate between intensive care and customary hospital care. As mentioned in Chapter 2, the actual benefit of this concept, however, has not been clearly established.

Concepts of Treatment in CCU

Although the basic concepts of treatment in coronary care units are essentially standardized, the application of these principles varies to some degree among institutions. For example, the concept of aggressive management of warning arrhythmias to prevent ventricular fibrillation is endorsed by all, but the extent of this practice differs in various coronary care units. In most medical centers antiarrhythmic drugs (e.g., lidocaine) are administered only after a warning arrhythmia has been identified, but some clinicians believe that prophylactic treatment should be used *routinely,* even before warning arrhythmias occur. This latter practice, although perhaps a safer method, carries a risk of producing undesirable side-effects from the drugs when in fact treatment may not be necessary at all.

A similar controversy exists about the management of mild (to moderate) heart failure. In some coronary units a very aggressive treatment program is initiated promptly, including vigorous diuretic therapy and the use of digitalis, vasodilators, and drugs to lower blood pressure resistance. Others believe this approach is overly aggressive and that the cautious use of diuretic agents alone is sufficient treatment, at least initially.

The reason for these (and other) differences in opinion about the extent of aggressive management is the concern of many cardiologists about the dangers of *overtreatment.* Although the value of preventive treatment of complications is undeniable, and remains the cornerstone of intensive coronary care, it is equally clear that overtreatment is a serious risk in itself. For instance, nearly all antiarrhythmic drugs act by depressing the myocardium, thus reducing myocardial pumping efficiency and increasing the likelihood of left ventricular failure. The overzealous use of diuretic agents and drugs to reduce venous and arterial pressures can produce hypotension and cardiogenic shock, totally defeating the purpose for which they were administered. This is not to say that aggressive management should be curtailed, but that overtreatment should be avoided. The ancient rule of medicine, *primum non nocere*—first do not harm—must never be forgotten.

4

The Coronary Care Unit:
Design, Equipment and Nursing Staff

A coronary care unit (CCU) is a specially designed and equipped facility staffed by highly skilled personnel who provide optimum care for patients with suspected or confirmed acute myocardial infarction. Many institutions have expanded the function of the CCU by admitting patients with other cardiac emergencies to the unit. Included in this latter group are patients with acute pulmonary edema, major arrhythmias unrelated to myocardial infarction, and those requiring pacemakers.

The object of this chapter is to discuss the design, equipment, and staff of an effective CCU.

DESIGN OF THE CCU

Because nearly all hospitals now have CCUs, little purpose would be served here by presenting a detailed description of the physical design of these specialized facilities. However, it is useful for nurses to understand some of the basic concepts and problems involved in planning a CCU. This knowledge is important particularly when the nursing staff is asked to participate in designing a new unit or remodeling an old one. Moreover, the physical layout of the unit influences patient care, and the nurse should appreciate this relationship. The following design factors are considered relevant.

1. Ideally the unit should consist of a series of individual private rooms. An open ward-type facility with curtains or partitions between beds is unsuitable for providing the peacefulness and serenity required in the overall treatment program. Furthermore, it is important that patients be unaware of each other so they are not affected by emergencies occurring in adjacent areas. Seeing a crisis elsewhere in the unit can be a devastating emotional experience. In the same vein, the unit should be designed in such a way that beds and litters can be moved to and from the individual rooms without the risk of disturbing other patients. This unobtrusive movement is particularly important when death occurs.

2. All beds should be directly visible (through glass windows) from a central nursing station. Direct visual observation is an integral part of coronary care nursing and it is thoroughly disadvantageous to rely on monitor surveillance as the prime means of patient assessment. In very large units more than one nursing station may be required to provide close observation of all patients. The optimal size of a CCU is four to six beds.

3. Patient's rooms should be at least 12×12 feet in size to allow adequate space for equipment and multiple personnel (particularly at the time of emergencies). Since many patients in the CCU are admitted because of suspected myocardial infarction and may not be desperately ill, it is important that the unit be attractively and cheerfully decorated. An outside window should

be present in each room; "inside" rooms are very depressing to patients. Provisions for noise control are essential, and acoustical materials for ceilings and floors should be used whenever possible. It is helpful to furnish rooms with clocks, calendars, a radio, and music so the patient does not become totally separated from his normal environment.

4. It is beneficial to locate the CCU at a site contiguous with (or nearby) the hospital's general medical intensive care unit. This arrangement allows for sharing of certain basic facilities and services (e.g., utility rooms, pantries, storage areas) that would otherwise require duplication. It also has the advantage of allowing the nursing staff to rotate between the units, thus facilitating staffing patterns and broadening the scope of clinical nursing experience. However, it is generally disadvantageous to combine the two specialized units into one facility, particularly since a general intensive care unit is usually much too hectic a setting for patients with acute myocardial infarction. In all, a separate CCU adjacent to a medical intensive care unit is perhaps the most effective and practical design plan. An alternative (but lesser used) arrangement is to locate the CCU close to the emergency ward of the hospital. This proximity permits patients to be transferred directly from the admission area to the CCU without any delay while preserving continuity of assessment and care.

5. In the design plan it is worthwhile to provide certain additional rooms near the CCU for purposes other than patient care. Of special importance are the following areas:

    a. Waiting room for families. Because of the abrupt and critical nature of cardiac emergencies it is understandable that families gather and remain near the patient for prolonged periods. Unless provisions are made to accommodate these visitors in a separate room outside the unit, disturbance and congestion at the nurses' station and patient care areas usually results. This family waiting room should have adequate telephone facilities, both for outside calls and for communicating with the nursing staff in the CCU.

    b. Nurses' lounge. Since nursing personnel must be in continuous attendance within the unit it is important that a room be allocated within the unit for the nursing staff. This lounge should include bathroom facilities, lockers, and comfortable furniture.

    c. Physicians' consultation room. Although certainly less essential than the two areas just described, a separate room for the use of

physicians has proven very useful in many institutions. This space provides not only an office for the physicians but sleeping quarters as well when necessary.

6. Effective air conditioning and ventilation systems are mandatory not only for patient and nurse comfort but also for proper upkeep of the monitoring equipment. Many monitoring systems and other equipment are heat-sensitive, and proper room temperatures must be maintained to ensure satisfactory function.

7. Multiple, separately fused electrical outlets are absolutely essential and should be considered in the early stages of planning. Approximately eight grounded outlets are required for each bed. Electrical grounding within the unit must have unquestionable integrity. Unless true and effective grounding is provided, there is danger of patient electrocution, particularly when several electrical devices are used simultaneously. Grounding that consists of no more than connecting a wire to a convenient water or heating pipe is wholly inadequate, and a three-pronged plug by itself is not a real safety measure. No compromise can be made with the need for a proper grounding circuit.

    Because of the increasing use of major electrical equipment within units (including portable x-ray machines), 220-volt lines should be included in the electrical system. An emergency power supply should also be available in the event of electrical failure of the primary circuit.

8. Effective communication and alarm systems are of great importance. The objective of the system should be to permit the nursing staff to summon help instantly and directly. The usual hospital communication network, which involves the circuitous chain of dialing the operator, paging physicians, and returning the call to the unit results in too much delay. A special alarm signal (or code) which bypasses the customary route is very desirable at each bedside.

9. In addition to the specialized equipment described in the following section, each room should be furnished with the following items:

    a. Hydraulic bed. A manually operated hydraulic bed is preferable to an electric bed in a CCU. Electric beds pose the potential threat of electric shock to the patient. Also, changing the patient's position with an electric bed is too slow a process in times of emergency.

    b. Toilet facilities. A "pullman" toilet or a bedside commode should be kept near each bedside. Bedpans are undesirable for patients with acute myocardial infarction because of the physical effort expended in their use. A portable toilet requires minimal space and can be brought directly to the bedside.

c. Blood pressure apparatus. A wall-mounted sphygmomanometer is required next to each bed. The ready accessibility of this instrument is advantageous because of the frequency with which blood pressures must be recorded.

d. Hangers for intravenous solutions. At least two metal rods with hooks should be suspended from the ceiling above each bed to hang intravenous solutions. These hangers are less cumbersome than floor standards and do not obstruct access to the patient.

EQUIPMENT FOR A CCU

To fulfill its objectives a CCU must contain equipment for detecting, assessing, and treating complications of acute myocardial infarction (and other cardiac emergencies). The type of equipment depends to a large degree on the role and function of the unit. For instance, a CCU that serves as a research or teaching facility or a referral center may be equipped with computerized systems and sophisticated instruments that are unnecessary in other settings. The following discussion focuses on the basic equipment considered necessary in an up-to-date CCU.

Equipment for Detection

Cardiac Monitoring System

The most important detection instrument in the CCU is the cardiac monitor used to identify arrhythmias on a continuous basis. A separate monitor, consisting of an oscilloscope, a rate meter, an alarm mechanism, and a write-out device, is required for each patient. (The specific details of cardiac monitoring are discussed in Chapter 6.) In some CCUs the monitors are placed at each bedside with "slave" oscilloscope, rate meter and write-out device) at each bedside, along with a central oscilloscope, alarm nursing station with the "slave" attachments at the bedside. Probably the best arrangement for most CCUs is to have an individual monitor (with an oscilloscope, rate meter and write-out device) at each bedside, along with a central oscilloscope, alarm system, and write-out module at the nurses' station. Alarm sounds are heard only in the nurses' station, rather than at the bedside, thus avoiding patient anxiety during false or true alarm situations. Otherwise, the same information is available to the nurse when at the bedside or nurses' station.

Electrocardiographic Machine

In addition to the monitoring system, the unit requires one or more ECG machines for obtaining 12-lead ECGs for diagnostic purposes. The machine is also used to document arrhythmias seen on the oscilloscope when the monitoring equipment does not include a direct ECG writeout device.

Equipment for Assessment

Hemodynamic Instruments

To assess the clinical status of patients with cardiogenic shock or left ventricular failure effectively it is often necessary to measure pressures directly in veins and arteries. Apparatus for this purpose should be on hand in the CCU. The equipment includes manometers, transducers, hemodynamic catheters, and appropriate tubing for determining central venous, intraarterial and pulmonary artery pressures.

Blood Gas Determinations

Arterial blood gases (and to a lesser degree, venous blood gases) are used to assess tissue oxygenation and metabolism, particularly in the presence of circulatory failure. Needles, syringes, and collecting tubes for blood gas studies should be readily available in the CCU.

Equipment for Treatment and Resuscitation

Defibrillator

A defibrillator must be available at all times, readily accessible to each bed. (In the past it was considered judicious to keep a defibrillator at every bedside, but with the present ability to prevent ventricular fibrillation, in most instances, one defibrillator per patient is no longer required.) However, coronary care units with more than four beds should contain at least two defibrillators. In addition, a portable, battery-operated defibrillator should be available to terminate ventricular fibrillation that may develop while patients are being transported to or from the CCU.

Cardioverter

A cardioverter, used to terminate certain rapid-rate arrhythmias (such as atrial tachycardia) should be kept at a central site in the CCU at all times. Most often, cardioverters are incorporated into defibrillators, making a separate cardioverter unnecessary.

Pacemakers

Battery-operated pacemakers for temporary cardiac pacing should be readily available in the CCU. Also required is an assortment of different-sized pacing catheters for transvenous insertion.

Respirators

Respiratory assistance equipment should be kept permanently in the unit. Of the many mechanical respirators now available, perhaps the most useful in a CCU is the pressure-cycled machine which inflates the patient's lungs until a preset pressure has been reached. In addition to mechanical respirators, manual breathing bags are essential.

Crash Cart

A mobile cart which contains all supplies, equipment and drugs needed for cardiac emergencies and resuscitation attempts must be ready for use at all times in the CCU. This cart should be easily movable, constructed of heavy gauge stainless steel, with a low center of gravity to prevent tipping. Preferably the cart should contain three or more shelves, the topmost of which serves as a work area. Separate drawers for drug storage are located between the first and second shelves. The equipment, drugs and supplies customarily contained in a crash cart are noted in Table 4.1. (Some units have adopted a drug system in which all necessary drugs are kept in a locked box on the cart. The box is easily opened during an emergency and, once used, is returned to the pharmacy to be checked and refilled. This plan assures that all drugs have been replaced and are available for the next emergency.)

Oxygen Supply

A dependable oxygen supply piped in from a central source to each bedside is mandatory. Face masks and nasal cannulas for oxygen delivery, along with humidification bottles, should be available for immediate use.

Aspiration Equipment

An effective system for aspirating and suctioning nasotracheal secretions should be located in each patient area. A laryngoscope, nasotracheal tubes, and endotracheal tubes are also required.

Tourniquets

Part of the treatment program for acute left ventricular failure is to reduce the work of the heart by applying tourniquets to the extremities in order to diminish the amount of blood returning to the heart. Either plain rubber tubing or a rotating tourniquet machine can be used for this purpose.

Automatic Timing Device

Because it is critically important to know precisely how much time has elapsed after the onset of a lethal arrhythmia, it is useful to have an automatic timer in the CCU. The nurse activates the device at the bedside by pushing the alarm signal as soon as a death-producing arrhythmia is identified.

Bed Board

Either a board or a cafeteria tray should be kept at each bedside for use during cardiopulmonary resuscitation. Without firm support behind the patient's thorax, external cardiac compression may be ineffective.

Prepared Trays

Sterile packages (trays) for venous cutdown, urinary catheterization, tracheostomy, and other procedures should be kept in readiness.

DRUGS FOR THE CCU

Because medications usually have to be administered at a moment's notice in cardiac emergencies, all necessary drugs and fluids must be immediately available in the CCU. A specific list of drugs for the unit should be established, and an adequate supply of these preparations kept on hand at all times. The responsibility for checking the inventory and reordering should be assigned to the head nurse or her designate. (In some hospitals pharmacy personnel undertake this responsibility.)

It is essential that the drugs be stored in a precise, orderly way so every nurse in the unit knows exactly where to find a particular item without having to search for it. The importance of this theme cannot be overemphasized: every second counts in a life-threatening emergency.

Although physicians have individual preferences about the specific drugs that should be stocked in the CCU, the basic drug list does not vary greatly at different hospitals. The drugs and intravenous solutions stocked in the CCU at the Presbyterian-University of Pennsylvania Medical Center are given in Table 4.2.

Table 4.1 Equipment and Supplies for a Crash Cart

Top Shelf

    Defibrillator
    Electrode paste
    Syringes (3, 5, 10, and 50 cc)
    Needles (18, 20, 21, and 25 gauge)
    Intracardiac needles (3.5 inch needle, 19 gauge)
    Alcohol sponges (one jar)
    Labels
    IV tray containing:
        intravenous tubing, adaptors and solusets
        3-way stopcocks
        armboards (1 short, 1 long)
        Betadine ointment
        1″ cloth tape and 1″ adhesive tape
        blood collection tubes (all types)
        alcohol sponges
        tourniquets
        butterfly needles (#19, #21, #23)
        Angiocaths
        Intracaths
        Longdwell needles (#16, #18, #20)
        4 × 4 dressings

Shelf 2

    Ambu bag and tubing
    Venous cutdown tray
    CVP manometers and tubing
    Prep tray containing:
        1 Kelly clamp
        1 forcep
        1 scissor
        1 scalpel with blade
        sterile gloves (2 of each size)
        sutures
        barriers
        1 stopcock
        1 fenestrated drape
        1 disposable tray
    Intubation tray containing:
        airway resuscitube
        padded tongue blades
        laryngoscope with #2 or #3 blades and extra bulbs and batteries
        stylette
        Universal adaptors
        T-tubes
        Lidocaine 4% (40 mg/ml) 50 ml with atomizer
        1″ adhesive tape
        4 × 4 gauze squares
        lubricating jelly
        McGill forceps
        rubber-tipped hemostat
        endotracheal tubes (#36, #32, #28)
        suction catheters (14 f)
        10 cc syringe
        bottle of Benzoin

(*continued next page*)

Table 4.1 Equipment and Supplies for a Crash Cart (*continued*)

Shelf 3

Pacemaker and pacing catheters
Tracheostomy set
5% Dextrose in water —500 cc
5% Sodium bicarbonate solution—1000 cc
Blood administration set

Side of Cart

Flashlight
Sphygmomanometer
Stethoscope
Clipboard with pencil containing:
    complete inventory of all crash cart supplies
    form for nurses to sign after checking and restocking cart each shift

Back of Cart

Resuscitation board
Portable IV pole

In Drawer (or in Medication Box)

Aminophylline (0.5 Gm/20 ml)	3 ampules
Atropine sulfate (1 mg/ml)	3 ampules
Bretylol (50 mg/ml)	2 ampules
Calcium chloride (100 mg/ml)	5 ampules
Calcium gluceptate (90 mg) (4.5 mg/ml)	4 ampules
Dexamethasone (4 mg/ml)	1 tubex
Dextrose 50% (25 GM/50 ml)	2 syringes
Digoxin (0.5 mg/2 ml)	2 ampules
Dilantin (100 mg/2 ml)	2 syringes
Dobutamine (Dobutrex) (250 mg)	2 vials
Dopamine (200 mg/5 ml)	4 ampules
Edrophonium chloride (10 mg/ml)	2 ampules
Epinephrine (adrenalin) (1 mg/ml) (1:1000)	1 30 ml vial
Epinephrine (adrenalin) (1 mg/10 ml)	4 syringes
Heparin (1000 U/ml)	1 10 ml vial
Isoproterenol (Isuprel) (1 mg/5 ml)	4 ampules
Lasix (10 mg/ml)	4 2 ml ampules
Levarterenol bitartrate (Levophed) (4 mg/4 ml)	6 ampules
Lidocaine (100 mg/5 ml)	4 syringes
Lidocaine (2 Gm/10 ml)	4 pin top vials
Lidocaine (1 Gm/5 ml)	2 pin top vials
Mannitol (12.5 Gm/50 ml)	4 vials
Naloxone (Narcan) (0.4 mg/ml)	2 ampules
Phenobarbital (130 mg/ml)	1 vial
Procainamide (Pronestyl) (100 mg/ml)	3 10 ml vials
Propranolol (Inderal) (1 mg/ml)	2 syringes
Sodium bicarbonate (10 mEq/10 ml)	5 syringes
Sodium bicarbonate (50 mEq/50 ml)	5 syringes
Sodium chloride for injection (30 ml)	2 vials
Valium (5 mg/ml)	4 vials
Water for injection (30 ml)	2 vials

Table 4.2. Drugs Stocked in the CCU at the Presbyterian-University of Pennsylvania Medical Center

Antiarrhythmic Agents
Atropine sulfate
Bretylium (Bretylol)
Diphenylhydantoin (Dilantin)
Disopyramide phosphate (Norpace)
Isoproterenol (Isuprel)
Lidocaine
Nifedipine (Procardia)
Potassium chloride
Procainamide (Pronestyl and Procan SR)
Propranolol HCl (Inderal)
Quinidine sulfate
Verapamil (Calan and Isoptin)

Anticoagulants
Heparin
Warfarin sodium (Coumadin)

Anticoagulant Antagonists
Protamine sulfate
Vitamin K_1 oxide (Mephyton)

Antiemetics
Prochlorperazine (Compazine)
Trimethobenzamide HCl (Tigan)

Antihypertensive Agents
Aldomet
Arfonad
Clonidine HCl (Catapress)
Hydralazine (Apresoline)
Metoprolol tartrate (Lopressor)
Sodium nitroprusside (Nipride)

Bronchodilators
Aminophylline

Coronary Dilators
Isosorbide dinitrate (Isordil)
Nitroglycerin
Nitroclycerin IV (Nitrostat)
Nitroglycerin ointment (Nitrol ointment)
Transdermal nitroglycerin (see also nifedipine and verapamil)

Digitalis Preparations
Deslanoside (Cedilanid-D)
Digoxin

Diuretic Agents
Furosemide (Lasix)
Mannitol
Thiazides

(continued next page)

Table 4.2. Drugs Stocked in the CCU at the Presbyterian-University of
Pennsylvania Medical Center (*continued*)

Electrolytes
    Calcium gluconate
    K-Lyte Cl
    Potassium chloride
    Sodium bicarbonate

Hypnotics and Sedatives
    Amytal sodium
    Brevital
    Chloral hydrate
    Flurazepam HCl (Dalmane)
    Phenobarbital

Intravenous Solution
    Dextran 6%
    Dextran 10%
    Dextrose 5% in saline 0.9%
    Dextrose 5% in ¼ strength saline
    Dextrose 5% in ½ strength saline
    Dextrose 5% in water
    Dextrose 50%
    Normal saline 0.9%

Narcotics
    Codeine sulfate
    Hydromorphone (Dilaudid)
    Meperidine HCl (Demerol)
    Morphine sulfate
    Pentazocine (Talwin)

Narcotic Antagonist
    Maloxone HCl (Narcan)

Steroids
    Hydrocortisone (Solu-Cortef)
    Methylprednisolone (Solu-Medrol)
    Prednisone

Tranquilizers
    Chlordiazepoxide HCl (Librium)
    Diazepam (Valium)
    Hydroxyzine pamoate (Vistaril)

Vasopressor (and Inotropic) Agents
    Dobutamine (Dobutrex)
    Dopamine HCl (Intropin)
    Epinephrine
    Glucagon
    Levarterenol bitartrate (Levophed)
    Metaraminol bitartrate (Aramine)
    Phenylephrine HCl (Neo-Synephrine)

Miscellaneous
    Benedryl
    Cimetidine (Tagamet)
    Lomotil

THE STAFF OF THE CCU

It is absolutely essential that the care of patients in
a coronary unit be delegated to a *team* of physicians
and nurses. In fact, the team approach is the most
distinguishing characteristic of the coronary care
concept. Because all members of the team understand
the aims of care and recognize their respective
responsibilities and functions, the effectiveness of the
system of care is markedly enhanced. Furthermore, a
team effort develops clarity of communication and a
mutual respect among the individual members. Unless the physicians and nurses in a CCU function as
an organized team, the ultimate result of the entire
program will prove very disappointing.

The ideal CCU team is composed of a director, attending physicians (and, in many hospitals, the intern and the resident staff), and a group of nurses specially trained in the principles and practices of coronary care nursing.

Director of the Unit

As with any successful team effort, one person must be in charge and serve as its responsible member and representative. Ideally, the director is a cardiologist or an internist who has the knowledge, dedication, interest, and time to coordinate the whole program. The general duties and responsibilities of the director are to: 1) assume authority and responsibility for establishing basic policies of the unit regarding admission of patients, length of stay in unit, physicians' privileges, and other administrative decisions; 2) establish an overall plan of care for patients in the unit and delegate specific duties to the respective members of the team; 3) work cooperatively with the nurse-instructor and participate in the training program of the CCU team; 4) be responsible for the selection of equipment and supplies used in the unit; 5) serve as liaison between the attending staff, hospital administration, and members of the CCU team concerning problems that may arise; 6) assume command of patient care in critical situations if the attending physician is not immediately available; 7) evaluate periodically the effectiveness of the unit; and 8) serve as a consultant to the attending physician upon request.

In some hospitals the overall responsibility for the proper functioning of the CCU is shared by a committee comprised of the director of the unit and representatives from the nursing service, hospital administration, and medical staff. The advantage of this plan is that all parties participate in making decisions that may affect their respective departments.

Attending Physicians

It is generally agreed that the care of the patient in the CCU should be supervised by his own physician. The director of the unit and the other members of the team essentially assist the attending physician but do not displace him or assume his role. However, it is essential that the attending physician be willing to delegate some of his normal responsibility to the other team members. In particular, the attending physician must transfer certain authority to the nurse so she can assume a decision-making role on her own when the situation demands.

The delegation of authority from one physician to another in the CCU has broad implications, and the extent of this practice varies considerably among hospitals. In some institutions this delegation of authority involves no more than an agreement that any physician who happens to be present at the time of a catastrophe may assume command (e.g., defibrillate a patient of another physician). In other hospitals the director of the unit (or a committee of physicians) is empowered to act not only in the event of emergencies but also if the general treatment program prescribed by the attending physician fails to meet the care standards of the unit.

Attending physicians should participate in the ongoing training program for nurses (and house officers). Their presence at team conferences is especially important when the patients to be discussed are under their care.

The Intern and Resident Staff

In many hospitals interns and resident physicians become part of the coronary care team as delegates of the attending physician. It should be recognized that these house officers are in training and that their primary function is not to replace the attending physician in the direct care of patients; their assignment to the CCU is meant to be an educational experience.

It is customary practice for a house officer to be notified when the CCU nurse detects a change in the patient's clinical status or if a life-threatening problem develops. The decisions the house officer makes at these times often mean the difference between life and death. In many instances the house officer has time to confer with the attending physician or the unit director before deciding on a course of action, but with catastrophic situations the resident physician alone makes the ultimate decision of treatment; therefore his role is vitally important to the success of the entire program. Certain aspects regarding house officers' responsibilities are worth considering, particularly as they relate to the team approach.

The unique role of the CCU nurse and her status on the team should be carefully explained to the house staff by the director of the unit. As might be anticipated, the traditional physician-nurse relationship is changed in this setting, where the nurse assumes duties and responsibilities far beyond those generally expected of nurses. Not infrequently, because of their constant exposure to the problems related to myocardial infarction, CCU nurses become extremely competent in the detection and management of arrhythmias and other complications, and the wise house officer will recognize the value of their judgment and experience.

An on-call schedule for the house staff should be posted daily in a conspicuous site so the nurse knows which physician to call for advice or for emergencies during each shift. Preferably two physicians should be listed for both day and night tours. This type of call system is more effective than having the nurse sound a general alarm in catastrophic situations, which may be answered by any physician who happens to be nearby. General alarms tend to create confusion, with the sudden assemblage of several members of the house staff but without one person responsible for making decisions.

House officers and the nursing staff should make daily patient rounds in the unit together. In this way patient problems that may not be apparent to individual members of the team may be identified and solved. This form of communication is fundamental to effective care.

The Nurse Members of the Team

The success of the coronary care system depends above all on the competence of the nurse members of the CCU team. As noted, unless nurses are adequately trained for their role and are delegated authority to make and carry out therapeutic decisions based on their own observations and judgment, coronary care is merely a token gesture.

For optimum effectiveness a CCU should maintain a ratio of one professional nurse for every two or three patients at all times. Thus a four- to six-bed unit requires two nurses per shift—or a total nursing staff of at least 10 or 12 professional nurses for full coverage (including relief during illness, vacations, and days off). This high quota of nurses may be unrealistic for many hospitals. In this circumstance, licensed practical nurses can be employed to assume some of the lesser duties of the professional nurse. However, it is essential that at least one professional nurse be present in the CCU at all times; the responsibility of the unit must never be delegated to a licensed practical nurse, even for a few minutes. This is not to say that highly motivated practical nurses cannot provide valuable assistance in patient care, but it does mean that duties and responsibilities of coronary care nursing are so encompassing that none but specially trained professional nurses should undertake them. When practical nurses are included as members of the CCU team, they should participate in relevant portions of the training program offered to professional nurses.

Nursing in a coronary care unit (CCU) requires skills, knowledge, and judgment beyond that which can be acquired in a basic nursing school curriculum. Consequently, additional training is necessary to prepare nurses (even those with extensive general duty experience) for their specialized role in the CCU. Before describing the details of this instructional program, it is pertinent to consider some of the most important qualifications (personal and professional) for coronary care nursing.

SELECTION OF NURSES FOR THE CCU

Despite hospital staffing problems, CCU nurses must be deliberately selected for their role rather than accepted merely because of their availability or willingness to work in the unit; under no circumstances should nurses be forced or persuaded to work in a CCU against their desire. The underlying purpose of the selection process is to ensure that the members of the nursing staff are all well qualified and able to work together as a team in providing quality nursing care. In view of the time, effort, and cost involved in preparing CCU nurses for the responsibilities they will be asked to assume, it is important for prospective candidates to decide at the onset if they are qualified and suited for coronary care nursing. To this end, it is useful for the nursing director to establish a list of basic requirements for those who contemplate working in a CCU. This practice minimizes misconceptions about CCU nursing and reduces undue turnover; it also results in a stable, smoothly functioning unit. The following personal and professional qualifications should be included among the selection criteria for CCU nurses.

Personal Qualifications

Emotional Stability

It must be recognized that patients admitted to a CCU are usually seriously ill and that the death rate among them is substantially higher than in other divisions of a hospital. The prospective CCU nurse should evaluate her personal reactions to working in this potentially depressing setting and make certain that she can cope with it. Also to be considered is whether making decisions instantly and assuming serious responsibility—inherent elements in coronary care nursing—are likely to produce adverse emotional effects. To be weighed and balanced against these emotional challenges is the sense of accomplishment and satisfaction that CCU nurses derive from saving lives through their own efforts—an experience that is probably unique in the nursing profession.

Social Maturity

Because intensive coronary care is a team effort, an ability to work closely with others is an essential attribute for CCU nurses. It is understandable that in a small, confined area like a CCU, where team members are together constantly, frictions may develop easily, particularly during stressful situations. Unless mature interpersonal relationships are maintained, the team's effectiveness is greatly weakened and the quality of care diminished.

In addition to working collaboratively with fellow nurses, CCU nurses must also maintain a secure, interdependent relationship with the physician members of the team. Unfortunately, some physicians are still unaccustomed to delegating authority to nurses, and problems may arise because of this. It is not uncommon, for example, for CCU nurses to become more proficient in interpreting arrhythmias than some physicians, thus challenging the physician's status and judgment. It takes considerable discretion and a mature approach for nurses to handle these situations.

Motivation

Although usually an exciting experience, coronary care nursing can become dull and routine if the nurse lacks enthusiasm for her work and the motivation to learn continually. The nurse should appreciate that nursing in a CCU is meant to be an ongoing learning experience—something to look forward to and enjoy. The degree of enthusiasm of the nursing staff correlates well with the quality of care offered. In fact, one of the most revealing characteristics of a superior CCU is a highly enthusiastic nursing staff.

Integrity

The importance of honesty in a CCU cannot be overemphasized. Errors are bound to occur at one time or another because actions often must be taken instantly and usual safeguards are bypassed. If the errors are recognized and reported immediately, corrective measures can be instituted. Thus total integrity on the part of all CCU personnel is mandatory. Those who cover up their mistakes or are fearful to admit them are ill-suited to work in a CCU.

Dependable Attendance

Nurses who are frequently ill or who are unable to comply regularly with the CCU time schedule for other reasons are poor candidates for coronary care nursing. Recognizing that the proper function of a CCU depends on an adequate nursing staff at all times, it is understandable that any absence or lateness can create a serious problem. This is particularly true in small coronary units where there is a limited number of nurses available as replacements.

Employment Commitment

In view of the time required to prepare CCU nurses (and for them to acquire enough experience to assume full responsibilities), it is only reasonable that candidates agree to remain employed for at least one year, unless some unforeseen circumstance arises. Lesser periods of employment weaken the stability of the CCU team and are defeating for all concerned.

Age

As a general rule, relatively recent graduates of basic nursing programs are the most adaptable and make the best adjustment to the demands required of CCU nurses. However, older nurses with excellent qualifications need not be excluded from CCU nursing solely because of their age. Indeed, the older nurse is often a distinct asset to the CCU staff, particularly if she is flexible and adapts relatively easily to the setting.

Professional Qualifications

Nursing School Record

All CCU nurses must be graduates of an accredited school of nursing, preferably a baccalaureate program. It is clear that a high ability to learn is an important requisite for nurses selected to work in a CCU. The specialized training program for CCU nurses includes many new concepts and skills which must be mastered quickly. Therefore nurses whose academic record in nursing school indicates a high level of intelligence and superior learning ability are apt to be the best candidates for coronary care nursing.

Dedication to Bedside Nursing

Because coronary care nursing is concerned almost entirely with direct patient care, it is essential that CCU nurses be dedicated to bedside nursing care and enjoy the nurse-patient relationship inherent in this role. Unless a nurse has a keen interest in direct patient care, working in a CCU is ill-advised. In fact, nurses who are more interested in the medical than the nursing aspects of coronary care are not apt to be the best candidates to work in a CCU.

Previous Nursing Experience

A particularly valuable asset for prospective CCU nurses is at least six months prior experience in caring for acutely ill medical patients in other settings. This background provides a foundation for the added duties and responsibilities of specialized coronary nursing.

PREPARATION OF THE CCU NURSE

After being selected to work in a CCU (according to the criteria just described), nurses must receive sufficient preparation to gain the skills and knowledge necessary to assume responsibilities in the unit. As mentioned previously, a nurse cannot function in a CCU solely on the basis of a basic nursing education program or previous general nursing experience.

Whenever possible, each hospital should conduct its own coronary care training program by appointing the most knowledgeable and best prepared CCU nurse as an instructor (and coordinator) of the program. When this is not feasible, cooperative programs with other hospitals in the area can be developed to serve the needs of the various institutions.

Although many methods may be used to prepare CCU nurses for their role, the overall education program can be considered in two phases: the basic orientation program and the continuing educational program.

The Basic Orientation Program

The customary training program for coronary care nursing involves a combination and integration of classroom instruction and clinical experience, with classroom teaching preceding clinical experience. The total program is usually given as a concentrated course of at least three weeks duration, but a less intensive course over a longer period of time is sometimes utilized. A clear schedule should be prepared in advance of the course, listing the time and place of lectures, the topics, and the speakers; similar preparation is necessary for the clinical experiences. A structured program of this type allows for proper staffing of the CCU during the instructional course, without depending on the orientees to provide nursing care when classes are scheduled. Because the background and previous experiences of the students may vary considerably, the design and objectives of the course should be tailored to meet the diverse needs of the class. This requires an evaluation of the nurses' knowledge and skills (usually determined by a preassessment test) before determining the course content.

By the completion of the orientation program the nurse should achieve the following objectives:

1. Use monitoring devices and other equipment required for assessment and treatment.
2. Assess the patient's physical and psychological status by bedside observation and appropriate examinations.
3. Institute measures designed to prevent complications.
4. Detect and interpret early signs and symptoms of complications.
5. Provide effective nursing care which meets the patient's physiologic, psychologic, and social needs.
6. Initiate emergency therapy and assess its effects.
7. Evaluate the results (both desired and untoward) of various means of intervention.
8. Determine patients' needs for instruction about rehabilitation, and start a teaching plan early in the course of hospitalization.
9. Function as a member of the CCU team in planning, evaluating, and delivering patient care.

Classroom Instruction

Learning is facilitated when a student is an active participant in the program rather than a passive listener. Therefore it is desirable to minimize formal classroom lectures, which often involve very little interaction between the instructor and the student, and focus instead on conferences and demonstrations whenever possible. Several excellent teaching aids are available to complement the instructional program, including films, film strips, slides, audiotapes, videotapes, and programmed instructional books. A typical outline for classroom instruction is presented below.

Topics for Classroom Instruction and Discussion

1. *Introduction to the concept of intensive coronary care:* rationale, prevention of complications; physician-nurse team approach to care; tour of CCU
2. *Anatomy and physiology of the heart:* cardiac chambers and valves; coronary circulation; cardiac hemodynamics
3. *Heart sounds:* sites of auscultation and normal heart sounds; significance of abnormal sounds
4. *Coronary heart disease:* the problem; risk factors; pathophysiology; approaches to combating the problem
5. *Acute myocardial infarction:* the patient's history; physical findings; diagnosis; enzyme and other laboratory studies; complications of the attack; clinical course
6. *Cardiac nursing care:* comprehensive care to meet the patient's changing needs; methods of clinical assessment; physical and psychological care; patient instruction and rehabilitation
7. *Electrocardiography and electrophysiology:* basic principles; monitoring leads and other

ECG leads; ECG wave forms; the normal ECG

8. *Arrhythmias:* classification; identification; interpretation; relative dangers
9. *Drug treatment of arrhythmias:* specific drugs; anticipated effects; side effects; nursing role
10. *Electrical treatment of arrhythmias:* defibrillation; elective cardioversion; temporary cardiac pacing; permanent cardiac pacing
11. *Lethal arrhythmias:* emergency treatment program; cardiopulmonary resuscitation (demonstration and practice with a manikin); emergency drugs; nursing role
12. *Left and right ventricular failure:* hemodynamics; clinical assessment; drug therapy; nurse's rule in therapy
13. *Cardiogenic shock:* hemodynamic measurements; clinical assessment; intraaortic balloon pumping; the nurse's role
14. *Other complications of acute myocardial infarction:* ventricular rupture; thromboembolism; papillary muscle dysfunction; pericarditis
15. *Assisted respiration and oxygen therapy:* indications; methods; problems
16. *Blood gas studies:* normal values and significance
17. *Fluid and electrolyte balance:* clinical signs; replacement therapy; use of diuretics
18. *Rehabilitation of the cardiac patient:* assessing needs; follow-up care; teaching based on needs of patients and families.

Clinical Experience

Clinical training in coronary care nursing is obtained for the most part at a nurse-to-nurse level, with an experienced CCU nurse serving as the preceptor. This plan involves much more than simply assigning the student to work in a CCU under the supervision and observation of the preceptor. Instead, the program should consist of a planned, orderly sequence of learning activities designed to prepare the nurse for specific duties and responsibilities. These clinical activities should be scheduled to follow the classroom discussion of the particular subject. However, this is not always possible, and the clinical program must be flexible so that each day's plan can be adjusted according to circumstances within the unit. For instance, if on the learner's third day in the unit, a patient requires a temporary pacemaker, it is logical to provide clinical experience with cardiac pacing then, rather than at a later scheduled time.

The clinical program usually covers a three week period, but can be extended, as necessary, to meet the needs of individual nurses. Throughout this period, it is wise to assign the trainee to work with one particular nurse during this nurse's tours of duty. This plan provides consistency and continuity in the clinical program and allows for individualized progress. Aside from this direct form of clinical training, it is important to provide the trainee with additional practical experience, involving specialized techniques and skills required by CCU nurses. The following methods may be used to attain these necessary skills:

Electrocardiographic Techniques

To become adept at recording 12-lead ECGs, it is useful for the nurse to spend a day or two in the hospital's Heart (ECG) Station. By recording many ECGs here, the technique can be learned promptly. Particular attention should be given to the methods used to obtain high quality (distinct) ECGs.

Venipuncture and Intravenous Infusions

Many nurses are not experienced in collecting blood samples (for laboratory studies) or in starting intravenous infusions, both of which are essential duties within the CCU. These skills can be acquired by having the nurse accompany laboratory technicians and the "IV team" as they make their rounds throughout the hospital. Also, experience can be gained through inservice programs by the nursing department.

Use of Respiratory Equipment

Valuable practical experience in the use of respiratory equipment can be obtained by assigning the learner temporarily to the inhalation therapy department. Included in this experience are the use of positive-pressure machines, manual breathing bags, and mechanical respirators, as well as various methods of oxygen administration. In addition, the orientee can learn the procedure for collecting arterial blood samples for blood gas determination, a common study among patients receiving inhalation therapy. (In some hospitals nurses only assist in collecting arterial blood samples, while in others the procedure is actually performed by the nursing staff.)

The Technique of Precordial Shock

Unquestionably the most unique experience for the beginning CCU nurse is the use of a defibrillator to terminate ventricular fibrillation. A machine that delivers 7000 volts of electricity has frightening implications. Because the same equipment is used in terminating other, nonfatal arrhythmias (e.g., atrial fibrillation) on an elective basis, it is extremely beneficial if nurses are allowed actually to give the precordial shock, called cardioversion, under the supervision of a physician, in these nonemergency situations. In this way the nurse becomes familiar with the equipment she later will use on her own if death-producing arrhythmias occur.

Cardiopulmonary Resuscitation

It is mandatory that every nurse be able to perform closed-chest compression and mouth-to-mouth ventilation in a wholly effective manner (according to the American Heart Association's standards). To this end, each nurse should take a certified basic life support course conducted by the local Heart Association or by a nurse-instructor who is certified by the American Heart Association.

Simulated Emergencies

As a means of achieving optimum efficiency during emergency situations, simulated catastrophes ("fire drills") can be staged, using a manikin as a "patient" who has suddenly developed ventricular fibrillation or asystole. Just as if a true emergency had occurred, a physician member of the team is called and all the team members fulfill their particular roles in resuscitating the "patient." This includes using all equipment (except for actually turning on the defibrillator) and administering intravenous therapy, according to the sequence used during real emergencies. (To avoid needless waste, outdated drugs and intravenous fluids are used for this latter purpose.) When the practice session is completed, an evaluation should be made by the entire team so that learning is achieved by all.

CONTINUING EDUCATIONAL PROGRAM

It is important to realize that the basic training plan just outlined is only an introduction to coronary care nursing, and that to achieve greater skill and competence nurses must continue to learn (and apply) new concepts and techniques. To this end, each hospital should develop a continuing education program for the CCU nursing staff. By participating in this ongoing learning program, the nurse increases her knowledge and the quality of nursing care in the unit improves steadily. Some of the methods used to conduct an effective ongoing educational program are described below.

Team Conferences and Medical Rounds in CCU

Team conferences, in which nurse and physician members of the coronary care unit team meet jointly, have proved to be useful and popular teaching exercises for the unit's staff. The meetings, which usually consist of case presentations or discussions of policies and practices within the unit, should be scheduled once a week with the unit director presiding. These conferences provide an opportunity for mutual learning and are extremely worthwhile. Equally valuable are the informal conferences held after daily medical rounds in the CCU. These meetings permit nurses and physicians to share their observations of individual patients and to develop a unified approach to patient care. Medical rounds are meant to enhance the knowledge of all team members, with physicians and nurses learning from each other.

The format we employ for team conferences involves a case history presentation given by a house officer, nurse, or attending physician, after which the members of the team describe their observations about the patient's clinical course. The treatment program is reviewed and the group identifies special problems. The following is an excerpt from one of our team conferences.

RESIDENT PHYSICIAN: Mr. Scott is a 48-year-old man who was admitted to the unit yesterday afternoon following an episode of typical substernal pain along with vomiting and sweating. On admission the pulse was 120/minute, but there were no signs of left ventricular failure. Other than the chest pain, which by then had persisted for an hour, his condition was quite stable. He was given 75mg Demerol, after which the pain disappeared. The ECG showed marked elevation of the ST segments in the precordial leads typical of acute anterior wall infarction. Monitoring revealed sinus tachycardia but no other arrhythmias. The first CPK enzyme level was markedly elevated with a high MB fraction. There wasn't much question about the diagnosis. I haven't seen him since late last evening, but he was doing quite well then. I should add that the patient is a known diabetic who apparently has been reasonably well controlled with insulin.

DIRECTOR: Dr. Edwards, as the patient's physician, could you tell us a little more about his history? Did he have known coronary disease in the past?

ATTENDING PHYSICIAN: Although this man has never had angina and an ECG 6 months ago was normal, I am not really surprised that he had a coronary. He would really be considered a high risk candidate. In addition to the diabetes, he smokes two packs of cigarettes a day, has an elevated serum cholesterol, and is 20 pounds over-weight. Unfortunately, I have been unable to get him to change his ways. Furthermore, his father died of a coronary at age 51.

DIRECTOR: We would all agree this man was looking for trouble. Now, Jan, could you tell us about his course since admission?

NURSE: In general, his condition hasn't changed much during the night. He did have one other episode of chest pain about 8 PM, and he was given an additional injection of Demerol. He didn't sleep well, but he has not been dyspneic nor does he have any other complaints this morning. The night nurse, however, was concerned about his pulse rate. It has remained between 100 and 120 since admission, and none of us is sure why this sinus tachycardia has persisted.

DIRECTOR: That is an important observation. We have a patient who seems stable but has a rapid heart rate. What do you make of this, John?

RESIDENT PHYSICIAN: Many patients have sinus tachycardia. It may be due to temperature elevation or anxiety, or it may reflect an early sign of impending heart failure.

DIRECTOR: Quite right. What do you think is causing this patient's tachycardia?

RESIDENT PHYSICIAN: If it persisted all night and he was restless, I would be suspicious that we may be seeing early left ventricular failure.

NURSE: That is what we suspect too.

DIRECTOR: Has a chest film been taken this morning?

SECOND NURSE: Yes, I called for the report just before the conference, and the interpretation was early left ventricular failure.

ATTENDING PHYSICIAN: I just examined his chest, and there were no rales present.

DIRECTOR: That would not be unusual. The x-ray findings and the persistent tachycardia often precede clinical failure.

Nursing Conferences

Nursing conferences offer another means for providing continuing education. The main objective of these meetings is to allow the nursing staff as a group to identify and seek solutions to particular nursing problems encountered in the unit. The success of this learning experience depends on a free and active exchange of ideas and opinions. Therefore the conferences should be scheduled at times that permit maximum attendance without depleting the nursing staff of the unit. An excerpt from a nursing conference follows:

MODERATOR: Mr. Clark was admitted yesterday with an acute myocardial infarction. He has not had any chest pain since admission and his course has been uneventful—no problems at all. We've noticed, however, that he has become increasingly upset about having his vital signs checked every few hours, and I thought it might be worthwhile to discuss this situation.

NURSE ONE: He certainly does get upset. As I walked into the room to take his blood pressure, he sat up in bed and said, "You're going to take my blood pressure *again?* I feel all right. Why is it necessary to check me so often?"

NURSE TWO: What did you say?

NURSE ONE: I told him we routinely check the blood pressure of each patient every few hours as a means of preventing complications. I tried to reassure him that his condition was stable and that there were no complications.

NURSE TWO: Didn't that help?

NURSE ONE: I guess not because Mary had the same experience with him at 8 o'clock.

MODERATOR: Why do you think he reacts this way?

NURSE THREE: Perhaps he believes his condition is worsening and we aren't telling him about it.

MODERATOR: That's one explanation, but I wonder if there isn't more to the problem than that?

NURSE TWO: I've seen other patients who question everything the nurse does and seem to resent it. Usually these patients have great anxiety, and complaining to the nurse is their way of seeking further reassurance.

NURSE ONE: If that's the case, we should try to reassure him more often, not only after he complains about vital signs.

MODERATOR: I think that would be a good plan.

NURSE THREE: I hope you're right—since I'm just coming on duty.

Ward Rounds After Transfer From CCU

Because nurses working in a CCU are involved in the care of patients with myocardial infarction for a period of only 4 or 5 days (the acute phase), they have little opportunity to observe the subsequent course of the illness. This is a disadvantage since patients in the CCU usually ask many questions about the remaining period of hospitalization and the program after discharge. In order to respond intelligently to these questions, it is important for CCU nurses to obtain a complete picture of the overall management of acute myocardial infarction. What medications are used during the subacute phase of hospitalization? What activities are permitted and when? Do the emotional responses noted initially (e.g., anxiety or depression) disappear after transfer from the CCU? What instruction does the physician give the patient at the time of hospital discharge? This type of information can be gained readily if CCU nurses make ward rounds with the attending physician after patients have been transferred from the CCU. A schedule should be established so that each nurse has the opportunity to participate in these rounds at regular intervals.

Physicians' Lectures

A lecture series given by physicians in different specialties is a valuable component of an ongoing educational program. The presentations should provide advanced, in-depth information; they should not review basic material already covered in the orientation program. It is desirable for the nursing staff to suggest and select the subjects to be discussed. Examples of various lecture topics (and speakers) for the series include the following:

Emotional Aspects of Myocardial Infarction—Psychiatrist

• Clinical assessment of the patient • Methods of coping • Intervention techniques • When is psychiatric consultation needed? • The nurses' own emotional responses • Emotionally induced cardiac invalidism

Electrocardiography—Cardiologist

• Interpretation of complex arrhythmias • His bundle electrograms • The ECG diagnosis of myocardial infarction • Monitoring leads • Electrical axis of the heart • Bundle branch blocks

Diagnostic Methods—Cardiologist

• Echocardiography • Cardiac scanning • Other noninvasive techniques • Cardiac catheterization • Stress testing

Assisted Respiration—Anesthesiologist

• Mechanical respirator therapy • Complications of artificial respiration • Oxygen toxicity • Interpreting blood gas studies • Intermittent positive-pressure breathing

Pathology of the Heart—Pathologist

• Current concepts of atherosclerosis • Complications of myocardial infarction • Enzyme studies and size of infarction • Interpretation of laboratory studies • Papillary muscle dysfunction

Heart Surgery—Cardiac Surgeon

• Coronary artery bypass graft surgery • Ventricular aneurysm surgery • Permanent pacemaker implantation • Intraaortic balloon pumping in cardiogenic shock

Drug Therapy—Pharmacist

• New drugs for use in CCU • Actions and side effects of cardiac drugs

5

Coronary Care Nursing

Intensive coronary care in the final analysis is a system of specialized nursing. Indeed, the number of lives saved in a coronary care unit (CCU) is directly related to the competence of the nursing staff; no other element of coronary care is as important. To define this specialized nursing role clearly it is appropriate first to outline the overall duties and responsibilities of the CCU nurse and then consider specific aspects of nursing care from the time of admission to discharge from the unit.

AN OUTLINE OF NURSING DUTIES AND RESPONSIBILITIES

The primary goals of coronary care are to preserve life, prevent complications, and restore the patient to his maximum functional capacity (physically and emotionally). To achieve these objectives the nurse members of the CCU team must assume the following responsibilities.

I. Continuous Assessment of the Patient's Clinical Status

A. By Means of Electrocardiographic Monitoring

Because arrhythmias are the most common cause of death after acute myocardial infarction, it is absolutely essential that the heart rate and rhythm be monitored continuously in all patients in the CCU. The nurse must be able to identify arrhythmic disorders, assess their relative danger, and decide what action to take when an arrhythmia develops. Much of the success of intensive coronary care depends on this nursing responsibility.

B. By Direct Observation of the Patient

Cardiac monitoring provides information only about the electrical activity of the heart; the remaining aspects of cardiac performance are assessed by other means. To evaluate the heart's function as a pump a series of planned observations at the bedside must be made. To this end, it is essential that the nurse examine the patient carefully at regular intervals to detect signs or symptoms of left ventricular failure and cardiogenic shock. In fact the detection of all complications except arrhythmias depends on direct observation of the patient. This nursing duty should not be overshadowed by cardiac monitoring.

C. By Means of Hemodynamic Monitoring

In patients with advanced left ventricular failure (or other circulatory complications) it is often necessary to measure venous and arterial pressures repeatedly in order to assess the severity of the problem and the effects of treatment. This type of monitoring—called hemodynamic monitoring—involves the insertion of long, indwelling intravenous or intraarterial catheters (by the physician) and the measurement and recording of the pressures at frequent intervals by the nurse.

Hemodynamic monitoring requires technical skill; but far more important, the nurse must be able to interpret the findings so that the treatment program can be altered accordingly.

II. Anticipation and Prevention of Complications

A. Intravenous Infusions

Because of the unpredictable nature of acute myocardial infarction and the threat that a serious arrhythmia (or other complication) may develop suddenly, it is standard practice to establish and maintain a "keep open" intravenous line in every CCU patient. In this way intravenous drugs can be administered instantly in critical situations. It is the duty of the CCU nurse to start the intravenous infusion, verify the patency of the system, and control the rate of flow.

B. Oxygen Therapy

CCU nurses are permitted to start oxygen therapy at their own discretion. The need for oxygen is determined by the patient's clinical condition. In addition to its use in circulatory failure, oxygen is administered as a preventive measure (in the hope of improving myocardial oxygenation) when ischemic chest pain or arrhythmias develop.

C. Treatment of Warning Arrhythmias

One of the fundamental objectives of coronary care (as explained in Chapter 3) is to prevent ventricular fibrillation and ventricular standstill by treating warning arrhythmias. When a warning arrhythmia is recognized the nurse must anticipate the treatment program and prepare appropriate antiarrhythmic drugs for immediate use. In keeping with this preventive approach, CCU nurses are authorized to administer intravenous drugs (e.g., lidocaine or atropine) when necessary. Depending on the particular policies of a CCU (discussed subsequently) a specific order may be required in each instance, or, under coverage of a standing order, the nurse may administer the drug on the basis of her own clinical judgment when dangerous arrhythmias occur.

D. Cardiac Pacing

The prevention of ventricular standstill is based primarily on the insertion of a temporary transvenous pacemaker when advanced heart block exists. The pacing catheter is positioned by the physician with the assistance of a nurse (either in the CCU or a catheterization laboratory). Thereafter the nurse must determine if the pacemaker is functioning properly at all times and, if necessary, identify sources of malfunction. These are important responsibilities because abrupt failure of a pacemaker (e.g., as the result of battery failure or a disconnected wire) can be disastrous.

III. Emergency and Resuscitative Treatment

A. Defibrillation

Although preventive measures certainly reduce the risk of ventricular fibrillation, the fact remains that this death-producing arrhythmia can develop at any time. The preservation of life after the onset of ventricular fibrillation depends in nearly all instances on the ability of the CCU nurse to recognize the arrhythmia and terminate it immediately by means of precordial shock (defibrillation). This nursing responsibility is of supreme importance.

B. Cardiopulmonary Resuscitation

When sudden death occurs because preventive treatment is ineffective or cannot be accomplished in time, the final hope for survival is cardiopulmonary resuscitation by means of external cardiac compression and mouth-to-mouth ventilation. This technique maintains the circulation, allowing corrective procedures to be attempted. Every nurse—indeed all personnel in the CCU—must be proficient in performing effective cardiopulmonary resuscitation.

C. Assisted Respiration

Mechanical respirators are sometimes required in the treatment of advanced circulatory failure to provide adequate tissue oxygenation. Although in most hospitals respiratory therapists operate and maintain this equipment, the CCU nurse must be familiar with the ongoing operation of mechanical respirators and must be able to recognize problems that occur during their use. Also necessary is the ability to use a manual breathing bag to assist respiration.

D. Rotating Tourniquets

Although no longer a frequent method of treatment, rotating tourniquets are still used in the management of acute left ventricular failure (pulmonary edema). The object of applying tourniquets to the arms and legs in this circumstance is to reduce venous return to the heart as soon as possible, before drug therapy has time to be effective. Initially, the nurse tightens the tourniquets on three of the four extremities (except where IV fluids are being administered) and then, every 15 minutes, loosens one tourniquet and tightens another, on a rotating basis in a clockwise direction. Care must be taken to palpate the distal pulses of the extremities each time a tourniquet is tightened to avoid arterial constriction from an overly tight band. When rotating tourniquets are discontinued, only one tourniquet at a time is loosened so that the vascular system is not burdened with a large volume of venous blood from all of the extremities at once.

IV. Diagnostic Procedures

A. Twelve-Lead Electrocardiograms

In other units of the hospital electrocardiograms (ECGs) are recorded by technicians from the heart station, but in the CCU nurses usually assume this duty. The reason for this practice is that ECGs must be taken so frequently in the CCU that enormous time would be wasted calling a technician on each occasion. Also, ECGs are often required at a moment's notice, for example, during an episode of angina, when ECG signs of myocardial ischemia may appear briefly. Furthermore, experienced CCU nurses can often detect changes in the ECG that may influence clinical decisions. Because the manner in which an ECG is recorded can affect its interpretation, it is important for nurses to master the technique of producing effective tracings. (In this regard, it is helpful to mark the electrode sites for the precordial leads on the patient's chest wall so that these same locations will be used with subsequent recordings.)

B. Laboratory Studies

In many CCUs laboratory technicians draw all blood samples for diagnostic purposes—while in others CCU nurses take on this responsibility. This decision depends for the most part on local circumstances, but in either case CCU nurses should be very skillful in this technique, especially since laboratory studies are required so often in emergency situations among patients in a CCU.

C. Arterial Blood Gases

To evaluate oxygen (and other gas) concentrations arterial blood samples are required. The arterial puncture and aspiration of blood is usually performed by a physician. Nursing duties include preparation of the syringe (with heparin), placing the blood sample in a container of ice, and sending the specimen immediately to the laboratory for blood gas analysis. (As noted previously in some institutions, CCU nurses are delegated authority to perform arterial puncture for blood gas studies, but this is not a standard nursing practice at present.)

V. General Nursing Care

In addition to their specialized duties, CCU nurses are expected to provide high level general nursing care to patients in the unit. The nursing care plan for the coronary patient should be very flexible; establishing rigid routines for carrying out nursing procedures is ill-advised. Preferably, the primary nurse who admits the patient to the CCU should develop the nursing care plan, and take responsibility for it during the patient's stay in the unit. The plan (as described later in this chapter) should include specific nursing objectives, nursing interventions, and an evaluation of the outcomes. The primary nurse communicates this plan to the other nurses in the unit who will assume the care of the patient in her absence and invites suggestions about revising the plan according to ongoing evaluation of the outcomes.

VI. Emotional Support

High on the list of nursing responsibilities are the identification and management of anxiety, depression, and other emotional responses that may affect the patient's clinical course and ultimate rehabilitation. The nurse should be able to recognize verbal and nonverbal clues of emotional stress, and understand the basic mechanisms for helping the patient to cope with his problems. (Because of its special importance, the subject of emotional support is considered separately in this chapter after the sections on admission procedure and subsequent care of patients in the CCU.)

VII. Communication

As a member of the CCU team who constantly attends the patient, the nurse must communicate with the patient and his family, and with physicians, nurses, and other hospital personnel involved in his care. The specific responsibilities involved in this communication are:

a. To explain to the patient (and a family member, if present) the objectives of intensive coronary care, the reasons for various procedures, and how they are accomplished. Above all, the nurse should answer questions about the illness in direct, understandable terms.

b. To apprise the family of the patient's clinical condition and progress, to allay their fears, and to enlist their cooperation.

c. To serve as a liaison between the physician, the patient, and the family, particularly in clarifying misconceptions of the plan of care.

d. To advise the physician of the patient's clinical status and to report any meaningful changes as soon as they occur.

e. To present succinct, comprehensive reports to the other members of the nursing staff about the condition of each patient (with the use of the nursing care plan) so that there will be effective continuity of care.

VIII. Collection and Recording of Data

A. Nursing History

A sometimes tedious but always important nursing duty is to obtain and record pertinent information about the patient's personal health habits, social history, and other factors that influence nursing care. A representative form for recording these facts is shown in Figure 5.1. Pertinent information from the nursing history should also be recorded on the Kardex for day-to-day nursing care plans.

B. Admission Summary

It is essential for the nurse to summarize the patient's clinical condition at the time of admission in order to establish a base line for comparison. These findings are usually reported on a separate admission note (Figure 5.2); however, in some CCUs these data are included in the nursing history form described above.

C. Documentation of Arrhythmias

Whenever a significant arrhythmia is observed the nurse should record an ECG strip from the cardiac monitor to document this disorder. Other ECG strips—called rhythm strips— are recorded at regular intervals, for example, hourly in acutely ill patients, for purposes of comparison. All of the strips should be analyzed by the nurse, and the recordings then placed in a folder for future reference. These serial tracings are very useful in detecting progressive changes in arrhythmias that might otherwise go unnoticed.

D. Drug Therapy

The dosage, time of administration, and effects of all cardiac drugs must be noted specifically. This information is extremely important in assessing whether changes are necessary in the treatment program.

E. Nursing Notes

Like medical notes, nursing notes are meant to provide an ongoing account of the patient's illness. To this end, the nurse should record clinical observations, interventions, future plans, and other information pertaining to nursing care. In many hospitals, nursing notes are recorded in a standardized way, using the S.O.A.P. format (Subjective Objective findings, Assessment, and Plan of care), and are included in the progress notes of the patient's chart, along with notes written by physicians.

IX. Education of Students and Other Nurses

An important responsibility of all CCU nurses is to serve as preceptors for student nurses (who usually spend a brief period in the unit) and for new staff nurses joining the CCU team. Not only does the teaching benefit others, but it also enhances the preceptor's own learning.

X. Patient Education

Although detailed, structured teaching of patients (and their family members) is not usually attempted during the acute phase of the illness, there is much that the CCU nurse can do in assessing learning readiness and in providing information which is appropriate at the time. Experience has shown that patients remember very few facts taught in formal teaching programs during the crisis stage of an illness; however, they do benefit from answers to questions. By responding to the patient's questions or cues in a simple but informative manner, the nurse can start an educational process that can be developed throughout the hospital course.

In order for the nursing staff to know what teaching has been started, a record of the subjects taught should be maintained. When the patient is transferred from the CCU to another unit, this teaching record should be transferred with the patient's chart. The recording of such information on a patient education form provides consistency and continuity of teaching throughout hospitalization and helps with discharge planning. A patient education recording form designed for this purpose is presented in Figure 5.3.

Nursing History

Patient's Name _____

Admitting Diagnosis _____

Date of Admission _____ Time _____

Attending Physician _____

    Notified by _____ Time _____

House Officer _____

    Notified by _____ Time _____

Mode of Arrival _____ Accompanied by _____

Responsible Family Member _____ Telephone _____

Informant Other than Patient _____ Telephone _____

Language Spoken _____

Medications Before Admission:

    Cardiac _____

    Other _____

    Last Dose _____

Medications Removed from Patient's Bedside? _____

    Taken home by family _____

    Stored in nurse's station _____

Known Allergies? _____

Personal Information:

    Glasses _____ Contact lenses _____ Hearing aid _____

    Dentures _____ : Upper _____ Lower _____ Partial _____

    Customary activity: Limited _____ Unlimited _____

    Diet: Unrestricted _____ Restricted _____ Type _____

    Sleep pattern: Hours at night _____

                Hours during day _____

                Requires sedatives? _____

                Number of pillows _____

    Bowel pattern: Frequency _____

                Laxatives? _____ Type _____

                Last B.M. _____

    Bladder pattern: Frequency _____

                Nocturia? _____

General Observations:

    Patient's level of understanding _____

    Reliability of information _____

    Hygiene _____

    Skin: Integrity _____ Rashes? _____

          Pressure sores? _____ Ulcers? _____

    Deformities or abnormalities _____

_____

_____

_____

Other Pertinent Information _____

_____

_____

Nursing History Obtained by _____

Figure 5.1. Nursing history.

Nurse's Admission Summary

Name _____ Age _____ Sex _____

Date of Admission _____ Time _____

Diagnosis _____

Past History:

    Known angina _____ Previous infarction _____

    Hypertension _____ Diabetes _____ Respiratory _____

    Other diseases _____

    Previous hospitalizations _____ Here _____ Other _____

Emergency Drugs Before Admission to CCU and Time Administered _____
_____

Condition on Admission:

    Chest pain _____

    Dyspnea _____

    Diaphoresis _____ Skin color _____

    Mental status _____

    BP _____ Pulse _____ Respirations _____Temperature _____

Cardiac Rhythm _____
    (*Attach rhythm strip to back of this sheet*)

Summary of Clinical Condition _____
_____

Laboratory Studies

	Ordered	Performed	Nursing Comments
CBC _____			
Urinalysis _____			
BUN _____			
Blood Sugar (____ hours p.p.) _____			
CPK _____			
SGOT _____			
LDH _____			
Electrolyte panel _____			
Prothrombin time _____			
ATPP _____			
Other _____			
ECG (12-lead) _____			
Chest x-ray _____			

Figure 5.2. Nurse's admission summary.

Topics	Date and Teacher	Reinforcement given (date)	Need for further teaching	
			Yes	No
Part 1. CCU Period				
1. Purpose of CCU				
2. Cardiac monitoring				
3. Constant IV				
4. Regulations of unit (visiting, etc.)				
5. Activities permitted				
6. Length of stay				
7. Oxygen				
8. Reporting chest pain				
9. ECGs, x-rays, laboratory studies				
10. Diet				
11. Myocardial infarction (introduction)				
12. Preparation for transfer from CCU				
Part 2. Post CCU Period				

1. Normal heart and circulation
   a) chambers
   b) circulation
   c) coronary arteries				

2. Coronary risk factors and their control (relevant to patient)				

3. Myocardial infarction
   a) collateral circulation
   b) healing process
   c) expectations
   d) complications				

4. Progression of activities during hospitalization				
5. Medications during hospitalization				

6. Diet therapy
   a) purpose
   b) foods to include and exclude				

7. Emotional responses				
Part 3. Preparation for Discharge				

1. Medications (list)
   a) purposes, side effects
   b) schedule				

2. Activity schedule
   a) general
   b) work
   c) sexual				

3. Medical follow-up
   a) appointment
   b) symptoms to report
   c) alteration of risk factors				

4. Psychosocial aspects (expectations)				
5. Community resources				

Figure 5.3. Patient Education Record.

XI. Legal Implications of Coronary Care Nursing

Coronary care nurses are delegated authority to perform certain skills that ordinarily might be considered outside the sphere of traditional nursing practice. Some of these skills and duties fall into a gray area, somewhere between medical and nursing care, with overlapping responsibilities. The authority given to CCU nurses to act on their own, when necessary, is fully justified, indeed mandatory, since having to wait for the arrival of a physician to initiate emergency care, for example, might jeopardize the patient's life and, as such, is incompatible with optimal care. Moreover, CCU nurses have been specially prepared for their role, and the skills they perform are in keeping with their training. Nevertheless, it is absolutely essential that written policies listing these skills be approved by the medical staff of the hospital; this formal authorization should be kept in the CCU at all times. In addition, a copy of the list, signed by the attending physician, is placed in the patient's chart as part of the orders for patient care. Although the duties of CCU nurses vary according to circumstances at different hospitals, the responsibilities listed in Figure 5.4 are usually included in the policy statement that authorizes nurses to perform these skills.

ADMISSION OF PATIENTS TO CCU

Admitting a patient to the CCU involves a sequence of steps, the final order of which is determined by the nurse. Certain procedures are of overriding importance and demand immediate action; others, although essential, have a lower priority. The critical factor in establishing priorities is the patient's clinical condition (and needs) at the time of admission.

Nurses' Responsibilities in CCU*
Overall Policies

CCU nurses may fulfill any of the following responsibilities:

1. Identify and interpret arrhythmias

2. Administer oxygen therapy

3. Start and maintain intravenous infusions

4. Perform defibrillation for ventricular fibrillation and symptomatic ventricular tachycardia

5. Perform cardiopulmonary resuscitation

6. Use equipment for assisted ventilation

7. Apply rotating tourniquets for pulmonary edema

8. Draw blood samples for laboratory studies

9. Administer lidocaine and atropine intravenously, in accordance with standing orders regarding emergency treatment of arrhythmias. (For example, inject lidocaine (1 mg/kg body weight) as an IV bolus dose if 3 or more PVCs occur consecutively or if the frequency of PVCs exceeds 6 per minute.)

10. Administer prescribed intravenous medications.

Signed _____ M.D.

Date _____

*This list of responsibilities, although representative, is by no means all-inclusive or suitable for every hospital. For instance, in some hospitals the list may include several lesser skills, such as recording 12-lead electrocardiograms; while in other institutions, where nurses are permitted to draw arterial blood samples (for blood gas studies), this advanced skill would be included in the list of responsibilities.

Figure 5.4. Nurses' Responsibilities in CCU.

For patients who are not in acute distress on arrival the primary goal of the admission process is to institute as quickly as possible a program for preventing complications while at the same time attempting to allay the patient's fears. In contrast, when complications already have developed and patients are in acute distress on admission, initial efforts must be channeled toward combating the existing problem (e.g., acute left ventricular failure, cardiogenic shock or major arrhythmias) and preventing further complications. The admission procedure for patients in both of these categories is described in the following pages.

Patients Not in Acute Distress

1. Initiate Cardiac Monitoring and Record an ECG Strip from the Monitor

The first step in the admission of any patient with suspected acute myocardial infarction is to attach electrodes to the chest and begin cardiac monitoring. Because death-producing arrhythmias can develop at any time, especially during the immediate hours after the attack, it is essential to institute ECG monitoring immediately, regardless of the patient's clinical condition. (The procedure for cardiac monitoring is described in detail in Chapter 6.) Once cardiac monitoring has been instituted an ECG strip should be recorded from the monitor. This rhythm strip documents the ECG pattern on admission and serves as a base line for future comparison. After this first ECG strip has been interpreted, it is attached to the Nurse's Admission Summary.

2. Explain the CCU Concept to the Patient

Being admitted to a CCU is a frightening experience for patients and the nurse must attempt to allay fears from the onset. One of the best ways of helping patients is to explain why and how each procedure (or test) is being performed. For example, while attaching the electrodes for cardiac monitoring, the nurse should briefly describe the function of the monitor, emphasizing its role in preventing arrhythmic complications through continuous nursing assessment and appropriate intervention. So that the patient does not become awed by the importance of the machine, the nurse must make it clear that cardiac monitoring is only one aspect of coronary care, and not the entire program. Detailed descriptions of procedures during the stressful period of admission should be avoided. Simple, non-technical explanations that can be reinforced, if necessary, usually serve the purpose very well.

3. Inquire About Presence of Chest Pain

A fundamental principle of coronary care is to relieve ischemic chest pain as soon as possible. This concept applies to pain that still persists at the time of admission or to recurrent chest pain that develops during the CCU period. Since ischemic pain is a subjective sensation, the nurse must inquire specifically about its presence. The patient should be advised to notify the nurse promptly if and when chest pain occurs. The severity of the pain pattern can be assessed by asking the patient to rank the discomfort on a scale of 1 to 10. Depending on the extent of the pain, the nurse may decide to administer an ordered narcotic to obtain prompt relief of this distressing symptom.

4. Start an Intravenous Infusion

Soon after admission, the nurse should start an intravenous infusion of 5% glucose in water. (Because the intravenous line must remain in place throughout the patient's stay in the CCU, it is advantageous to administer the infusion through a flexible, indwelling venous catheter (intracath), rather than through a rigid needle.) The line is kept open at all times so that intravenous medication can be given without delay during emergency situations. To prevent overloading of the circulation by excessive infusion of fluids, a microdrip system and regulator should be used routinely. The usual flow rate is 15-60 microdrops per minute.

5. Assess the Patient's Clinical Condition

Even though a patient appears comfortable and is not in acute distress, early signs or symptoms of complications may nevertheless be present. One of the main objectives of the initial clinical assessment is to determine if there is any evidence of a beginning complication (particularly early left ventricular failure or cardiogenic shock). This is accomplished by questioning the patient about his symptoms and by physical examination (as described in Chapter 7). In addition, as part of the assessment, information must be obtained about the patient's past medical history (including pre-existing diseases, medications, and allergies) which may influence the treatment program. These facts should be recorded carefully on the admission summary sheet (Figure 5.2).

6. Notify the Physician

After high priority procedures and the initial clinical assessment have been completed, the nurse should communicate with the physician, apprising him of the patient's clinical status on admission. The nurse's observations and findings are extremely important because they influence the physician's decisions about the initial treatment program.

7. Record a 12-Lead ECG

Unless an ECG was obtained in the emergency department or physician's office just before admission, a full (12-lead) ECG should be recorded in the CCU by the nursing staff. This initial tracing is used for comparative purposes with subsequent ECGs to establish the diagnosis (and location) of acute myocardial infarction. Usually, an ECG is recorded at least once a day while the patient is in the CCU, particularly if the electrocardiographic pattern is unstable or if the diagnosis remains uncertain. In the event a patient develops recurrent chest pain after admission, the nurse should record a full ECG during (or soon after) the episode.

8. Assist the Physician in the Physical Examination of the Patient

The nurse's presence at the bedside during the physician's examination serves several useful purposes. Especially important is that it provides an opportunity for the physician and nurse to evaluate the patient together and to compare the findings of this examination with those of the initial assessment. Any significant changes in blood pressure, pulse rate, cardiac rhythm, or other clinical signs that may have developed in the interim are of considerable importance in planning the treatment program. Also, the physician's evaluation can be used as a point of reference for the staff in assessing and comparing subsequent changes on the patient's clinical status.

9. Arrange for Laboratory Studies

In most CCUs a routine set of laboratory studies are ordered for all patients admitted with a suspected myocardial infarction. The tests usually include a complete blood count, urinalysis, serum enzymes, and a 6/60 screening panel (electrolytes, glucose, urea nitrogen). If anticoagulant therapy is contemplated, a prothrombin time (PT) or activated partial thromboplastin time (APTT) is ordered. In addition, the physician may request several other studies for purposes of diagnosis or clinical assessment, including chest x-rays, arterial blood gases and hemodynamic measurements, for example. The nurse should arrange for each of these procedures and, when indicated, assist in performing them.

10. Start the Treatment Program As Ordered By the Physician

Although standard orders are sometimes used initially for patients who are not in acute distress on admission, it is nevertheless essential that the physician discuss the proposed management of each patient with the nursing staff. The specific aims of therapy and any anticipated problems should be considered at this time. Drug treatment must be started promptly and the time of administration recorded carefully.

11. Explain the Situation to the Family

The great concern of a family for a patient with acute myocardial infarction and the worry of the patient about his family must always be recognized. The patient is one of the family and cannot be set apart simply because he is in a hospital. With this in mind the nurse should provide a general description of the purpose of the unit to family visitors and explain the type of care the patient will receive. In many CCUs families are given prepared brochures which describe the monitoring system, visiting hours, and other pertinent information regarding the patient's stay in the unit. It is a mistake to view the family as burdensome; indeed every effort should be made to enlist their cooperation. Reassuring the family is often every bit as important as reassuring the patient.

Patients in Acute Distress

1. Initiate Cardiac Monitoring

Although the clinical picture of patients in acute distress is usually dominated by signs of acute left ventricular failure or cardiogenic shock, it is critically important that cardiac monitoring be started immediately in order to detect and terminate lethal arrhythmias that are particularly likely to occur in this circumstance. If several nurses are available, emergency treatment of pump failure can be started concurrently; otherwise cardiac monitoring should precede other therapy.

2. Start Oxygen Therapy and Place the Patient in an Upright Position

The most effective method for administering oxygen in this situation is by means of a tight-fitting face mask with a flow rate of 8-10 liters of oxygen per minute. An oxygen concentration of at least 60% can be achieved with this technique. (By contrast, a two-pronged nasal cannula with an oxygen flow rate of 6-8 liters per minute usually provides an oxygen concentration of only 30-40%.) By positioning the patient in an upright (high Fowler's) position, the diaphragm descends, fluid tends to drift to the bases of the lungs, and breathing improves.

3. Start an Intravenous Infusion

An intravenous line should be established as soon as possible, using an indwelling venous catheter. This conduit, which is kept open at all times with a micro-drip infusion of 5% glucose in water, is used to administer intravenous drugs required in the treatment programs, and for emergency purposes in combatting sudden arrhythmias.

4. Assess the Patient's Clinical Status

Patients admitted to the CCU in acute distress often have a hectic course, and their clinical condition may change very rapidly. Therefore it is important to establish base line clinical findings for comparison as soon as possible. Clinical signs that should be assessed and recorded by the nurse at this time include blood pressure, pulse rate, cardiac rhythm, respiration, findings of left ventricular failure, skin color, sweating, mental status, and urinary output.

5. Notify the Physician Promptly

That a patient is in acute distress at the time of admission indicates that a serious complication of acute myocardial infarction has already developed and that a program of therapy must be started without delay. Indeed, the sooner treatment is initiated in these critical circumstances, the better the chance for survival. For this reason the nurse should advise the physician immediately that the patient has been admitted in acute distress.

6. Assist the Physician with Assessment Procedures and Order Diagnotic Tests

Hemodynamic measurements and other procedures are frequently required to assess the severity of the patient's condition or to develop a treatment plan. The assistance of a nurse is necessary in performing most of these procedures (e.g., insertion of an intraarterial line or a Swan-Ganz catheter). Laboratory studies, such as arterial blood gases, should be arranged for promptly by calling or paging a laboratory technician.

7. Begin the Treatment Program As Ordered by the Physician

No time can be wasted in starting treatment for patients in acute distress. In fact, the nurse can facilitate treatment by anticipating the equipment and drugs that will be needed in the management of particular complications and preparing them for use. The specific nursing role for each complication is described in the following chapter.

8. Inform the Family of the Situation

A member of the nursing staff should be readily available to keep the family informed about the patient's condition and to explain how his needs are being met in the CCU.

SUBSEQUENT CARE OF PATIENTS IN THE CCU

The preventive regimen started at the time of admission is continued throughout the patient's stay in the CCU. The main objective of nursing care during this period is to *anticipate* problems. Included in this anticipatory care are the following measures.

Cardiac Monitoring

Constant vigilance is essential if warning arrhythmias are to be detected and lethal arrhythmias prevented. This does not imply that it is necessary to watch the monitor incessantly, but it does mean that the nurse must always be aware of the heart rate and rhythm. For sudden changes in the heart rate to be recognized instantly, the alarm system of the monitor should be utilized to its fullest advantage (as explained in Chapter 6). Although death-producing arrhythmias are most likely to develop within the early hours after myocardial infarction, it can never be assumed that the risk period has passed, even though the cardiac rhythm appears stable.

Clinical Evaluation

The use of monitors and hemodynamic equipment is meant to complement direct nursing care, not replace it. Careful evaluation of the patient's clinical condition at regular intervals is mandatory. Basically the assessment consists of eliciting symptoms, measuring vital signs, and examining the patient for signs of heart failure. As a general rule the evaluation is conducted every 2 hours during the first 8 hours after admission (or until the patient's condition is stable), and then every 4 hours thereafter.

Chest Pain

As part of the assessment process the nurse should specifically inquire about the recurrence of chest pain. Also, the patient should be instructed to notify the nurse promptly whenever chest pain develops. Depending on the intensity and duration of the pain (along with associated clinical findings) the nurse must decide whether to administer nitroglycerin or an analgesic. As mentioned previously, one helpful method of judging the severity of chest pain is to ask the patient to rank the discomfort on a scale of 1 to 10. This ranking provides some guide for comparison of the intensity of pain episodes. When angina occurs, the nurse should record the pulse and blood pressure during and after the attack. Usually the heart rate and blood pressure increase just before angina develops and rise further during the chest pain episode. If the chest pain persists for more than a few minutes an electrocardiogram should be recorded to determine whether additional myocardial injury has occurred.

Preparation for Emergencies

Despite all efforts at prevention, unexpected catastrophes can and do occur in patients with acute myocardial infarction. In these circumstances survival hinges on split-second decisions and actions. Not only must the nursing staff itself be prepared for these emergencies, but it is absolutely essential that all resuscitative equipment and supplies be ready for instant use. Machines—particularly defibrillators—should be tested regularly to verify that they are functioning properly.

Intake and Output

Maintaining fluid balance is an important aspect of coronary care. For example, overhydration and underhydration pose serious threats to circulatory efficiency, particularly in the presence of left ventricular failure or cardiogenic shock. Also, the effectiveness of diuretic therapy is determined primarily by urinary output volume. In order to assess fluid balance adequately, the nurse must not only maintain accurate records of fluid intake and output but also relate these findings to the patient's clinical status.

Activity and Cardiac Rehabilitation

One of the mainstays of the treatment program for acute myocardial infarction is to reduce the workload of the heart in order to decrease myocardial oxygen demands. For this reason it was customary in the past to confine patients to complete bed rest in the CCU during the acute phase of the illness. This practice is now changing, and complete bed rest is no longer considered a necessity. Experience has shown that immobility causes weakness, loss of muscle tone, and increases the risk of certain complications, such as pulmonary atelectasis. Therefore, unless the patient's clinical condition dictates otherwise, the following activities are encouraged, particularly after the first day or so: washing hands and face, brushing teeth, comb-

ing hair, self feeding, and simple exercises of the extremities. On the other hand, activities demanding sustained muscle tension, such as straining at stool, should be avoided since isometric muscle contraction substantially increases cardiac work. In addition, patients with uncomplicated myocardial infarction are usually permitted to sit in an arm chair for increasing periods of time after the first day. With a properly designed chair, which supports the head, arms and lower legs, the energy expenditure is only slightly more than bed rest. During and after these activities the nurse should ascertain the blood pressure, heart rate, and the development of arrhythmias. Should any significant changes occur or if the patient experiences angina or dyspnea, the degree of activity must be curtailed.

Guidelines for exercises and other activities for patients with uncomplicated myocardial infarction are presented in Figure 5.5.

Maintaining a Serene Atmosphere

Physical and emotional rest can be achieved only in a setting conducive to these needs. Ideally the CCU is the quietest place in the hospital. The nursing staff must make every effort to maintain a calm, serene atmosphere by providing care in an efficient, unhurried manner and, also, by controlling noise, avoiding commotion, and reducing traffic in the unit. Scheduling visiting hours to meet the needs of the patient and his family, and limiting the number of visitors in a room to one or two at a time, are helpful measures. In addition, it is worthwhile as part of the nursing plan to include deliberate rest periods for the patient in which he can relax without interruption. During these periods the room should be darkened to minimize distractions.

Elimination

Patients should be allowed to use a bedside commode (or pullman toilet) for urination and defecation. Indeed the physical effort involved in using these facilities is much less than that expended with a bedpan. Male patients may stand at the bedside to void. Bedpans are required only if patients are desperately ill and cannot get out of bed. Stool-softening drugs and mild cathartics are useful in easing bowel movements and preventing straining. Enemas should be avoided because rectal stimulation may induce undesirable cardiovascular reflexes.

Diet

Because many patients experience nausea and vomiting during the first day (particularly if narcotics have

Guidelines for Exercise and Activities for Uncomplicated MI Patients

Exercises	Activities
Step 1 (Usually Day 1)	
Deep breathing q. 2 h.	Feed self with bed at 45° angle
Passive range of motion exercises (5 times each extremity) b.i.d.	Partial personal care
	Bedside commode
Active foot circles q.h. when awake	Dangle with arms and feet supported
Footboard exercises q. 4 h. when awake	
Step 2 (Usually Day 2)	
Passive range of motion exercises (5 times each extremity) b.i.d.	Sit up in chair 20 minutes, t.i.d.
	Shave and comb hair
Repeat Step 1	Brush teeth
	Bedside commode
	Partial self bath with assistance
	Feed self
	Light reading
Step 3 (Usually Day 3)	
Active range of motion exercises (4 times each extremity) b.i.d.	Bathe self at bedside
	Sit in chair for meals and feed self
	BRP (if bathroom is near)
	Light reading
	Watch TV
Step 4 (Usually Day 4)	
Walk in room 20 minutes, t.i.d.	Bathe self
	Up in chair ad lib
	Feed self while sitting in chair
	BRP
	Diversional activities

Figure 5.5. Guidelines for Exercise and Activities for Uncomplicated MI Patients.

been administered), a liquid diet is usually ordered initially. After the gastrointestinal symptoms have subsided and the patient's appetite has returned, the choice of diet depends to a large degree on the philosophy of the individual physician about the need for rigid sodium (and cholesterol) restriction at this stage of the illness. As a general rule, a 1-2 gm sodium diet is prescribed. Many patients find low-sodium diets unpalatable and therefore do not eat their meals. The nurse should assess the adequacy of the patient's nutrition and assist him in selecting foods he will enjoy. Low-sodium diets can be made tastier by using flavors such as lemon, thyme, vinegar, and sodium-free spices. Coffee, tea, and other caffein-containing beverages are generally excluded from the diet during the CCU period. Also to be avoided is iced water (or any iced drink); it is believed that the chilling effect of these drinks may affect the cardiac rate and rhythm through reflex mechanisms.

Prevention of Thromboembolism

Venous stasis predisposes to clot formation in the lower extremities and therefore measures designed to prevent pooling of venous blood in the legs are important, particularly in elderly patients and those with complications demanding bed rest, in whom the risk of thrombosis is greatest. Antiembolic stockings are helpful in this respect and should be used in all high-risk patients. Also, patients must be instructed not to cross their legs at the calves because the pressure thus exerted may hinder venous circulation. Another prevention measure is to place a foot board at the end of the bed against which the patient can extend his feet; this exercise promotes the return of venous blood. (Further details of the nursing role in preventing thromboembolism are described in Chapter 7.)

Medications

The nurse must carefully observe the clinical response to all medications administered. Has the drug achieved its desired effect? Are there any side effects? These observations strongly influence subsequent decisions about treatment, and therefore repeated assessment is essential. (The actions and side effects of cardiac drugs are described in Chapter 16.)

TRANSFER FROM CCU

In the absence of serious complications patients are transferred from the CCU to regular hospital quarters usually after the fourth or fifth day. Leaving the protective setting of a CCU is often a disquieting experience for the patient. The source of this apprehension is readily understandable: no longer will the patient be under constant surveillance and protected from sudden death. Furthermore, the abrupt interruption of the close relationships between the patient and the CCU team may lead to a sense of loss and abandonment. There are several ways to help the patient adjust to this transition.

1. A day or two before transfer the nurse should advise the patient that his condition has improved to a point where intensive care will no longer be needed. Being moved from the unit is an indication that the clinical course has been satisfactory and that the acute phase of the illness has passed. Repeated reassurance along these lines is often necessary to convince the patient of the safety and desirability of the change.
2. It is also wise to tell the patient that apprehension on his part about being transferred is a normal reaction, one that most patients experience. Allowing the patient to express his feelings and to ask questions is a very helpful approach.
3. Introducing the patient to the head nurse of the floor to which he is being transferred is a valuable method of demonstrating continuity of care. The introduction should be made while

the patient is still in the CCU, not on arrival in the new ward.
4. After transfer is accomplished, a nurse from the CCU should visit the patient in his new quarters. The psychological effects of transfer often do not become apparent until after the patient is situated in his new surroundings; seeing a familiar face offers a sense of security.
5. To avoid the problems associated with the sudden termination of coronary care, some hospitals utilize intermediate (step-down) units to bridge the gap between intensive and regular nursing care. These units serve as halfway houses; a patient is kept under surveillance but not with the same intenseness as the CCU. As an alternative, cardiac monitoring can be continued after transfer from the CCU by means of telemetry. This permits the patient to be assigned to an ordinary hospital room and be ambulatory, while still being monitored.
6. A concerted effort should be made to maintain continuity of patient teaching plans after transfer from the unit. In some institutions CCU nurses make follow-up visits for this purpose; in others, staff nurses assume this responsibility. In either case it is important for the nurse to review the patient education form (as shown in Figure 5.3) to note which subjects have already been discussed with the patient.

EMOTIONAL SUPPORT OF THE PATIENT

An extraordinarily important part of coronary care nursing is to help the patient manage (and cope with) the profound emotional stress that accompanies acute myocardial infarction. This intervention is essential not only for compassionate reasons (inherent in all nursing care), but also because emotional stress can adversely affect the clinical course and eventual outcome of the illness. For example, severe anxiety during the early days after acute myocardial infarction is a serious threat since it results in a rapid heart rate, a rise in blood pressure, and an increase in the oxygen demands of the myocardium. These emotionally induced cardiac effects (medicated through the sympathetic nervous system) may lead to life-threatening complications, including heart failure, pulmonary edema, lethal arrhythmias, and extension of the size of the original infarction. Furthermore it has been reported that the patient's emotional adjustment during the coronary care period significantly influences rehabilitation and long-term survival. Some studies indicate that patients who adjust poorly while in the coronary unit are less likely to return to work and more prone to develop another myocardial infarction than those who make good adjustments during the early stages of hospitalization. In light of these facts it is understandable that the management of emotional problems is a major nursing responsibility in a coronary care unit. Although professional nurses are well prepared to identify and resolve emotional reactions to illness (indeed very few health disciplines emphasize these principles as strongly), the psychological effects of acute myocardial infarction are unique in many ways and demand special attention. Before describing the basic elements of the nursing role, it is pertinent to mention some of the factors that contribute to the severe stress the patient with acute myocardial infarction encounters initially, and to consider the most common emotional responses observed in the coronary care unit.

Sources of Emotional Stress

Experiencing a myocardial infarction is a terrifying feeling from the very start. The realization that death may be imminent, the unrelenting chest pain, the dependence on others to provide help, the rush to a hospital (usually by ambulance), and the looks of anguish on the faces of relatives or friends are just a few of the many fears that immediately confront the patient; but this is only the beginning of his ordeal. As soon as the patient reaches the coronary care unit (or while still in the emergency ward) he encounters other unexpected threats, and his burden of fear mounts. Monitoring electrodes are attached to his chest, an intravenous infusion is started, oxygen is administered, injections are given, blood samples are drawn, and unfamiliar nurses, physicians, and technicians hurriedly enter and leave his room. The thought, "Am I dying?" runs through the patient's mind. The coronary unit itself contributes to his terror: the room is small; strange machines encircle him; he sees bottles, syringes, tubes, and needles; he hears the sounds of the equipment and the voices of the staff. Thus from the moment of the attack the patient is subjected to an enormous *sensory overload,* both internal and external, over which he has no control.

Added to this already formidable problem is the fact that the patient is inadequately prepared, if at all, for this sudden sensory overload. Unlike many illnesses in which the patient can anticipate some of the fears and frights he will experience, acute myocardial infarction occurs suddenly and unexpectedly, and therefore precludes adequate preparation. Because of this lack of preparation, the patient's fears are intensified greatly.

Another factor that contributes to the profound psychological stress of acute myocardial infarction is that the patient does not have the opportunity, at least at first, to mobilize his emotional resources and attempt to resolve ("work through" as psychiatrists say) the stressful situation. He is preoccupied with more crucial thoughts, particularly survival, and consequently other problems are of much less importance.

The combination of marked sensory overload, inadequate preparation for this stress, and inadequate opportunity to mobilize emotional resources to reduce the stress represent the three characteristic features of an overwhelming emotional experience. It is readily understandable that patients with acute myocardial infarction face great difficulty in maintaining emotional equilibrium, particularly during the acute phase of the illness.

Emotional Responses to Acute Myocardial Infarction

The severe stress associated with acute myocardial infarction provokes a wide variety of emotional responses. Fundamentally, patients attempt to cope with the stress by relying on defense mechanisms that have served them in the past with other crises. Because each person responds according to his own psychological makeup, the behavioral pattern among patients in a coronary care unit is by no means constant. Nevertheless there are certain predictable emotional responses, the most common of which are described below.

Anxiety

The emotional response observed most often during the coronary care period is anxiety (which for practical purposes is synonymous with fear). The degree of anxiety is influenced by many psychosocial factors and varies considerably among patients. Psychological studies suggest that the main source of anxiety is the prospect of sudden death. Consequently, signs of anxiety are most likely to be noted during the early days of hospitalization, when recurrent symptoms develop (e.g., chest pain or shortness of breath), or when special procedures are required (e.g., insertion of a temporary pacemaker or cardioversion). Curiously, perhaps there is no definite relationship between anxiety and the seriousness of the illness. It appears that anxiety depends more on how the patient perceives the threat to his life rather than on the severity of the infarction itself.

Anxiety is often difficult to identify in patients with acute myocardial infarction because many of them attempt to hide or deny the fact that they are anxious (as explained below). Objective evidence of anxiety is probably a more reliable clue to the problem. Patients who are anxious usually appear tense, apprehensive, fidgety, restless, and seem unable to relax.

Sweating is frequently apparent on the palms of the hands and the axillae. Particularly important from a nursing standpoint is that patients with anxiety repeatedly seek reassurance in one way or other. For example, they may ask the nurse time and again about coronary disease, monitoring, laboratory tests, and methods of treatment—all in an effort to be reassured. What may appear to be intellectual curiosity is usually a sign of anxiety.

Denial

Many patients attempt to cope with emotional stress by means of denial. There are two principal forms of denial: denial of fact and denial of meaning. Denial of fact means that the patient does not acknowledge that he has actually had a heart attack. He attempts to pass off or minimize the event by saying, for example, "I am sure it's not a heart attack, nobody in my family had heart disease," or "we are going on vacation next week." Denial of meaning, probably the more common mechanism, is defined as a conscious or subconscious effort to deny the emotional feelings (e.g., anxiety or depression) associated with acute myocardial infarction and hospitalization. The patient does not admit his fears and, in fact, often displays an optimistic attitude. Both forms of denial are a reaction against reality posed by the illness.

Denial usually can be recognized by statements the patient makes, in conjunction with the way he acts. For instance, the patient may tell the nurse that he feels well and is not upset, yet it is evident that he is sweating and has a look of fear in his eyes. Threatening to sign out of the hospital against advice is a manifestation of severe denial.

Depression

It is understandable that patients generally become despondent when they begin to consider the implications of a heart attack. They realize that their activities, earning capacity, and way of life may be affected drastically. This is a normal response and is of concern only when the depression is prolonged or severe.

Patients often deny depression just as they do anxiety; therefore the problem may not be readily apparent. However, moderate or severe depression has characteristic signs: disinterest in the surroundings, a sad look, slow speech, listless behavior, loss of appetite, insomnia, and crying.

Anger

Some patients react to the emotional stress of their illness by becoming angry. The anger, either openly expressed or hidden, may be self-directed, aimed at the family, at the CCU staff, or at God. Self-anger is often expressed by the question "Why me?" Anger directed toward the family may take the form of criticism; and if directed at the nursing staff, by repeated complaints about the quality of care. In dealing with an angry patient, the nurse may be inclined to respond with anger. This reaction intensifies the problem rather than helps it. Instead, the nurse should attempt to understand the behavior, and accept the expressions of anger as a manifestation of emotional conflict, while helping the patient work through these emotions.

Nursing Intervention

Explanation and Clarification

One of the most useful methods of helping the patient adjust to the emotional stress of acute myocardial infarction is to explain his illness to him. The main object is to dispel common misconceptions about heart disease and its consequences. The patient's concept of a heart attack is usually grossly distorted and therefore many of his fears are unrealistic and unwarranted. For example, patients commonly believe that even if they recover from a heart attack they will have to take medication for the rest of their lives, or curtail their sexual activity. To combat these fears the nurse should offer repeated explanations about various aspects of myocardial infarction, always attempting to identify and clarify any misconceptions the patient may have. It is important to answer the patient's questions in a forthright manner. By avoiding a question or simply saying, "You will have to ask the doctor," the nurse can indirectly intensify the patient's anxiety (as well as block any further discussion).

Fostering Optimism

As noted, patients with acute myocardial infarction frequently deny their emotional feelings as a means of coping with stress. In many cases it may be beneficial to allow the patient to continue to use this defense mechanism, at least up to a certain point. Certainly this is not to say that the CCU team should ever let the patient believe that he has not in fact suffered a heart attack, or lie to him about the seriousness of his condition; but it does imply that allowing the patient to maintain an optimistic outlook by means of denial may be advantageous. In fact some studies have shown that patients who can effectively deny anxiety or depression during the acute phase of the illness have a better chance for survival than nondeniers. From a practical standpoint this suggests that it may be helpful to foster the patient's optimism by treating him with the conviction that recovery is fully anticipated. In other words, the CCU team should emphasize survival and recovery rather than risks and dangers. (It is important to point out that this concept applies to the management of acute myocardial infarction, but not necessarily to all other illnesses.)

Reassurance

The nurse can provide reassurance in two ways: by her own demeanor and by talking to the patient in the most encouraging fashion possible. Patients become more confident when the nurse acts in a calm, positive, efficient manner. If the nurse appears tense and anxious (a normal reaction in many instances) the patient's anxiety level is bound to increase. It is very reassuring for the patient to learn of any evidence of progress toward his recovery. For example, if it is apparent that the patient is able to tolerate increased activity without difficulty, the nurse should deliberately comment on this fact, and indicate that it represents a good sign. Broad promises such as, "Don't worry, everything will be all right," serve little purpose and should be avoided. It is also important for the nurse to offer the patient a hopeful outlook for the future, and make him aware that most patients can lead useful, productive lives despite myocardial infarction. It is helpful to emphasize that normal activities after recovery from a heart attack are beneficial rather than dangerous.

Listening

By listening attentively and demonstrating genuine interest the nurse can assist the patient to ventilate his feelings and fears. Expression of emotions is often, in itself, an effective form of therapy, since by describing his fears the patient may recognize the sources of the problem, and be able to deal with them. However, the nurse should not prod the patient to discuss his emotions since many times, particularly during the acute phase of the illness, the patient is not able to sort out his feelings. In expressing his feelings, the patient may give cues suggesting some spiritual need. This need should not be minimized or neglected (as sometimes happens in intensive care settings) since it may have deep significance to the patient. In this circumstance, the nurse should arrange for a member of the clergy to visit the patient, or deal with this need if she feels prepared to do so.

Anticipating Emotional Reactions

It is very helpful for patients to understand that many of the emotions they experience are normal, anticipated responses. The nurse can assist the patient by letting him know that being depressed, for example, is a common reaction during the coronary care period. The intensity of emotional reactions can often be reduced if they are anticipated.

Drug Therapy

As a general rule it is useful to administer tranquilizers during the first few days of hospitalization. However, the dosage should be adjusted so that the patient is not constantly drowsy or sleepy. Antidepressant drugs should not be used in patients with acute myocardial infarction because they may produce adverse cardiac effects.

Nursing Care Plan

In order to provide efficient, individualized nursing care, a nursing care plan should be developed for each patient, preferably by the nurse admitting the patient. The use of a nursing care plan has several major benefits. First, it gives direction to the nursing staff by setting goals and indicating how to achieve them. Second, it provides for consistency and continuity of care. The care plan allows nurses on each tour of duty to follow the same pattern of care, and to concert their efforts. Third, a nursing care plan facilitates communication among other members of the health care team. By reviewing the instructions offered to the nursing staff regarding patient care, and noting the outcome of various interventions, others involved in treating the patient can obtain a clear picture of the overall goals of the CCU team.

The most important characteristic of a good nursing care plan is that the information it provides should be valuable for any nurse assuming the care of the patient. Therefore, the plan must be kept up-to-date through repeated evaluation of outcomes and through appropriate revisions. Although there are a variety of forms used to record nursing care plans, the simplest method involves a prepared form (Kardex) with separate columns to list the problem, the objectives in solving it, nursing interventions, frequency of interventions (time intervals), and the outcome. By reading across these columns the nurse responsible for the care of the patient at a particular time can immediately understand the situation. Identifying information about the patient is usually recorded at the bottom of the Kardex so that it can be easily seen in a flip chart. An example of a portion of a nursing care plan for a patient with acute myocardial infarction is demonstrated in Figure 5.6.

Nursing Care Plan for a Patient with Acute Myocardial Infarction

Date	Problems	Objectives	Nursing Interventions	Time	Outcomes
10/24	Chest pain	There will be no complications from chest pain	Evaluate chest pain Ask patient to rate on scale from 1 to 10 Give ordered morphine sulfate 15 mg PRN Q 4 hrs. Record a full ECG during and after chest pain Start O$_2$ Check BP and pulse during and after pain episode	Whenever it occurs	One episode at 9 p.m. on 10/25 relieved by morphine sulfate No signs of ischemia on ECG No change in BP and pulse
10/24	Arrhythmias	There will be no complications from arrhythmias	Maintain cardiac monitoring Record and interpret rhythm strips Report significant arrhythmia to M.D. Follow CCU protocol for serious arrhythmias	Continuously Q 2 hrs. Whenever they occur	In NSR 10/24 Isolated PVCs on 10/25
10/24	Anxiety	Anxiety will be relieved	Introduce yourself Orient patient to CCU concept and routines Allow patient to verbalize fears and concerns Give ordered sedative	On adm. PRN	Pt. expressed anxiety about his job Relaxes at 10 p.m. on 10/24
10/25	Inadequate knowledge of M.I.	Meet the patient's learning needs	Assess readiness to learn Answer questions honestly If ready, explain about an M.I. Record progress on teaching plan		On a.m. of 10/25, pt. asked about a heart attack. Nurse answered questions briefly. Pt. needs reinforcement of information.

Room #26A   Admitted 10/24   Name: JAMES C. SMITH   Diagnosis: AMI   Age: 51   Doctor: Harris

Figure 5.6. Nursing Care Plan for a Patient with Acute Myocardial Infarction.

6

Cardiac Monitoring

Central to the coronary care concept is continuous electrocardiographic monitoring of the heart. Indeed, without the ability to detect warning and lethal arrhythmias, intensive coronary care would have little advantage over regular hospital care. Therefore it is essential that all coronary care nurses fully understand the principles and methods of cardiac monitoring, and be able to utilize this procedure to its fullest advantage.

Curious as it now seems, as late as 1960 arrhythmias were not considered to be a particularly common complication of acute myocardial infarction. However the reason for this erroneous impression is understandable: there was no practical method available until that time for detecting arrhythmias on a continuous basis; instead, arrhythmia detection depended for the most part on routine electrocardiograms (recorded perhaps once or twice a day) and on physical examination. Because of the intermittent nature of these observations the majority of arrhythmias went unnoticed, and more than 40% of deaths from acute infarction were due to arrhythmic complications. Then electronic equipment was developed (as a byproduct of space age engineering) which permitted a *continuous* display of the patient's electrocardiogram. With these instruments, appropriately called cardiac monitors, it became possible to observe the heart's electrical activity at all times and in this way identify arrhythmic disturbances the instant they occurred. Cardiac monitoring became the cornerstone of intensive coronary care.

THE BASIS OF CARDIAC MONITORING

Each heartbeat is the result of an electrical stimulus. This impulse, which originates normally in a specialized area of the right atrium, called the sinoatrial node, is conducted through a network of fibers within the heart (the conduction system) and finally stimulates the myocardium to contract. This same electrical force spreads outward from the heart and reaches the surface of the body, where it can be detected with electrodes attached to the skin. The purpose of the cardiac monitor is to pick up the electrical signals generated by the heart and display them on a screen (oscilloscope) in the form of a continuous electrocardiogram. By analyzing the electrocardiographic wave forms, any disturbance in cardiac rate, rhythm, or conduction can be identified (as explained in subsequent chapters).

MONITORING EQUIPMENT

There are dozens of different types of cardiac monitors currently available. While these machines vary in size, design, dependability, elegance, and cost, their fundamental components are the same. A basic monitoring system works in the following way:

1. Electrodes applied to the patient's chest wall pick up the electrical impulses initiated by the heart.

2. These original waves are too small to be seen on the monitor screen, and for this reason they are directed through an amplifier where their height is increased about 1000 times.

3. The amplified impulses pass through a magnetic field (galvanometer), where a series of wave forms are established. These deflections, reflecting each phase of the heart's electrical activity, comprise an electrocardiogram.

4. The electrocardiogram is then displayed continuously on an oscilloscopic screen (similar to a small television screen). The size, position, and brightness of the electrocardiogram can be adjusted as necessary to obtain the clearest "picture."

5. In addition, the monitor counts each heartbeat and displays the average heart rate per minute on a rate meter. (Actually, the machine counts the electrical waves associated with ventricular activation, called R waves, and not the ventricular contractions themselves.) With each heartbeat a light (pulse light) flashes and a sound ("beep") is heard. (The "beeper" may be turned off if the sound is annoying.)

6. Integrated with the rate meter is an alarm system, which sounds a loud audio signal and causes a light to flash if the patient's heart rate falls below or exceeds present levels. For example, if the lower-limit alarm is set at 50 per minute and the upper limit at 120 per minute, any decrease or increase in the heart rate beyond this particular range will cause the alarm to be triggered. Thus the onset of slow-rate or fast-rate arrhythmias can be recognized immediately, even though the nurse may not be observing the monitor at the time.

7. A direct write-out mechanism provides a printed record of the electrocardiogram seen on the oscilloscope. This documentation (in the form of a rhythm strip) permits precise identification of an arrhythmia and is also valuable for comparing electrocardiographic changes over a period of time. The recording can be obtained on demand as well as automatically (whenever the alarm system is triggered.)

A diagrammatic representation of a basic cardiac monitor is shown in Figure 6.1. In addition to these fundamental components cardiac monitors may also include a variety of accessory devices.* Perhaps the most useful of these additional modules are those designed to enhance the detection of early warning signs of lethal arrhythmias. (As noted previously, the underlying theme of intensive coronary care is to *prevent* lethal arrhythmias by recognizing and treating

warning arrhythmias.) That it may be difficult to specifically identify a transient warning arrhythmia from the electrocardiographic pattern seen on an oscilloscope screen can be readily appreciated: the electrocardiogram moves across the screen rapidly, and the observer has only one fleeting glance of the pattern with no chance to analyze it in detail. The most popular mechanisms used to facilitate arrhythmia detection are memory systems and components to hold or "freeze" the oscilloscopic pattern for closer inspection.

Memory systems are designed to store and play back the electrocardiogram of the preceding 15-60 seconds (or more). This "instant replay" technique is useful in two circumstances. First, if a transient arrhythmia is noted on the oscilloscope but there is insufficient time to activate the direct write-out device, the episode can be recaptured and recorded by using the memory system. Second, if an observer is not near the monitor when an alarm is triggered, the memory mechanism will replay the events that *preceded* the occurrence. Hold or "freeze" devices stop the movement of the electrocardiogram across the oscilloscopic screen, keeping a particular pattern in place until it can be interpreted. These modules do not print out an electrocardiogram (from which precise measurements can be made), and for this reason they may be less useful than direct write-out or memory mechanisms.

THE OPERATION OF CARDIAC MONITORS

Four steps are involved in cardiac monitoring: 1) attaching electrodes to the patient's chest wall; 2) connecting the wires from the electrodes to the monitor (by way of a "patient" cable); 3) adjusting the monitor to obtain an effective electrocardiogram; 4) setting the high-rate and low-rate alarm system at desired levels. Each of these aspects will be discussed separately.

Electrodes and Their Attachment

Electrodes serve to pick up the heart's electrical signals at the skin surface. It is apparent that unless

---

*In recent years there has been an attempt to make monitoring equipment more and more sophisticated by adding various accessories to the basic system. Some of these additions are valuable and improve monitoring capabilities, but others are no more than unnecessary luxuries. It is unwise to assume that a monitor will necessarily be more effective or do a better job just because the machine has a large number of dials, knobs, switches, or lights; indeed our own experience indicates exactly the opposite.

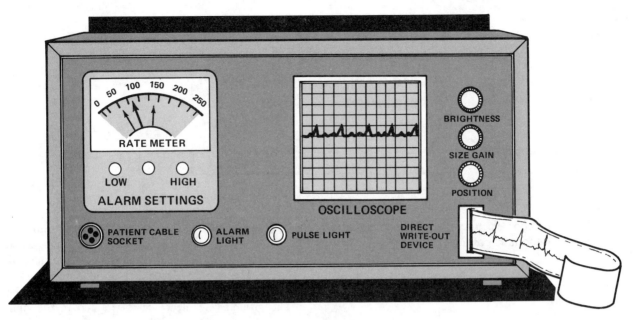

Figure 6.1. Diagram of basic cardiac monitor.

the signals are detected accurately the remaining phases of cardiac monitoring will have little meaning. Therefore the electrodes themselves and the manner in which they are applied to the skin is of critical importance.

Three basic types of electrodes have been used for cardiac monitoring. Although two of these devices have become for the most part obsolete, it is nevertheless worthwhile to discuss them in order to understand the fundamental problems associated with electrodes and their application.

The first monitoring electrodes, called direct-contact electrodes, were round metal plates about 1.5 inches in diameter, which were anchored to the skin by layers of adhesive tape. Because of high electrical resistence between the skin and large electrode surface, it was necessary to apply a layer of conductive jelly (gel) at the interface before the electrodes were attached. These direct-contact metal electrodes presented several problems. First, they had to be changed 2-3 times each day because the electrode gel would dry quickly under the adhesive tape blanket. Second, the electrodes were annoying to patients because they were cumbersome and produced skin irritation. Third, cleaning and preparing the electrodes, and taping them in place, wasted much nursing time and posed a serious handicap in emergency situations. Above all, the electrocardiographic patterns were often of poor quality: not only was it difficult to maintain direct contact between the electrodes and the skin, but the large surface area of the electrodes picked up extraneous electrical currents within the skin itself, thus distorting the electrocardiogram.

In an effort to get rid of most of these difficulties many coronary care units began to use hypodermic needles as electrodes. Small, 0.5-inch 25-gauge, metal hubbed needles were inserted directly under the skin surface for this purpose. In principle, needle electrodes were splendid: electrode gel was not required, contact with the skin was perfect, electrical interference was minimal, and the needles could be placed very rapidly in emergencies. Unfortunately, however, these electrodes were difficult to keep in place, and many patients found them uncomfortable.

The third form of electrode was the disc type or "floating" electrode. These electrodes differ from direct-contact electrodes in that they are deliberately separated from the skin by a built-in "spacer" (Figure 6.2). Conductive gel is placed in the spacer, and the electrode is then attached to the skin by means of a surrounding ring of adhesive material. The main purpose of separating the electrode from the skin is to reduce local electrical interference at the skin surface, thus improving the quality of the electrocardiogram. In addition, disc electrodes do not have to be changed more than once a day since the electrode jelly remains moist in the spacer. Furthermore, these electrodes are lightweight, simple to apply, and seldom annoy the patient.

At present, nearly all CCUs use a modified version of the basic disc electrode. These electrodes are prepackaged, pregelled, and disposable. Their principal advantage is that they greatly shorten the time for electrode placement and permit cardiac monitoring to be instituted without delay. By peeling off a paper backing from a porous adhesive pad, the gel-filled electrode is immediately ready for use. Moreover, the electrodes can often remain in place for several days since the gel does not dehydrate and seldom produces skin irritation. Equally important is that there is less

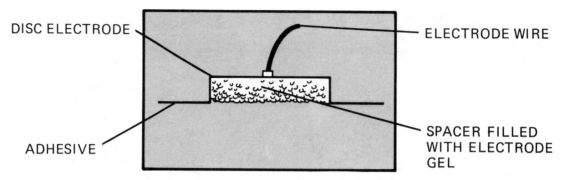

Figure 6.2. Disc-type or "floating" electrode.

likelihood of poor electrocardiographic signals, resulting from too much or too little gel.*

Location of Electrodes

Three electrodes are required for cardiac monitoring. Two of these serve to detect the heart's electrical activity; the third is a ground electrode, which carries off ("grounds") extraneous electrical currents from sources other than the heart. (With some monitoring equipment four or even five electrodes may be used; the purpose of these additional electrodes is to permit multiple electrocardiographic views of the heart by simply turning a lead selector dial.)

In positioning the electrodes on the chest wall the object is to select locations that will provide the clearest electrocardiographic wave forms, permitting arrhythmias to be identified readily. The two most common positions are the so-called conventional position and the modified chest lead position.

With the conventional position (Figure 6.3), the right (R) electrode is placed on the right side of the sternum below the clavicle and medial to the pectoral muscles. The left (L) electrode is situated at the level of the lowest palpable rib on the left side of the chest in the anterior axillary line. The ground (G) electrode is placed at the lower right rib cage area, opposite the left (L) electrode. With the electrodes in these positions the monitor records the electrical activity between the R and L electrodes. This particular path (or lead) normally produces the tallest ventricular complexes (R waves) and is chosen primarily for this reason.

With the modified chest lead (MCL) position the right (R) electrode is placed in the fourth interspace at the right border of the sternum (or over the sternum itself). The left (L) electrode is located near the left shoulder, just under the outer portion of the clavicle. The ground (G) electrode is situated in the right shoulder area. Because the electrical path between the R and L electrodes in this position is different than that of the conventional lead, the resultant electrocardiographic pattern is also different (as will be explained in Chapter 8).

The choice of electrode positions is a matter of individual preference. Some clinicians believe that the MCL position may be more useful in identifying certain arrhythmias; others favor the conventional position. However, strict reliance on one method for all patients is ill-advised. The nurse should select the position that provides the clearest and most informative electrocardiogram for each individual patient.

Attachment of Electrode to Skin

Proper attachment of the electrodes to the skin is undoubtedly the one most important step in effective cardiac monitoring. Unless there is excellent contact between the skin and the electrodes, the electrocardiographic wave form will be distorted and artifacts will appear. In addition, the electrodes must be anchored firmly to prevent movement or displacement. The procedure for attaching electrodes is as follows:

1. Prepare the skin areas designated for electrode placement.
   a. If necessary, chest hair should be shaved in 4-inch areas around the intended electrode sites.
   b. The area is cleansed with alcohol to remove skin oils and tissue debris, and then rubbed dry with a towel or gauze sponge. With some electrodes mild abrasion of the skin is recommended in order to lower skin-to-electrode impedance. The abrasion may be performed

---

*More than 50 companies now manufacture disposable, pre-gelled electrodes. It should not be assumed that all electrodes are essentially the same in terms of function; in fact, despite their simple appearance, electrodes differ considerably in design, materials and methods of production. Since the quality of monitoring depends greatly on the effectiveness of the electrodes, it is worthwhile for each CCU to test several different electrodes to determine which provides the best monitoring performance.

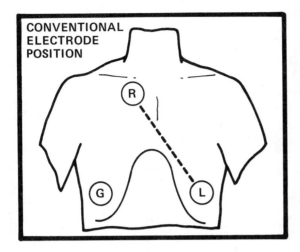 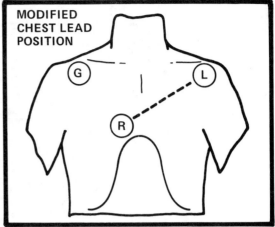

Figure 6.3. The two most common monitoring leads.

with an abrasive pad or, simply, with a gauze sponge.

c. If the chest wall is damp or wet with sweat, the electrode sites should be dried thoroughly so the adhesive pad will adhere to the skin. (If sweating continues and the area cannot be kept dry, an antiperspirant spray can be used and a thin coat of tincture of benzoin applied to the peripheral area.)

2. Prepare the electrodes for use and apply to skin.
    a. When pregelled, disposable electrodes are used, the sealed package is opened just before the electrode is applied. (If the foil package remains open too long, the conductive gel may dry.)
    b. The protective paper covering is peeled from the electrode, exposing the adhesive backing and the gel-covered disc. Avoid contact with the adhesive surface as much as possible.
    c. The electrode is attached by simply pressing the adhesive foam pad firmly to the skin surface. Do not press the gelled portion of the electrode since the gel may be squeezed out and interfere with adhesion.
    d. If the electrodes are not pregelled, conductive jelly is placed in the spacer before application. Excessive amounts of jelly should be avoided because the conductive medium may spread and interfere with the adhesion of the electrode.

3. Change electrodes as necessary.
    a. Pregelled disposable electrodes may remain in place for several days. However, if the electrocardiographic pattern becomes less distinct (due to drying of the electrode gel), if the patient is diaphoretic, or if skin irritation develops, the electrode must be changed and reapplied.

    b. Nondisposable electrodes are generally changed at least once a day. When these electrodes are changed, freshly cleaned electrodes should be used rather than adding more gel to the used electrode.

Connecting the Wires from the Electrodes to the Monitor

The signals detected by the electrodes are transmitted to the monitor through an electrical cable known as the patient cable (in contrast to the monitor cable, which goes to a wall socket for electrical power). The electrodes are connected to the patient cable by means of thin wires, 12-18 inches in length. These connecting wires—called lead wires—snap on or clamp on to the electrodes; the other end of the wire plugs into a receptacle on the patient cable. The receptable has designated openings for the respective electrode wires. Depending on the monitoring equipment being used, one opening is marked either R (right) or RA (right arm). The second opening is designated L (left) or LA (left arm). The third opening is identified as G (ground) or RL (right leg). Figure 6.4 illustrates these openings.

The following steps are involved in connecting the electrodes to the patient cable and then to the monitor:

1. After the electrodes are firmly attached to the skin, the connecting wires are clamped or snapped into place on the electrode. (When snap connectors are used it is advisable to attach the connecting wires to the electrodes before electrode placement: this avoids applying pressure to the positioned electrode, which could squeeze gel onto the adhesive area.)

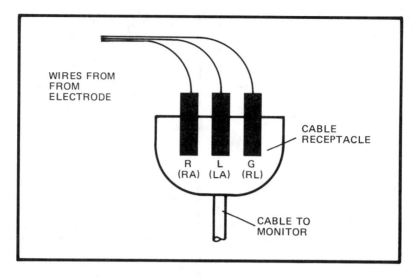

Figure 6.4. Connections for electrode wires.

2. When the contentional electrode position is used for monitoring the wires from the right (R), left (L), and ground (G) electrodes are inserted into the corresponding R, L, and G terminals of the cable receptacle.
3. In contrast, when the modified chest lead position is used, the electrode wire from the right (R) electrode is inserted in the L opening, and the wire from the left (L) electrode into the R opening. In other words, the R and L electrode wires are placed in a reversed position in the receptacle. The ground (G) electrode is placed in the G terminal.
4. After verifying that all connections are secure, position the connecting wires and the patient cable so that there is no tension on the electrode wires. The patient cable receptacle is then pinned to the patient's gown.
5. The monitor end of the patient cable is then inserted into the cable socket of the monitor.

Adjusting the Monitor

If the electrodes have been applied properly and all wires connected securely, the electrocardiographic pattern appearing on the oscilloscopic screen should be clear and distinct. Failure to obtain clear signals is due, in most instances, to faulty technique during the first two steps of the monitoring procedure or to external electrical interference (as described in the following pages).

Even with flawless technique, three monitor adjustments may be necessary: brightening (or darkening) the display, centering the pattern on the screen, and adjusting the height of the wave forms, particularly the waves of ventricular activation (R waves).* The amplitude of the ventricular complexes is of great importance because if these waves are too small the rate meter will not recognize and count them and therefore the heart rate will appear falsely low. In this circumstance the height (gain) control dial is adjusted to increase the amplitude of the wave forms. If the height of the waves cannot be increased sufficiently by adjusting the dial, the electrode positions must be changed to obtain a greater electrical potential. An alternative method of augmenting wave height is to switch the electrode wires in the cable receptacle. For example, by placing the wire from the R electrode in the G terminal and vice versa, a different electrical lead will be recorded, which may produce taller waves.

Setting the Alarm System

As noted previously, the high- and low-rate alarms are integrated with the rate meter and are triggered when the heart rate displayed on the meter falls below or exceeds predetermined levels. The alarm limits should be set according to the patient's prevailing heart rate. If the patient's heart rate is between 60 and 100, it is customary to set the low alarm at 50 per minute and the high alarm at 140 per minute. However, if the heart rate is either very low or very fast, the range for the alarm settings should be narrowed. For instance, if the patient's rate is 50 per minute, the low-rate alarm should be set at 40 and the high-rate alarm at about 80. In this way the observer

---

*The exact methods for making these adjustments may vary with different monitors; therefore it would be impractical to attempt to describe a uniform set of instructions. The manufacturer's manual, provided with the equipment, explains these procedures in detail and should be studied carefully.

would be alerted to even slight rate changes, which may be very significant in this situation.

Because of false alarms (described in the following paragraphs), there may be a temptation to set the alarm limits widely apart (e.g., 40-180) or, worse, to turn off the alarm mechanism entirely. This practice defeats the purpose of the alarm system and should *never* be adopted.

PROBLEMS WITH CARDIAC MONITORING

Many different problems may be encountered during cardiac monitoring; some of these are due to limitations of the monitoring system itself, but the great majority are the result of improper technique. The most common difficulties are discussed here.

False High-Rate Alarms

The alarm system is dependent on the accuracy of the rate meter. In principle, the meter is meant to count the average number of heartbeats (ventricular complexes) per minute; but most meters are not this specific and actually count *all* high deflections on the electrocardiogram, assuming that these are ventricular waves. Unfortunately, contraction of skeletal muscles also produces tall waves (called muscle potentials), which the rate meter is unable to distinguish from ventricular complexes. Consequently, if a patient turns in bed, moves his extremities suddenly, or has a muscle tremor—all of which may produce rapid, tall muscle potentials—the rate meter will misinterpret these spikes as heartbeats and cause a *false* high-rate alarm (Figure 6.5).

Attempts have been made to control this problem by adding electronic filters to "absorb" muscle potentials and by programming rate meters to count only waves of a particular configuration rather than all tall

spikes. Despite these measures, false high-rate alarms are still common occurrences in actual practice.

One simple method for reducing interference from muscle potentials is to place the electrodes in positions that are not directly over large muscle masses (e.g., not over the pectoral or shoulder muscles).

False Low-Rate Alarms

Any disturbance in the transmission of electrical signals between the skin surface and the monitor can produce a false low-rate alarm. This problem is caused most often by ineffective skin-electrode contact resulting from separation of an electrode, profuse sweating, or drying of the conductive jelly. Disconnection of an electrode wire (or the patient cable) is another common source of false low-rate alarms. In all of these situations no electrical activity will be transmitted to the rate meter and oscilloscope, and it might appear at first glance that the heartbeat has stopped (Figure 6.6). The danger of mistaking this technical error for ventricular standstill is obvious and of serious consequence. To prevent this particular problem specific alarms have been incorporated in some monitoring systems to distinguish "lead failure" from lethal arrhythmias.

False low-rate alarms can also occur if the ventricular waves are not tall enough to activate the rate meter. For example, if an arrhythmia develops in which every other ventricular complex is oriented in an opposite direction to the normal beats (R waves) and is of reduced amplitude (Figure 6.7), the rate meter may not be able to detect the smaller complexes. In the electrocardiogram in Figure 6.7, the actual heart rate is 64 per minute; however, if the rate meter detected only the taller upright waves, just 32 beats per minute would be counted. This would create a *false* low-rate alarm. This problem can be corrected by either increasing the amplitude of the complexes or by changing the lead position.

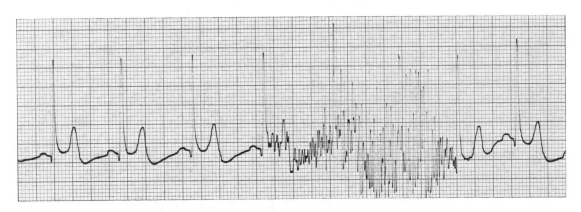

Figure 6.5. False high-rate alarm caused by muscle potentials.

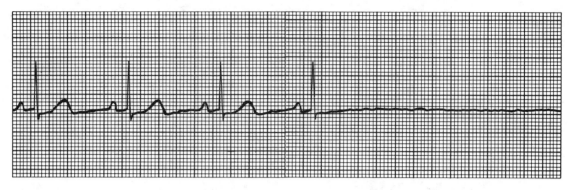

Figure 6.6. False low-rate alarm caused by "lead failure."

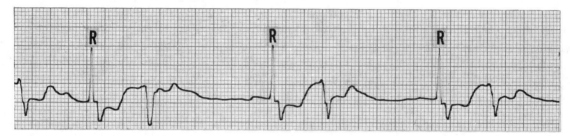

Figure 6.7. False low-rate alarm caused by ventricular waves not tall enough to activate the rate meter.

Electrical Interference

Electrical current from external sources, such as power lines or other electronic equipment, may create interference with the monitor signal. This form of interference appears on the oscilloscopic screen as a series of fine, rapid spikes (60 per second because alternating current has 60 cycles per second) which distort the base line of the electrocardiogram. The effect of electrical interference is shown in Figure 6.8A. Note the difference in clarity of the pattern once the interference from external voltage had been eliminated (Figure 6.8B). Electrical interference may arise from improper grounding of equipment or from loose connections.

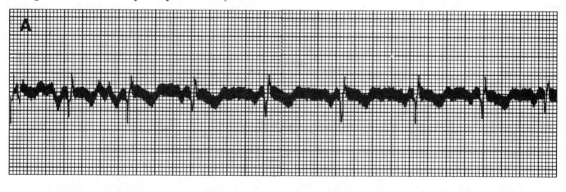

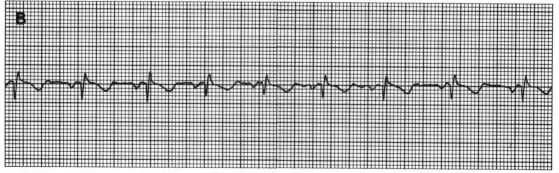

Figure 6.8.(A). Electrical interference from an external source such as a power line. **(B).** Pattern is clear after interference is eliminated.

When electrical interference occurs, the first step is to determine if electrode contact is secure and if all connecting wires are firmly in place. Failure to eliminate interference with these measures suggests improper grounding of other electrical equipment being used. Frequent or persistent electrical interference may indicate a defect in the wiring system in the CCU. (An electrical engineer should be consulted in this circumstance, particularly since the problem may represent an electrical hazard to the patient.)

Wandering Base Line

At times the electrocardiographic pattern displayed on the oscilloscope may wander up and down on the screen (Figure 6.9). This movement, called a wandering base line, makes it difficult to identify arrhythmias, particularly when part of the pattern moves completely off the screen. These excursions are generally produced by motion of the patient (e.g., turning in bed) or simply by respiration. When the problem is caused by body movement, the fluctuation is transient and can be corrected by adjusting the "position" dial to center the electrocardiogram. A wandering base line caused by respiratory motion usually has a cyclic pattern related to inspiration and expiration. In such cases the electrodes should be repositioned away from the lowest ribs to minimize the effect of chest wall movement.

Skin Irritation

Because electrodes must remain attached to the skin for several days, inflammatory reactions at these sites are not uncommon. This skin irritation may develop from the adhesive that secures the electrodes or from the conductive jelly. Disposable electrodes are less likely to produce skin reactions because the adhesive material is usually hypoallergenic and the gel less irritating. If inflammation does develop about the electrode site, the area should be treated with an emollient or anesthetic cream, and the electrode repositioned a few inches away. Regardless of the electrode used it is important to examine the electrode sites at regular intervals to determine if skin irritation is present.

Electrical Hazards

Until recently there were no uniform safety standards for electronic equipment, and therefore with some monitors (particularly older models) patients may be exposed to electrical hazards. The main threat is that leakage current may pass from the monitor to the patient, particularly when more than one piece of equipment is being used. For example, if a temporary transvenous pacemaker has been positioned in the heart, leakage current from the monitor may travel down the pacing catheter to the heart and induce ventricular fibrillation! It is mandatory that all electrical equipment be designed in a way to avoid electrical hazards of this kind. Moreover, the grounding system within the coronary unit must be wholly effective in its purpose. As a safety precaution, electrically powered beds should not be used for patients who are being monitored.

COMPUTERIZED ARRHYTHMIA MONITORING

Many coronary care units now utilize computer systems to detect, analyze, and record arrhythmias. The

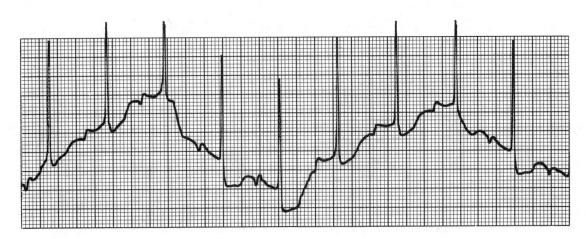

Figure 6.9. Wandering base line.

main advantage of computerized arrhythmia monitoring is its ability to identify *warning* arrhythmias more accurately than conventional cardiac monitoring, thus allowing preventive treatment to be started as soon as possible. Several studies have shown that even under the best of circumstances a high percentage of serious ventricular warning arrhythmias go unnoticed in coronary care units. This inaccuracy is not surprising since the detection of warning arrhythmias with customary cardiac monitoring depends for the most part on nurse surveillance of the electrocardiographic patterns of several patients on multiple screens; also, most of these arrhythmias are transient in character and do not trigger high- or low-rate alarms. Because nurses have scores of other responsibilities in the CCU and cannot (and should not) spend their time observing monitors constantly, many significant arrhythmic events are never recognized, particularly those that last for only a few beats. Even if cardiac monitoring is accomplished by having a nurse or specially trained technician sit in front of a bank of monitors (as is the case in some CCUs) the error rate may still be substantial because of human fatigue and monotony. In addition to this fundamental flaw in warning arrhythmias, conventional electrocardiographic monitoring represents a time-consuming, arduous, and repetitive nursing task, especially in large CCUs, and in this sense

detracts from direct patient care. In principle, computerized arrhythmia monitoring can alleviate both of these problems to the benefit of the patient and the nurse.

The basic procedure for computerized monitoring is essentially the same as for customary cardiac monitoring. The electrocardiographic signals picked up by the skin electrodes are displayed on monitor screens, and relayed to the computer system. The computer analyzes each beat as it occurs and classifies it as normal or a particular arrhythmic disorder. The computer program is designed to identify and tabulate several different types and classes of arrhythmias, and depicts these findings (along with the heart rate) on a separate screen in the form of an ongoing status report for each patient (Figure 6.10). The computer system stores this information and presents it graphically as an hourly trend (Figure 6.11 A & B).

The most significant feature of a computerized monitoring system is its alarm mechanism. Unlike ordinary cardiac monitors which trigger alarms only on the basis of high or low heart rates, computerized arrhythmia monitors are programmed to deliver visual and audible alarms for many other disturbances as well, especially warning arrhythmias. Alarm limits are set individually for each type of arrhythmia. If any of these limits are surpassed the respective alarm is activated and a rhythm strip documenting the event is

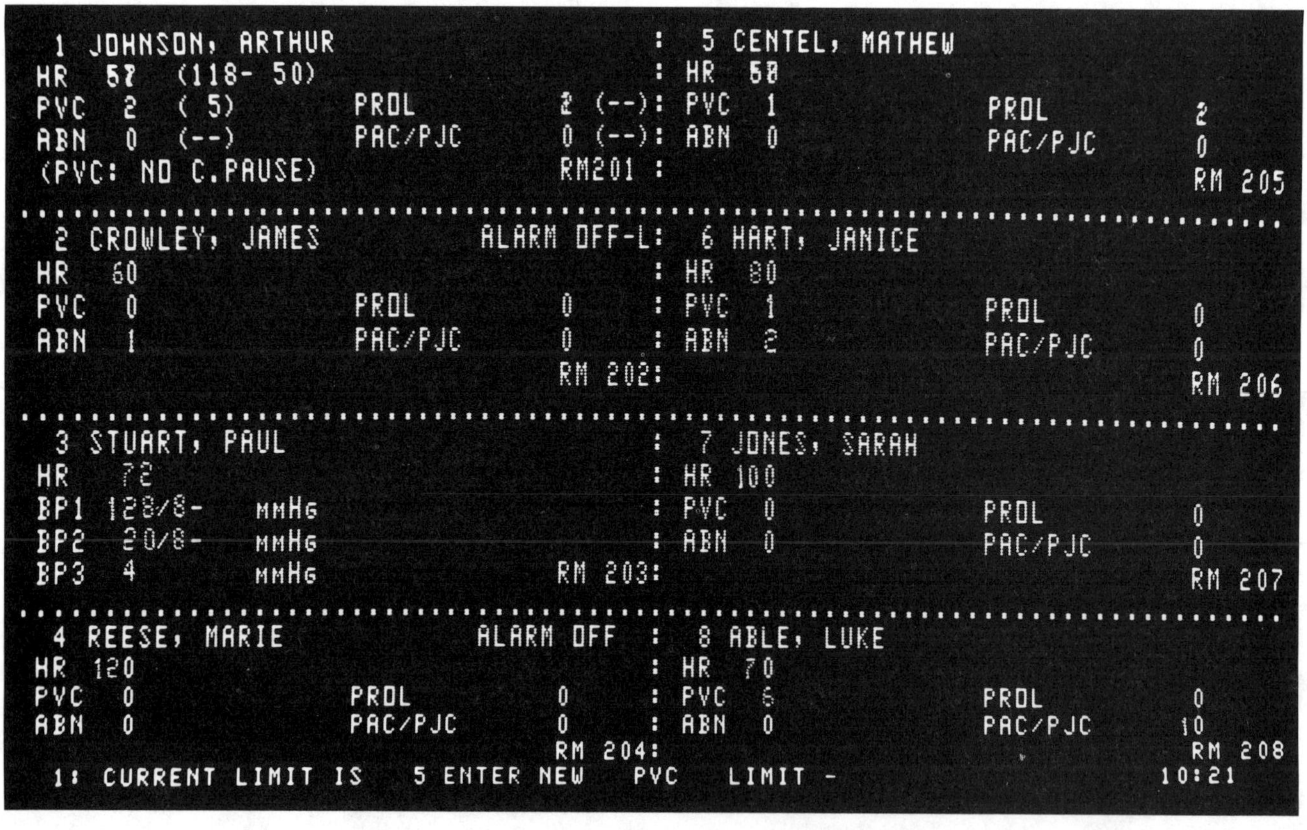

Figure 6.10. Computerized monitoring: status report.

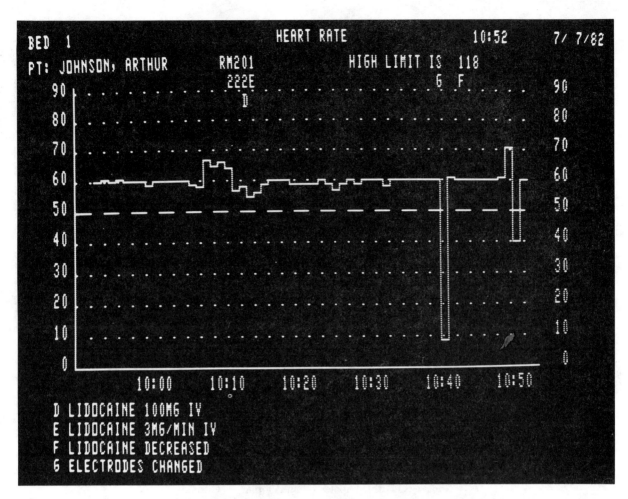

Figure 6.11 A. Computerized monitoring: heart rate trend.

produced. Printed across the top border of the electro-cardiographic strip is the patient's name, room number, time of the event, and the reason for the alarm (Figure 6.12). This added information simplifies and expedites the charting of arrhythmic events.

Despite the apparent advantages of computerized monitoring, most coronary care units continue to use standard cardiac monitoring equipment. There are several reasons for this decision. First, computerized monitoring systems are far more expensive than customary monitors and are usually designed to monitor 8 (or more) patients. Thus for smaller coronary units, automated monitoring is often a luxury. Second, conventional monitors are just as effective as computerized monitors in detecting *lethal* arrhythmias (e.g., ventricular fibrillation) or, for that matter, any other fast or slow rate arrhythmias that trigger the alarm system. Third, computerized monitors are not totally accurate or foolproof. Much of this latter problem stems from the fact that computers analyze arrhythmias on the basis of rigid mathematical criteria; therefore even slight variations in the configuration or timing of the ventricular (QRS) complexes, (which are of no clinical significance), may be misinterpreted as an arrhythmia. Accordingly, *false alarms* are relatively common with most computerized arrhythmia detection systems. Also, computer programs often experience difficulty in analyzing complicated arrhythmias, particularly if the shape of the waves varies greatly.

Nevertheless, computerized monitoring holds great promise, and it seems that as technology improves and costs are controlled this form of continuous surveillance will play an increasingly important role in coronary care units.

TELEMETRIC MONITORING

The heart's electrical activity can be recorded without direct wiring from the patient to the monitor. This method, called *telemetric* monitoring, can be utilized with conventional or computerized monitoring systems. It works as follows: the electrode wires are connected to a small battery-operated radio

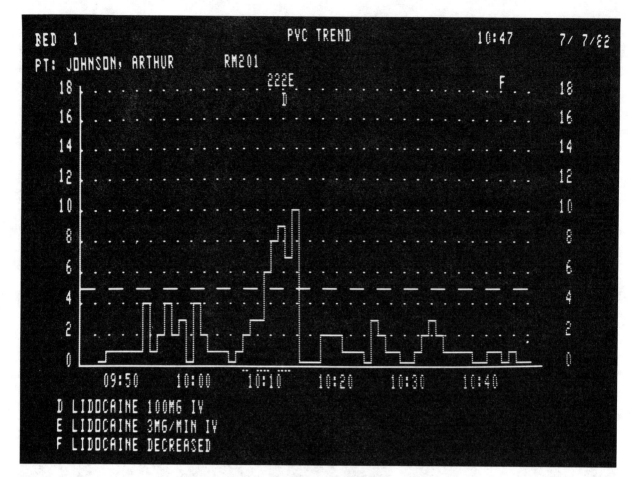

Figure 6.11 B. Computerized monitoring: PVC trend.

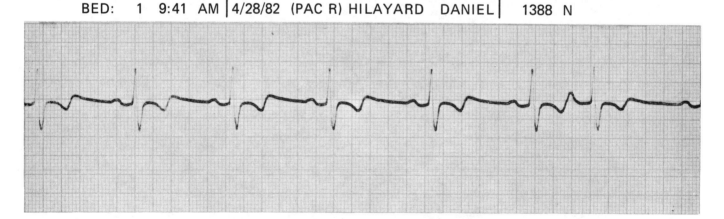

Figure 6.12. Rhythm strip produced by computerized monitoring system.

(FM) transmitter, about the size of a cigarette package, which is pinned on the patient's gown or worn about the neck. The transmitter sends the electrical signals to a receiver by means of a radio beam. The receiver then feeds the signals into the monitoring system. Telemetry has several advantages: the patient is not restricted by wires and can sit in a chair or use the bathroom without the risk of disconnecting the monitoring system. More important is that mon-

itoring can be accomplished even though the patient is no longer in the CCU; in fact, he can be on a different floor in the hospital, hundreds of feet away from the monitor. Many institutions use telemetric monitoring after patients have been transferred from the CCU, particularly among those who experienced serious arrhythmias during the acute phase and may be at high risk of developing recurrent problems. In this sense telemetry may be a suitable alternative to intermediate (step-down) coronary care units. The main disadvantage of telemetric monitoring is that the quality of the electrocardiographic signals is usually not as good as with direct wiring. Radio transmission is frequently distorted by steel beams, elevator shafts, and other structures within the hospital.

Electrocardiograms can also be transmitted by telephone so that monitoring can be accomplished from hundreds of miles away if necessary. The telephone number of the receiving station in the CCU (or emergency department) is dialed and a special transmitter sends the signals through the telephone line to the monitor. Rescue squads sometimes use telephonic monitoring when assistance or advice is needed from hospital personnel.

7

The Major Complications of Acute Myocardial Infarction and the Related Nursing Role

There are five death-producing complications of acute myocardial infarction: heart failure, cardiogenic shock, thromboembolism, ventricular rupture and, above all, arrhythmias.

The objective of intensive coronary care, as explained in previous chapters, is to prevent or successfully treat these complications; it is only in this way that lives can be saved. To achieve this goal it is essential to understand the mechanisms, clinical manifestations and methods of treatment of each complication, particularly in relationship to the nursing role.

HEART FAILURE

Acute myocardial infarction affects the pumping action of the heart in nearly all instances; however the degree of impairment varies greatly. The critical issue is whether the infarction produces *heart failure*. Heart failure, by definition, implies that the injured myocardium is unable to pump an adequate amount of blood to meet the metabolic demands of the body. Approximately 60% of patients with acute myocardial infarction develop clinical signs of heart failure during the acute phase of the illness. The greater the degree of heart failure, the higher the in-hospital mortality and the poorer the long-term prog-

nosis. In fact, with the present ability to prevent arrhythmic deaths, advanced heart failure and cardiogenic shock (collectively called power failure) have become the leading cause of death among patients treated in coronary units.

Left Heart Failure

The heart consists of two separate but closely related pumping systems: the *right* heart, the pump for the pulmonary circulation, and the *left* heart, the pump for the systemic circulation. The relationship of these two systems is shown in Figure 7.1.

Heart failure may involve the left heart, the right heart or both sides of the heart, depending primarily on the underlying type of heart disease. In patients with acute myocardial infarction, *left ventricular failure* is by far the most common form since it is the left ventricle that is injured in practically all cases. When right ventricular failure develops in this circumstance it is most often secondary to left ventricular failure. However, right ventricular failure can develop independently in patients with right ventricular infarction, but usually heart failure in this circumstance is mild and seldom of critical importance.

The primary cause of left heart failure after acute myocardial infarction is damage to the muscles of the left ventricle. The infarcted area and the surrounding

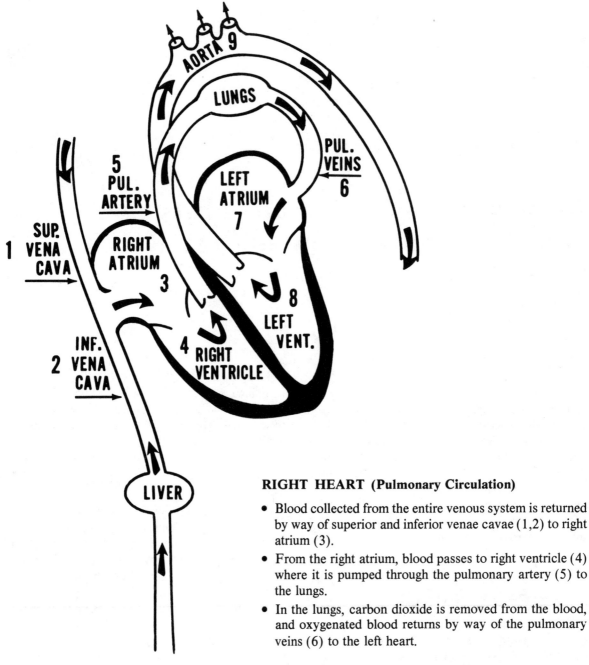

RIGHT HEART (Pulmonary Circulation)

- Blood collected from the entire venous system is returned by way of superior and inferior venae cavae (1,2) to right atrium (3).
- From the right atrium, blood passes to right ventricle (4) where it is pumped through the pulmonary artery (5) to the lungs.
- In the lungs, carbon dioxide is removed from the blood, and oxygenated blood returns by way of the pulmonary veins (6) to the left heart.

LEFT HEART (Systemic Circulation)

- Oxygenated blood from the pulmonary veins enters the left atrium (7) and passes to the left ventricle (8).
- Contraction of the left ventricle propels the blood through the aorta (9) into the systemic circulation.

Figure 7.1. Circulation through the left and right heart—schematic diagram.

zones of injury and ischemia do not contract normally; as a result the pumping ability of the left ventricle is reduced. This reduction in pumping performance is manifested by a decrease in the stroke volume and the cardiac output. *Stroke volume* is the volume of blood ejected from the ventricle with each contraction. *Cardiac output* represents the total volume of blood pumped from the ventricle per minute. The relation between stroke volume and cardiac output is expressed as follows:

Cardiac output = stroke volume × heart rate*

The decrease in cardiac output can be mild, moderate or severe, depending fundamentally on the size of the infarction. A marked fall in cardiac output, as usually occurs with power failure, is an ominous sign and is associated with a very high mortality.

Because of the reduction in pumping performance the left ventricle is no longer able to eject (empty) the volume of blood it receives from the pulmonary circulation (right heart). Consequently an excess amount of blood remains in the left ventricle after each contraction (systole). This residual volume gradually increases since the uninjured right ventricle continues to pump its normal quota of blood into the pulmonary circulation but the incompletely emptied left ventricle cannot readily accept the volume delivered to it. Therefore the pressure rises in the left ventricle during diastole (the interval between contractions in which the ventricles fill with blood). This elevation in *ventricular diastolic pressure* impedes the subsequent flow of blood from the pulmonary circulation into the left heart, causing the pressure to increase in the left atrium and, in turn, in the pulmonary veins and pulmonary capillaries. In effect, a backward pressure develops throughout the pulmonary venous system. The engorged (congested) veins and capillaries impose on the available air space within the lungs and also reduce the lungs' distensibility. More significantly, the increased pulmonary venous pressure forces fluid through the walls of the pulmonary capillaries into the lung tissues. This exudation of fluid into the lungs produces the clinical state known as *left ventricular failure.*

At first, the fluid collects in the interstitial tissues which surround the air cells (alveoli) of the lungs; it is called *interstitial edema.* This early manifestation of left ventricular failure does not produce specific symptoms nor can it be detected by physical examination of the chest. (Therefore the condition is also designated incipient or *subclinical* left ventricular failure.) The presence of interstitial edema can,

however, be identified by chest x-ray, as shown in Figure 7.2. (This is one of the reasons that x-ray examination of the chest is a standard procedure in most CCUs.) As left ventricular failure progresses, edema fluid is then forced into the alveoli themselves; this collection of fluid within the air space is called *alveolar edema.* Unlike interstitial edema, alveolar edema produces distinct signs and symptoms and therefore is described as *overt left ventricular failure.* The chain of events leading to overt left ventricular failure is summarized in Figure 7.3.

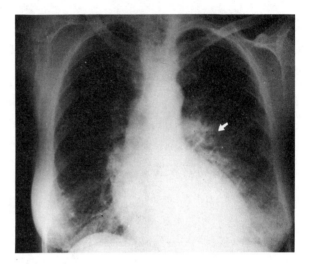

Figure 7.2. Xray film of chest demonstrating interstitial edema (arrow).

Before describing the clinical manifestations of left ventricular failure, it is important to point out that the cardiovascular system utilizes several compensatory mechanisms in an attempt to maintain an effective circulation and avert heart failure. One of the main compensatory mechanisms is an increase in sympathetic nervous system activity that occurs (through reflex means) as soon as cardiac output begins to fall. As a result of this sympathetic stimulation, the heart beats faster and the strength of myocardial contractions increases; both of these actions help to preserve an adequate cardiac output, at least temporarily. For example, if the stroke volume falls after acute myocardial infarction to 40 cc, but the heart rate increases to, say, 120/minute, cardiac output is maintained at a satisfactory level of 4800 cc (40 × 120) despite the reduction in ventricular pumping ability. Thus a rapid heart rate and several other characteristic signs of left ventricular failure (as described below) are actually compensatory mechanisms meant to limit the progression of heart failure. In addition to the indirect effects of the sympathetic nervous system, the heart itself attempts to compensate for its diminished pumping performance. This is accomplished as follows: when the residual volume and pressure in the left ventricle increase during

---

*If, for example, the stroke volume is 60 cc and the heart rate is 70/minute, the cardiac output is 4200 cc. Normally, the cardiac output at rest is about 4000-6000 cc. The normal stroke volume is 70-80 cc.

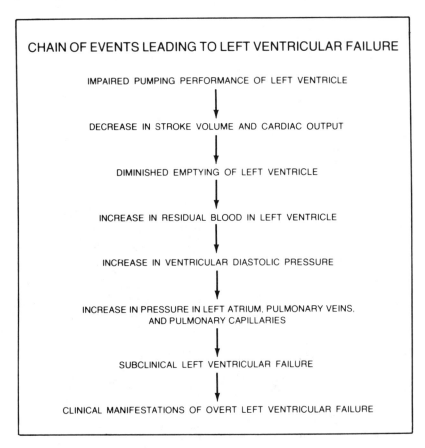

CHAIN OF EVENTS LEADING TO LEFT VENTRICULAR FAILURE

IMPAIRED PUMPING PERFORMANCE OF LEFT VENTRICLE

DECREASE IN STROKE VOLUME AND CARDIAC OUTPUT

DIMINISHED EMPTYING OF LEFT VENTRICLE

INCREASE IN RESIDUAL BLOOD IN LEFT VENTRICLE

INCREASE IN VENTRICULAR DIASTOLIC PRESSURE

INCREASE IN PRESSURE IN LEFT ATRIUM, PULMONARY VEINS, AND PULMONARY CAPILLARIES

SUBCLINICAL LEFT VENTRICULAR FAILURE

CLINICAL MANIFESTATIONS OF OVERT LEFT VENTRICULAR FAILURE

Figure 7.3.

diastole, the ventricle dilates and its muscle fibers stretch (lengthen). This stretching has a beneficial effect because the strength of ventricular contraction depends on the length of the myocardial fibers just before they contract (in much the same way as a rubber band contracts more forcefully when it is stretched fully). These (and other) compensatory mechanisms are effective up to a certain point, but finally they can no longer counteract the failing heart and, in fact, become self-defeating. At this stage, called *decompensation,* signs and symptoms of overt failure develop.

Clinical Manifestations of Left Ventricular Failure

Symptoms

Dyspnea. Shortness of breath (dyspnea) is the earliest and most common symptom of left ventricular failure. It results primarily from congestion of the pulmonary venous network which reduces the elasticity (distensibility) of the lungs and diminishes the available air space. The problem is intensified when alveolar edema develops because the edema fluid interferes with the exchange of oxygen and carbon

dioxide in the alveoli, causing a reduction in the oxygen saturation of the blood. At first, dyspnea occurs only on exertion and therefore may not be apparent except during physical activity (e.g., when the patient gets out of bed or washes himself). As heart failure worsens, dyspnea occurs even at complete rest. Mild dyspnea may be difficult for the observer to detect (since it is a subjective symptom), and for this reason the nurse should ask the patient specifically if he feels short of breath, particularly during activity.

Orthopnea. If dyspnea is present when the patient is in the recumbent position and is relieved by sitting up, the condition is called *orthopnea.* This more advanced form of dyspnea can be suspected when the patient requests extra pillows or asks that the head of his bed be raised. With severe orthopnea the patient may prefer to be propped straight up in bed or to sit in a chair. These positions relieve orthopnea by diminishing pulmonary congestion and improving the ventilatory capacity of the lungs.

Paroxysmal Nocturnal Dyspnea. For reasons that are not wholly clear, marked shortness of breath sometimes develops abruptly while the patient is asleep; hence the condition is called *paroxysmal* *nocturnal dyspnea.* These episodes of sudden dyspnea represent decompensation of the left ventricle following an acute increase in pulmonary venous congestion. The usual clinical story of paroxysmal nocturnal dyspnea is that about an hour or two after falling asleep the patient awakens *suddenly* with marked dyspnea and respiratory distress. He complains of suffocation, and great anxiety is usually evident. Paroxysms of coughing associated with loud wheezing accompany the dyspnea. (Because of the wheezing character of respiration, which resembles an asthmatic attack, the term cardiac asthma is sometimes used to describe the episode.) Breathing is improved in the sitting position, and most patients assume this posture immediately or attempt to leave the bed and reach a nearby window, believing that fresh air will help their breathing. The attack may subside after a few minutes in a sitting position or the episode may worsen progressively, with dyspnea, coughing, and wheezing becoming more intense. Although paroxysmal nocturnal dyspnea develops with dramatic suddenness in most instances, it is quite likely that subclinical left ventricular failure existed previously and progressed insidiously.

Acute Pulmonary Edema. The most advanced stage of acute left heart failure is *pulmonary edema.* This condition develops because of a massive accumulation of fluid throughout the alveolar and interstitial tissues of the lungs. The fluid interferes with oxygenation of the blood and results in *hypoxia* (a decrease in the oxygen content of the blood). Unless hypoxia is corrected, the vital organs become deprived of oxygen, irreversible arrhythmias develop, and death occurs.

The clinical picture of acute pulmonary edema is distinctive and seldom poses a problem in diagnosis. The characteristic features are severe dyspnea, orthopnea, incessant cough (producing frothy, blood-tinged sputum), and extreme anxiety. Cyanosis may be present, and gurgling sounds are audible from the respiratory tree. In conjunction with these obvious signs of respiratory difficulty, a rapid pulse rate and profuse sweating are noted. (The latter findings, as noted, are due to a marked increase in sympathetic nervous system activity.) The total picture leaves no doubt that the patient is in acute distress and that emergency treatment is essential.

Physical Signs

Rales. The cardinal physical sign of overt left ventricular failure is the presence of rales. These abnormal breath sounds are produced by fluid in the alveoli and can be detected by auscultation of the chest. At first, rales are usually confined to the bases of the lungs (basilar rales), but as left ventricular failure progresses the rales extend higher and higher in the lung fields. Thus the height of rales in the lungs provides a general index of the extent of heart failure. With acute pulmonary edema coarse, bubbling rales may be heard throughout the *entire* chest.

Gallop Rhythm. The second classic sign of left ventricular failure is a gallop rhythm which is identified by stethoscopic examination of the heart. Normally the heart has two distinct sounds described simply as the first and second heart sounds (or as S_1 and S_2). When the left heart fails and the ventricle dilates (in order to accommodate the increased diastolic volume) a third heart sound usually appears. Because the cadence of the three sounds resembles the sound of a galloping horse, the rhythm is descriptively termed a *gallop rhythm.* This extra heart sound (called S_3) occurs just after the second heart sound, as illustrated in Figure 7.4. It is heard best with the bell of the stethoscope placed over the apex of the heart. The presence of this type of gallop rhythm (known as a ventricular gallop) indicates dilation of the left ventricle and is a distinct sign of left ventricular failure even if rales cannot be heard.

There is a second type of gallop rhythm known as an atrial gallop. It differs from a ventricular gallop in that the extra heart sound is heard just before the first heart sound instead of after the second sound. In this circumstance the extra sound is called a fourth heart sound (S_4) to distinguish it from the S_3 of a ventricular gallop. An atrial gallop (also described as an S_4 gallop) is a less serious finding than a ventricular gallop (an S_3 gallop) and may sometimes occur even in the absence of left ventricular failure. It is believed that an atrial gallop is caused by resistance to ventricular filling during diastole.

Nonspecific Signs. Although rales and a ventricular gallop rhythm are the only two definite diagnostic signs of left ventricular failure, other physical findings usually develop when the heart fails. For example, tachycardia, sweating, a reduction in blood pressure, and restlessness are often observed during acute left ventricular failure. The latter signs are not specific indications of left ventricular failure, but they are usually part of the overall clinical picture. Moreover, these nonspecific findings may be the earliest manifestation of left ventricular failure and therefore are important diagnostic clues.

Treatment of Left Ventricular Failure

The underlying objective of the treatment program for left ventricular failure is to increase cardiac output. This can be accomplished (up to a certain

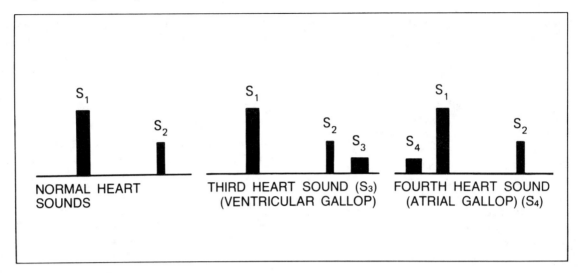

Figure 7.4. Normal heart sounds and components of a gallop rhythm.

stage, at least) by correcting or adjusting the four principal mechanisms that normally govern left ventricular performance (Figure 7.5). To this end, the following methods may be used singly or in combination:

1. Preload Volume Reduction

Since the injured left ventricle is unable to adequately empty (eject) the volume of blood it receives, a logical step in treatment (in fact, usually one of the first steps) is to reduce venous return to the heart. This method, called *preload volume reduction,* results in a decrease in the filling volume of the left ventricle and, in turn, a lowering of pulmonary venous pressure. These desirable hemodynamic effects serve to increase stroke volume (and cardiac output) and relieve pulmonary venous congestion.

The simplest means for reducing preload is *diuretic therapy.* By promoting fluid loss, diuretics diminish the circulating blood volume and thus, reduce venous

return to the heart. (The use of diuretic therapy is discussed in the next section on right heart failure.) In addition to diuretics, a second class of drugs, categorized as *vasodilating agents* or vasodilators, may also be used to lower preload volume, particularly when left ventricular failure is severe or not sufficiently responsive to diuretics alone. Vasodilating agents act by relaxing the tone and resistance of peripheral blood vessels, causing the vessels to dilate. Some vasodilators are designed to dilate the arterial system while others act predominately on the venous system; several of these agents exert a combined action (Table 7.1).

Preload reduction can be achieved by the use of vasodilators that act on the venous system. Nitroglycerin (administered sublingually, intravenously, or topically) and long acting nitrates (isosorbide dinitrate), the most commonly used agents for this purpose, expand the venous bed and allow large quantities of blood to pool in the peripheral veins. As a result of this venous pooling, the amount of blood returning directly to the heart is decreased substantially, thus reducing preload volume.

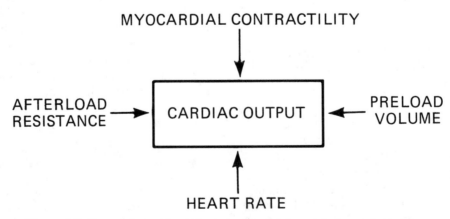

Figure 7.5. Four major mechanisms that regulate left ventricular performance.

Table 7.1. Vasodilators Used in the Treatment of Heart Failure

Agent	Main Sites of Action	Route of Administration	Usual Dose
Nitroglycerin	Venous	Sublingual (also: IV, ointment and transdermal)	0.4 mg
Isosorbide dinitrate	Venous	Sublingual Oral	2.5-10 mg 20-40 mg, q 6 hr
Hydralazine (Apresoline)	Arterial	Oral	50-100 mg, q 6 hr
Minoxidil (Loniten)	Arterial	Oral	10-40 mg daily
Phentolamine (Regitine)	Arterial	Intravenous	0.1-2 mg/minute
Sodium nitroprusside (Nipride)	Arterial and venous	Intravenous	25-200 μg/minute
Prazosin	Arterial and venous	Oral	5 mg, q 6 hr
Captopril (Capoten)	Arterial and venous	Oral	50-150 mg, q 8 hr

2. Afterload Reduction

In addition to preload reduction, another important method used in the treatment of (advanced) heart failure is to reduce ventricular *afterload.* Simply stated, afterload refers to the resistance against which the heart must pump to eject blood. This resistance (impedance), although dependent on other factors as well, can be loosely equated with the arterial blood pressure. In general, the higher the arterial blood pressure, the lower the volume of blood ejected by the ventricle (stroke volume). In other words, the stroke volume and cardiac output decrease when the injured heart meets increased resistance from the systemic arterial system. Furthermore, in working harder to overcome this resistance, the heart requires more energy and consumes more oxygen, which lead to a further decrease in cardiac output. Therefore it is highly desirable to reduce systemic vascular resistance (afterload) as a means of improving cardiac performance. Afterload reduction is accomplished primarily with arterial vasodilators (see Figure 7.6). However, agents with combined arterial and venous vasodilator action (e.g., prazosin or nitroprusside) are often used for this purpose since they permit concomitant reduction of afterload and preload. While this new concept of afterload reduction represents a major advance in therapy, its application may pose problems. For example, excessive lowering of the blood pressure (to hypotensive levels) with vasodilators—a not uncommon event—can compromise coronary artery blood flow and cause sudden deterioration of cardiac performance.

3. Strengthening Myocardial Contractility

Aside from unburdening the injured heart by means of preload and afterload reduction, the treatment program for heart failure also includes the use of digitalis (or other drugs) to increase the strength of myocardial contraction. The object of strengthening myocardial contractility is to improve ventricular emptying so that the residual volume of blood in the ventricle decreases, while the stroke volume and cardiac output increase. Although digitalis is usually very effective in treating overt heart failure, and has remained the standard drug for this purpose for years, its use in the earliest stages of acute myocardial infarction is still controversial. Some believe that the drug may provoke ventricular arrhythmias in this situation, and that it also increases the work (energy expenditure) of the heart; others feel that the benefits of digitalis therapy outweigh these potential risks.

4. Controlling Heart Rate

Cardiac output, as noted earlier, is a function of heart rate (cardiac output = stroke volume $\times$ heart rate). As a general rule, in patients with acute myocardial infarction, heart rates that are either too fast or too slow cause a reduction in cardiac output and may lead to or worsen heart failure. With fast rates (for example about 140/minute), the period of ventricular filling is shortened and therefore stroke volume falls. With slow rates (below 50/minute), cardiac output decreases because the stroke volume cannot increase sufficiently to counteract the slow rate. All of this means that, in principle, part of the treatment program should be directed at establishing an effective heart rate with drug therapy or cardiac pacing (as explained in subsequent chapters) to preserve cardiac output. Of the four determinants of left ventricular performance, rate control is the most difficult to achieve and maintain practically. For this reason, attempts to correct preload, afterload and myocardial contractility usually comprise the bulk of the treatment program.

Treatment of Acute Pulmonary Edema

The methods and sequence of treatment depend primarily on the severity of left ventricular failure and the urgency of the clinical situation. For example, with mild heart failure only diuretic therapy may be required; but with acute pulmonary edema, the most serious form of left ventricular failure, a combination of several methods of treatment is utilized. These methods are described below:

Morphine

Administration of this narcotic should be one of the first steps in the treatment program for acute pulmonary edema. Morphine has several beneficial effects in this circumstance: not only does it relieve the intense anxiety associated with pulmonary edema but, more significantly, it decreases the volume of blood returning to the heart by reducing venous tone, which causes pooling of blood in peripheral veins (vasodilator effect). At the same time, morphine depresses the respiratory center in the brain and thereby reduces the number of respirations; as a result of this respiratory slowing blood returning to the left ventricle from the pulmonary circulation is also decreased. Morphine sulfate is usually administered intravenously in pulmonary edema in doses of 4-10 mg.

Oxygen Therapy

During the period of respiratory embarrassment, the concentration (saturation) of oxygen in arterial blood is usually markedly reduced. Therefore it is essential to administer oxygen in order to preserve tissue function. The highest oxygen concentration is provided by the use of an intermittent positive-pressure apparatus which delivers 100% oxygen through a well-fitted face mask (with a nonrebreathing bag). Nasal catheters or cannulas deliver only 30-40% oxygen concentrations and therefore are the least desirable means of supplying oxygen in this

critical situation. Oxygen should always be humidified prior to inhalation to prevent drying of the airway. Humidification can be accomplished by bubbling oxygen through water. A 30% solution of ethyl alcohol may be used instead of water; it has the added advantage of reducing pulmonary secretions by its antifoaming action.

Diuretics

Rapid-acting diuretics, such as furosemide (Lasix) or ethacrynic acid (Edecrin), administered intravenously, usually produce dramatic clinical improvement; dyspnea abates within minutes, after which there is a copious diuresis. Theoretically these agents are effective because they promote excretion of fluid, thereby reducing the volume of blood returning to the heart. However, the extraordinary rapidity with which these drugs act in controlling pulmonary edema (even before diuresis occurs) suggests that other pharmacologic actions are also involved. It is believed that these agents have a direct effect on the venous system, causing the veins to dilate and hold a greater volume of blood. Furosemide (Lasix) is administered intravenously in doses of 40-80 mg. The usual intravenous dose of ethacrynic acid (Edecrin) is 50 mg. (Diuretic therapy is described in greater detail in the discussion of right heart failure.)

Vasodilators

Severe dyspnea, resulting from acute pulmonary edema can often be relieved promptly by the administration of 0.4-0.8 mg nitroglycerin sublingually. Nitroglycerin, as already explained, acts as a venous dilator and reduces preload volume substantially. Left ventricular filling pressure begins to fall within 2-3 minutes after nitroglycerin is given, and this beneficial effect lasts for 15 to 30 minutes. Isosorbide dinitrate (Isordil or Sorbitrate, for example), administered either sublingually or orally, produces the same effect, but the onset of action is somewhat slower (about 5 minutes) while the duration of action is much longer (2-4 hours). The proven effectiveness of both short- and long-term nitrate therapy has placed these drugs high on the list of methods used to treat acute pulmonary edema. After their initial action in decreasing ventricular filling pressure, nitrate administration is continued, at least during the period of hospitalization. The main limitations of nitrate therapy are the frequent occurrence of headaches (vasodilator effect) and excessive lowering of the blood pressure (postural hypotension). Consequently, titration of the dosage is essential to the successful management of heart failure. Vasodilators that act on both the arterial and venous networks, such as nitroprusside or prazosin, are usually reserved for patients with high arterial blood pressures or those who do not respond to preload reduction alone.

Digitalis

After years of acceptance as the cornerstone of the treatment program for left ventricular failure, digitalis has now been relegated a lesser role than before in the management of heart failure associated with acute myocardial infarction.* The demonstrated effectiveness of nitrates (as just discussed) in conjunction with diuretic therapy has diminished the emphasis on digitalis and the value of increasing myocardial contractility after myocardial infarction. This is not to say that digitalis has been abandoned (or should not be used) in this circumstance, but it implies that less difficult agents, particularly nitrates and diuretics, can control acute pulmonary edema on their own, and therefore should be used first. Current opinion— which remains divided—suggests that digitalis should not be administered routinely in acute pulmonary edema unless other methods are ineffective or unless the heart failure is accompanied by a rapid rate arrhythmia (e.g., atrial fibrillation). The use of digitalis, if necessary, after the first four days of acute myocardial infarction however, is uncontroversial. Digitalis is generally administered intravenously in the form of digoxin 0.25-0.5 mg, initially. The total dosage should not exceed 1.5 mg daily in patients with acute myocardial infarction, and lesser amounts may be adequate.

Bronchodilators

Acute pulmonary edema is accompanied by spasm of the bronchial tree. This bronchospasm (which creates the loud wheezing sounds heard during the acute attack) interferes with ventilation. In an effort to relieve bronchospasm, bronchodilator drugs are frequently used (in conjunction with oxygen therapy). The most popular drug for this purpose is aminophylline, which is administered intravenously in a dosage of 250-500 mg. The drug is diluted to 50 cc and injected slowly, over a 15-minute period. The dose may be repeated every 3-4 hours if needed. In addition to dilating the bronchioles, aminophylline also increases cardiac output and lowers venous pressure. The main disadvantage of the drug is that it may cause hypotension and arrhythmias, particularly

---

*The controversy about the use of digitalis in treating left ventricular failure only concerns acute myocardial infarction. With other causes of heart failure (e.g., valvular heart disease), digitalis remains a key therapy.

if it is injected too rapidly. To avoid these undesirable effects, aminophylline is often administered by rectal suppository (500 mg).

Rotating Tourniquets

In the unlikely event that the measures just described are not successful in promptly controlling acute pulmonary edema, rotating tourniquets may be employed. The application of tourniquets traps venous blood in the extremities and thereby reduces venous return to the heart. The tourniquets are applied to the extremities with a pressure sufficient to impede venous return but not great enough to interfere with arterial blood flow to the limbs (i.e., the distal pulses must always remain palpable). The pressure is released in one extremity every 15 minutes in a rotating fashion (to prevent tissue damage). When the acute episode has subsided, the tourniquets are removed, one at a time, at intervals of 15 minutes. Releasing all the tourniquets simultaneously may cause a sudden increase in venous return and again overload the pulmonary circulation.

Phlebotomy

The circulating blood volume can also be reduced by means of phlebotomy, during which 500 cc of blood is withdrawn into a vacuum-type bottle. This method is used only when all other means of treatment have failed, and is seldom required, especially since the emergence of vasodilator therapy which is the equivalent of a "medical" phlebotomy.

Other Measures

The actual methods of treatment of acute pulmonary edema vary with the clinical response. However, on some occasions the precise benefit (and risks) of a particular means of treatment cannot be determined without continuous *hemodynamic monitoring* (as explained in the section on cardiogenic shock).

Right Heart Failure

In acute myocardial infarction the right heart fails as a sequel to left heart failure; isolated right heart failure, as mentioned previously, is rare, except with right ventricular infarction. The sequence of events leading to right heart failure is outlined in Figure 7.6. When the left heart fails, significant backward pressure develops in the pulmonary veins and capillaries, as already noted. Therefore blood being pumped from the right ventricle through the pulmonary arteries

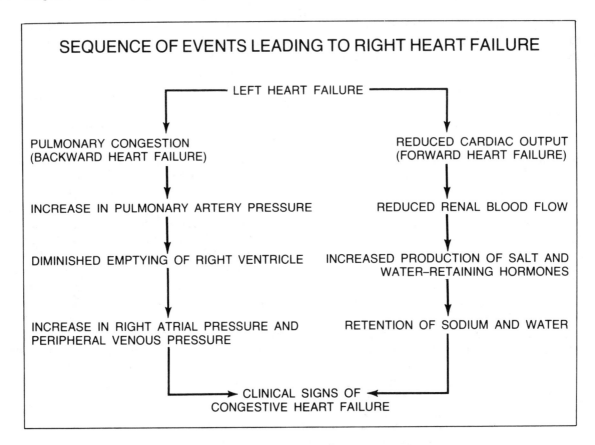

Figure 7.6.

meets resistance in the pulmonary capillaries, causing the pressure to rise in the main pulmonary artery. As the pulmonary artery pressure mounts, emptying of the right ventricle is impaired. The residual volume of blood within the right ventricle impedes the flow of blood from the right atrium. As a consequence, blood returning to the right atrium from the superior and inferior vena cavae meets resistance. This creates a backward pressure throughout the entire peripheral venous system, leading to congestion of the venous network. The clinical picture that results from this overloading of the venous system is called *congestive heart failure.*

Although this etiologic concept, described as *backward* heart failure, is logical and explains many of the clinical findings of right heart failure, it is certain that the problem of the failing heart is infinitely more complicated. For instance, it is well known that congestive heart failure is accompanied by the retention of sodium and water, and that kidney function is also disturbed. The latter changes cannot be explained fully on the basis of increased backward pressure, and it is apparent that renal and hormonal factors also contribute to the total picture of right heart failure. It is believed that the reduction in cardiac output that accompanies left heart failure results in a decrease in renal blood flow; this insufficiency of renal flow stimulates the production of

salt- and water-retaining hormones (e.g., aldosterone). This theory, called *forward* heart failure, implies that part of the problem of congestive failure develops independently of backward pressure. It is very likely that backward and forward heart failure coexist, and that the various clinical findings of right heart failure are a combination of both causes.

Clinical Manifestations of Right Heart Failure

The signs and symptoms of right heart failure are related fundamentally to the retention of water and sodium within the body. The end result of this fluid entrapment is an overloading of the venous system which produces the following clinical findings.

Distended Neck Veins

Increased venous pressure in the superior vena cava causes distention of the veins in the neck. If the veins remain distended when the patient is placed in a semiupright (45-degree angle) position, it is very likely that right heart failure is present. (Neck veins may distend in the absence of heart failure, but in this circumstance the veins empty immediately when the patient's head is raised; therefore observation of the neck veins should always be made with the patient in a semiupright position.) Neck vein distention is one of the earliest signs of right heart failure and certainly the easiest to detect.

Peripheral Edema

As the result of increased pressure in the venous system, fluid is forced from the capillaries into the subcutaneous tissues of the body. This fluid collection, called peripheral or subcutaneous edema, occurs primarily in the dependent areas of the body. In patients with acute myocardial infarction who are bedfast, the back (especially the sacral area) is dependent, and therefore edema is usually noted first in this area. (In patients who are ambulatory, the feet and legs are the usual sites of edema formation.) Rarely, peripheral edema is generalized and found throughout the entire body; this condition is called anasarca. The severity of peripheral edema is graded from 1+ to 4+. Mild edema (1+) is sometimes difficult to detect on physical examination; however, all forms of edema are accompanied by a gain in body weight. Therefore weighing the patient each day is a useful method of estimating the extent of edema fluid accumulation.

Pleural Effusion

Edema fluid may also accumulate in the pleural cavity. This collection is described as a pleural effusion. It usually develops along with peripheral edema but can occur independently. Large pleural effusions compress the lungs and therefore may produce (or intensify) dyspnea. The presence of a pleural effusion can be suspected if diminished or absent breath sounds are noted while listening to the patient's lungs. The diagnosis is confirmed by x-ray examination of the chest (Figure 7.7).

Enlarged and Tender Liver

Backward pressure in the inferior vena cava and hepatic veins causes venous engorgement of the liver. As a result the liver enlarges, becomes tender, and can be palpated on physical examination. Hepatic enlargement may produce discomfort in the right upper quadrant of the abdomen and is often accompanied by loss of appetite and nausea. When the liver is engorged, pressure applied over the right upper quadrant of the abdomen causes the neck veins to distend. This phenomenon, known as the *hepatojugular reflux*, is a diagnostic sign of right heart failure. Abdominal compression increases the amount of blood returning to the heart, thus raising venous pressure and intensifying neck vein distention be-

cause the right heart is unable to handle the increased blood flow.

Treatment of Right Heart Failure

Since right heart failure coexists with left heart failure (especially in patients with acute myocardial infarction), the treatment programs of the two conditions overlap and share certain common features. Nevertheless, the management of right heart failure is based on specific objectives that differ in direction and emphasis from left ventricular failure. The two goals in treating right ventricular failure are: 1) to improve cardiac performance and 2) to control sodium-water retention. The following measures are used in achieving these aims.

Improvement in Cardiac Performance

1. Reduction of Metabolic Needs of the Body. As stated previously, heart failure indicates that the cardiac output is insufficient to meet the metabolic demands of the body. Therefore it is highly desirable to reduce the body's metabolic needs, if possible, as a means of assisting the failing heart. Rest is one of the most effective ways to diminish the cardiac workload. Consequently, limitation of physical activity by bed rest or chair rest is a basic element in the treatment program. Total bed rest, however, is unnecessary, and patients can obtain adequate rest while sitting in a bedside chair. Also, patients should be permitted to use a bedside commode rather than a bedpan since the energy expenditure is less with a commode. Moreover, complete bed rest is undesirable because it tends to increase the risk of thromboembolism, as explained later in this chapter. Rest, as the first step in the treatment program, is often remarkably effective on its own in promoting diuresis, slowing the heart rate, and relieving dyspnea.

2. Vasodilator Therapy. Unloading the heart afterload resistance is a very useful adjunct in the treatment of congestive heart failure. However, vasodilators are not usually employed as an initial therapy in this situation; instead they are reserved for situations in which bed rest, diuretic therapy, and digitalis have not been effective. Arterial dilators (e.g., hydralazine), venous dilators (e.g., nitrates) or vasodilators with combined arterial and venous action (e.g., prazosin) may be utilized in this situation; the choice depends on the overall hemodynamic picture.

3. Digitalis. Although its use during the first few days after acute myocardial infarction is controversial (for reasons mentioned), digitalis therapy

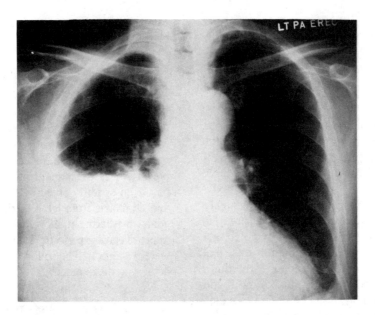

Figure 7.7. A very large pleural effusion in the right chest is noted in this x-ray film. In most instances pleural effusions are much less extensive than shown in this example.

remains a fundamental method of treatment for congestive heart failure. Digitalis is indicated when congestive failure develops after the acute phase of myocardial infarction or if heart failure persists despite diuretic therapy and sodium restriction.

Control of Sodium-Water Retention

1. Restriction of Sodium Intake. Right heart failure is characterized by the retention of sodium and water, which in turn produce overloading of the vascular tree. Consequently, it is highly important in treating congestive heart failure to rid the body of this excess of sodium and water, thus permitting a reduction in the circulating volume. To this end, restriction of sodium in the diet is essential. When clinical signs of right heart failure develops, sodium intake is usually limited to 1000-2000 mg per day (the average American diet contains more than 10,000 mg of sodium daily). Even when heart failure is not evident, many physicians prescribe low-sodium diets (e.g., 2000 mg) prophylactically for all patients with acute myocardial infarction.

2. Diuretic Therapy. Diuretics are highly effective in promoting the renal excretion of sodium and water and, through this mechanism, of reducing the circulating fluid volume. In fact, edema and other manifestations of heart failure are so readily controlled with diuretics in most instances that these drugs have become the initial means of treatment for congestive failure. Despite their ability to alleviate

heart failure, diuretics are not self-sufficient; they should be used in conjunction with rest, sodium restriction and, if necessary, digitalis and vasodilators. There are several classes of diuretic agents with varying degrees of potency:

Thiazide diuretics. These drugs, which are moderately potent, act by blocking the reabsorption of sodium in the tubules of the kidneys.* By inhibiting the customary return of sodium to the body, thiazide diuretics allow large amounts of sodium and water to be excreted in the urine. These agents are administered orally and usually promote diuresis within 2 hours. The effectiveness of their action can be assessed by carefully measuring the urinary output and fluid input, along with recording the patient's body weight daily. The main problem encountered with the use of thiazide diuretics is *potassium depletion.* This occurs because thiazides also block the tubular reabsorption of potassium, and therefore excessive amounts of potassium are excreted in the urine. The loss of potassium resulting from this drug-induced mechanism is of particular concern in patients with acute myocardial infarction because low potassium levels (hypokalemia) can increase myocardial excitability and cause serious ventricular arrhythmias. Also,

---

*Fluid filtered through the glomeruli of the kidneys normally contains a large quantity of sodium; however, most of this sodium is reabsorbed by the tubules of the kidney and returned to the bloodstream (in order to maintain an adequate sodium level in the body). Only the amount of sodium not reabsorbed by the tubules is excreted in the urine.

hypokalemia is dangerous in patients receiving digitalis since potassium depletion sensitizes the myocardium to digitalis and therefore predisposes to digitalis toxicity. Indeed, in the presence of hypokalemia even small doses of digitalis may produce digitalis toxicity. In addition to these adverse effects on the heart, hypokalemia also produces systemic signs and symptoms. With marked potassium depletion many patients develop lethargy, anorexia, mental confusion, and a decrease in urinary output. Hypokalemia can be determined by measuring serum potassium levels and, less dependably, by electrocardiographic (ECG) findings. If hypokalemia develops, replacement of potassium (either by intravenous infusion or orally, depending on clinical circumstances) is essential.

Furosemide (Lasix) and ethacrynic acid (Edecrin). These agents are the most potent diuretics available. They exert their effect in the same way as the thiazides: by blocking tubular reabsorption of sodium. They can be administered intravenously or orally and produce a rapid and profound loss of sodium and water, far greater than that achieved by the use of thiazide diuretics. Because of their extreme potency, which may produce marked hypokalemia and excessive fluid loss, these drugs should be reserved for urgent clinical situations (e.g., acute pulmonary edema) or heart failure that is refractory to the thiazide diuretics. Potassium replacement therapy is nearly always required in patients treated with furosemide or ethacrynic acid.

Aldosterone antagonists. As mentioned, congestive heart failure is accompanied by an excessive production of aldosterone, a hormone that causes the body to retain salt. Spironolactone (Aldactone) is an aldosterone antagonist and therefore promotes the excretion of sodium. This drug is far less potent than the thiazode diuretics; and its onset of action is very slow (usually 2-5 days). Consequently this diuretic is used in nonurgent situations, particularly if other forms of therapy have failed. The main advantage of aldosterone antagonists is that they do not cause significant potassium loss, thus minimizing the risk of hypokalemia.

Triamterene (Dyrenium). This drug, also a weak diuretic, increases the excretion of sodium by acting on the renal exchange mechanism. However, the urinary excretion of potassium is not affected by this agent, and therefore there is no danger of inducing hypokalemia. This potassium-sparing effect eliminates the need for supplemental potassium therapy.

3. Fluid Restriction. Usually it is not necessary to restrict fluid intake in patients with mild or moderate heart failure. However, with more advanced failure it is beneficial to limit water intake to 1000 cc daily. The reason for this restriction is that excessive water intake tends to dilute the amount of sodium in the body fluids and may produce a *low-salt syndrome* (hyponatremia). The latter condition is characterized by lethargy and weakness. It results most often from the combination of a restricted sodium diet, increased sodium loss during diuresis, and excessive water intake. The diagnosis of hyponatremia is established by measuring serum sodium levels.

Nursing Role in Heart Failure

The nursing role in the management of patients with heart failure has many facets. These can be grouped into three main categories: 1) detection of early heart failure, 2) evaluating the response to therapy, and 3) initiating emergency treatment for acute pulmonary edema. These nursing responsibilities are discussed below.

Detection of Early Heart Failure

There is good reason to believe that the earlier acute heart failure is treated, the better will be the result. Therefore recognition of the first signs and symptoms of heart failure is an important aspect in the total care of patients with acute myocardial infarction. Because the nurse (unlike the physician) is in constant attendance and has the opportunity to observe the patient's clinical course uninterruptedly, the detection of early heart failure has become an integral part of coronary care nursing. The nurse is expected to assess the patient's clinical status frequently and advise the physician of significant findings. This nursing evaluation should be based on planned observation, careful physical examination, and thoughtful analysis of the clinical data. The following signs and symptoms may indicate early heart failure:

Respiration. The onset of overt heart failure is often accompanied by a gradual increase in the rate of respiration; therefore an ongoing comparison of the number of respirations per minute may provide a valuable diagnostic clue. Dyspnea and orthopnea, the classic symptoms of left ventricular failure, cannot always be recognized by observation alone, especially with mild or early heart failure. Consequently, it is important to ask the patient (while vital signs are being obtained) if he feels short of breath. Is he more comfortable propped up in bed? Coughing, another manifestion of heart failure, should also be noted: Has the frequency of coughing increased? Is the cough productive of sputum?

Heart Rate and Rhythm. A heart rate persistently greater than 100 per minute is cause for suspicion of left ventricular failure. (This possibility becomes even more likely when other causes of tachycardia, such as temperature elevation or anxiety, are not present.) Other than observing the heart rate, monitoring the cardiac rhythm is also essential because arrhythmias develop very frequently during heart failure.

Sweating. Perspiration is another manifestation of early heart failure. It results from increased sympathetic nervous system activity that occurs when cardiac output falls. In this circumstance sweating is usually mild or moderate rather than drenching (as it is with acute pulmonary edema).

Restlessness and Insomnia. Although in many instances restlessness, anxiety and disturbed sleep patterns are the result of emotional turmoil, these symptoms may also represent subtle warnings of early left ventricular failure. The indiscriminate use of tranquilizers or sedatives without consideration of the underlying cause of the problem is unwise and may mask a useful clue to the early diagnosis of heart failure.

Physical Examination. Careful physical examination should be conducted by the nurse every 4 hours (when vital signs are ordinarily recorded) to detect evidence of heart failure. The following physical findings should be noted specifically:

1. Rales in the lungs. Indicate whether the rales are heard only at the bases of the lungs (mild failure) or if they extend higher in the lung fields (moderate failure).

2. Gallop rhythm. Is the extra sound an S_3 gallop (a definite sign of heart failure) or an S_4 gallop (a less specific sign)?

3. Distention of the neck veins (with the patient in a semiupright position).

4. Hepatojugular reflux (neck vein distention while pressure is applied over the liver area).

5. Peripheral edema, especially of the sacral area and back.

6. Abdominal tenderness in the right upper quadrant, resulting from venous engorgement of the liver.

Evaluating the Response to Therapy

After the treatment program for heart failure has been started it is essential to evaluate the patient's clinical status at regular intervals in order to determine what steps should be taken next. Should vasodilators be administered? Is digitalis therapy indicated? Is oxygen still necessary? Should the dosage of the diuretic agent be reduced? These are just a few of the questions that the physician must answer on the basis of the patient's response to treatment. As with the detection of early heart failure, repeated clinical assessment by the nurse is a major component of the overall evaluation of the treatment program. The nursing assessment includes the following details:

1. Recording vital signs (every 4 hours) with particular emphasis on changes in heart rate, respiration and blood pressure.

2. Examining the patient frequently to determine improvement or worsening of the clinical signs of heart failure.

3. Questioning the patient about changes in dyspnea and other symptoms that may be difficult to assess objectively.

4. Recording accurate intake and output measurements to assess fluid balance. Also, the patient should be weighed at the same time each day to detect fluid retention that otherwise might not be apparent.

5. Recognizing the side-effects of the various drugs used in the treatment program. Remember that many drugs affect the heart rate and blood pressure, causing changes in the vital signs. For example, beta-blocking agents (e.g., Inderal) usually slow the heart rate substantially and vasodilators (e.g., nitrates) may reduce blood pressure to hypotensive levels.

6. Monitoring the heart to identify arrhythmias that may result from heart failure itself or from drug therapy (e.g., arrhythmias caused by hypokalemia from diuretic therapy).

7. Organizing laboratory data (e.g., electrolytes and arterial blood gases) in an orderly way so that changes in results can be readily noted.

Initiating Emergency Treatment for Acute Pulmonary Edema*

1. Recognize the complication, examine the patient, and notify the physician promptly. The clinical picture of acute pulmonary edema is so distinctive that diagnosis is seldom a problem.

---

*The scope of nursing intervention in emergency situations as acute pulmonary edema varies considerably among hospitals. In hospitals that do not have house officers or other physicians in full-time attendance it is a common practice for the medical staff to adopt a standard program for emergency treatment which the nurse may initiate if a physician is not immediately available.

2. Administer humidified oxygen by means of a tight-fitting face mask. The flow rate should be adjusted to 8-10 liters per minute. Face masks are usually frightening to patients in respiratory distress, and the nurse should make it clear that the mask will not interfere with breathing. Intermittent positive-pressure ventilation may be ordered by the physician.

3. Raise the head of the bed so that the patient is in a sitting (Fowler's) position. This position facilitates breathing by lowering the diaphragm and allowing the lung capacity to expand.

4. Prepare and administer drug therapy as ordered by the physician (or in accordance with the standard protocol of the CCU). The customary treatment program involves the immediate administration of morphine and a rapid-acting diuretic.

5. Apply rotating tourniquets to the extremities in the event other measures have not produced improvement.

6. Observe the cardiac monitor for the development of arrhythmias. Reduced tissue oxygenation and electrolyte disturbances resulting from heart failure commonly precipitate serious arrhythmias during this period.

7. Arrange for the collection of arterial blood samples (for blood gas determinations), if ordered.

8. Help the patient to understand the treatment program. Acute pulmonary edema is an extremely frightening experience; most patients feel that death is near. The nurse should reassure the patient that prompt improvement can be anticipated after treatment is started. A calm, confident attitude is often the best form of reassurance. Each step in the treatment program should be explained briefly to the patient, particularly when the use of equipment (e.g., positive-pressure breathing devices) is involved.

CARDIOGENIC SHOCK

Cardiogenic shock is the most severe manifestation of impaired left ventricular pumping function; it occurs in approximately 15% of patients hospitalized with acute myocardial infarction. Until recently more than 80% of patients who developed the clinical syndrome of cardiogenic shock (also called power failure syndrome) could be expected to die during the period of hospitalization. Now there is hope that this awesome mortality can be reduced by the application of new methods of treatment.

The precise cause of cardiogenic shock is still uncertain, but it is known that this complication is associated with extensive destruction of the left ventricle. Autopsy studies have shown that in most patients who die of cardiogenic shock more than 50% of the myocardium is destroyed. This does not necessarily mean that all of the damage is produced by the initial infarction; it may be that the infarcted area continues to enlarge during the course of cardiogenic shock. As mentioned in Chapter 3, research studies now are being conducted to determine whether the extent of myocardial damage can be controlled by drug therapy administered within the first few hours after the attack. If it becomes possible to limit the ultimate size of an evolving myocardial infarction, the incidence of cardiogenic shock (and left ventricular failure) may decline.

The effects of this severe damage to the myocardium are depicted in Figure 7.8. As a result of extensive injury to the myocardium the stroke volume and cardiac output are reduced greatly. (This is accompanied by an increase in pressure in the left atrium, pulmonary capillaries, and pulmonary arteries, as noted in the discussion of left ventricular failure.) The marked decrease in cardiac output causes the systemic arterial blood pressure to fall (*hypotension*). In an effort to preserve effective circulation the small arterioles throughout the body constrict, in effect confining the circulating blood volume to the vital organs at the expense of peripheral tissues. This generalized *vasoconstriction*, mediated through the sympathetic nervous system, is beneficial at first; ultimately, however, it cannot compensate for the very low cardiac output, and sustained hypotension develops. When the systolic arterial blood pressure falls below a critical level, the vital organs fail to receive adequate amounts of blood and oxygen to sustain normal cellular metabolism; this is called *inadequate perfusion*. This generalized perfusion deficit affects all of the organs of the body and produces the clinical findings of cardiogenic shock. Of particular importance is the effect of inadequate perfusion on the heart itself: blood flow through the coronary arteries decreases during shock, and the myocardium is further deprived of oxygen. This impairs myocardial contractility of the uninjured segment of the ventricle and at the same time promotes additional tissue destruction (thus increasing the size of the infarction). Consequently the cardiac output falls even more, and a vicious cycle is created. In summary, cardiogenic shock develops because the damaged left ventricle is unable to maintain the cardiac output at a level necessary for adequate tissue perfusion.

Unless adequate perfusion can be restored promptly, the body cells deteriorate and die. Once the vital organs are destroyed in this way, treatment is to no avail and death must be anticipated; this latter state is called *irreversible shock*. The exact dividing line between irreversible and reversible shock is unknown,

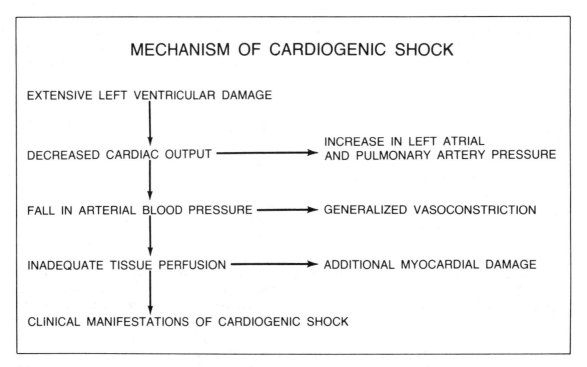

Figure 7.8.

but it appears that reversibility is related primarily to the duration of the perfusion deficit. It is believed that certain enzyme systems concerned with utilization of oxygen by the tissues are irreparably damaged during cardiogenic shock and that death occurs from this cause. The end stage of cardiogenic shock is associated with profound vasodilation (circulatory collapse) and, finally, the development of ventricular fibrillation or ventricular standstill, which are unresponsive to treatment.

Clinical Manifestations of Cardiogenic Shock

Inadequate tissue perfusion results in a combination of clinical findings which *collectively* define cardiogenic shock. In other words, underperfusion affects all of the major organs of the body, and therefore the clinical picture of cardiogenic shock is characterized by involvement of multiple systems. The most important manifestations of cardiogenic shock are as follows.

Hypotension

A marked decrease in arterial blood pressure is an outstanding feature of acute circulatory insufficiency. In nearly all instances the systolic blood pressure falls below 90 mm Hg. However, it must be clearly understood that hypotension by itself is not synonymous with cardiogenic shock. Unless hypotension is accompanied by other clinical findings of inadequate perfusion (e.g., diminished urinary output or mental

confusion, as described below), the diagnosis of cardiogenic shock is not justified. For example, if a patient has a blood pressure of 84/50 but the pulse rate is not rapid, urinary output is normal, and there is no evidence of mental confusion, it should not be assumed that cardiogenic shock is present. A more reasonable diagnosis of this condition is hypotension, a common occurrence in the early stages of acute myocardial infarction and of much less importance than cardiogenic shock.

When cardiogenic shock develops, the systolic pressure declines before the diastolic pressure; consequently it is not unusual to record a blood pressure, for instance, of 70/60 in this circumstance. The numerical difference between the systolic and diastolic pressures is called the *pulse pressure* (e.g., 120/80 = pulse pressure of 40 mm Hg). Since narrowing of the pulse pressure is frequently an early sign of cardiogenic shock, it is essential to measure the systolic and diastolic pressures precisely in order to detect insidious changes. When cardiogenic shock worsens, the diastolic pressure falls along with the systolic pressure; and often the blood pressure becomes unobtainable. (In assessing blood pressure levels it is necessary to realize that the customary cuff-stethoscope method of measurement may produce spuriously low readings, particularly in the presence of cardiogenic shock. Therefore when blood pressure readings are very low or cannot be obtained, *direct* blood pressure measurement may be required; this is accomplished by inserting an indwelling catheter into the arterial system and recording the intraarterial pressures directly.)

Mental Changes

One of the earliest features of cardiogenic shock is mental apathy and lassitude: the patient seems disinterested in his surroundings and often just stares into space. Other common findings that occur at the same time or later are disorientation, confusion, agitation, and restlessness. All of these mental changes reflect ineffective perfusion of the brain. As the shock state progresses, seizures may occur and finally coma develops.

Oliguria

As a result of diminished renal blood flow, the kidneys fail to function effectively and the urinary volume decreases markedly. With adequate perfusion the kidneys normally excrete at least 1 cc of urine per minute (or 60 cc per hour). During cardiogenic shock the urinary output falls below 20 cc per hour (*oliguria*), or it may cease entirely. This latter condition (*anuria*) is an ominous sign and generally signals irreversible shock.

Cold, Moist Skin

Because of peripheral vasoconstriction which usually accompanies cardiogenic shock, there is a marked reduction in blood flow to the skin. Consequently the skin becomes cold and pale. Along with this vasoconstrictive response there is an increase in sympathetic nervous system activity, which causes profuse sweating. The combination of vasoconstriction and sympathetic stimultion produces the cold, pale, clammy skin that characterizes cardiogenic shock.

Metabolic Acidosis

Adequate oxygenation is essential for normal cellular metabolism and function. In cardiogenic shock the supply of oxygen available to the tissues is drastically reduced. In an attempt to preserve cellular function and life the body employs a temporary, alternate metabolic pathway which does not demand oxygen; this is called *anaerobic* metabolism, in contrast to the normal *aerobic* pathway, which uses oxygen. The end product of aerobic metabolism is carbonic acid, which is excreted as carbon dioxide by the lungs; the end product of anaerobic metabolism is *lactic acid*. Unlike carbon dioxide, which is readily removed from the body, lactic acid cannot be excreted by the lungs or kidneys and therefore accumulates in the blood. This retention of lactic acid results in *lactic acidosis*. Lethal arrhythmias, which are refractory to treatment, develop in the presence of lactic acidosis and cause death.

Treatment of Cardiogenic Shock

Over the years a variety of methods have been used to treat cardiogenic shock. That the present mortality rate remains greater than 80% clearly indicates that no mode of therapy has been consistently successful in combating this complication. However, ongoing research has provided several important leads regarding an improved plan of treatment. The plan is based on the following concepts: 1) the earlier cardiogenic shock is recognized and treated, the greater is the chance for survival; 2) therapeutic decisions must be based on repeated assessment of the patient's hemodynamic status; 3) a standardized treatment program for all patients is self-defeating because the clinical course has many variations; 4) drug therapy should be selected and altered according to the hemodynamic and clinical response; 5) in many patients the main hope for survival rests with mechanical assistance of the failing circulation; 6) surgical treatment may be feasible if other measures have failed. According to these current concepts a logical approach to the treatment of cardiogenic shock should involve the following steps.

Early Recognition of Cardiogenic Shock

Because there is only a minimal chance for survival once cardiogenic shock reaches an advanced stage (e.g., complete cessation of urinary output), the primary focus of the treatment program must be directed toward early detection and treatment of the complication. Occasionally cardiogenic shock develops soon after acute myocardial infarction has occurred, but far more often the shock state evolves gradually, usually several hours after the attack. Consequently in most instances there is an opportunity to recognize the first clinical manifestations of shock. Early detection can be achieved only by planned, repeated observation of the patient's clinical condition. Any evidence suggesting impending shock, such as diminished mental alertness, a modest reduction in blood pressure, narrowing of the pulse pressure, a gradual decrease in urinary output, or coolness and paleness of the skin, is cause for prompt investigation of the patient's physiological status and the initiation of supportive treatment.

Hemodynamic and Physiologic Measurements

In order to assess the extent of the problem and to plan a logical treatment program for cardiogenic shock it is necessary to perform a few basic hemodynamic and physiologic measurements, all of which can now be accomplished quickly and safely at the bedside.

Arterial Blood Pressure. As noted, blood pressure recordings made with a standard sphygmomanometer are frequently inaccurate in the presence of cardiogenic shock. Therefore if the systolic pressure is low (e.g., less than 80 mm Hg) or if the pressure is difficult to obtain, it is advantageous to insert an intraarterial catheter (usually by way of the radial or brachial arteries) to permit *direct* blood pressure measurement. In this way the blood pressure can be determined precisely and monitored continuously. Furthermore, the arterial catheter can be used for other purposes as well, including collection of arterial blood samples (for blood gas studies) and measurement of cardiac output.

Pulmonary Artery Pressure. Left ventricular pumping performance can be determined indirectly by measuring the pressure in the pulmonary artery with a Swan-Ganz catheter. The basis of this measurement is as follows: As noted earlier, when myocardial contractility is impaired the ventricle cannot empty adequately and therefore the volume (and pressure) of blood in the left ventricle at the end of the filling period (diastole) increases significantly. This increase in *left ventricular end-diastolic pressure* (LVEDP) is one of the earliest and most important expressions of diminished left ventricular function. Therefore it is highly desirable to measure LVEDP as a means of evaluating the severity of cardiogenic shock, as well as the effects of treatment. However, *direct* measurement of LVEDP is a formidable procedure. The catheter must be inserted into a surgically exposed artery and threaded backward through the aorta and the aortic valve, and into the left ventricle. The procedure is performed in a cardiac catheterization laboratory with the use of fluoroscopy. Furthermore, placing a catheter in the left ventricle is hazardous in patients with acute myocardial infarction because of the risk of inducing myocardial irritability and ventricular fibrillation. In 1970 it was shown that LVEDP could be measured *indirectly* by means of a balloon-tipped catheter (Swan-Ganz catheter) inserted into the pulmonary artery by way of a peripheral vein. Unlike direct left ventricular catheterization, this method is safe and simple, and can be performed at the patient's bedside.

The procedure for monitoring pulmonary artery pressure (PAP) involves the use of a double-lumen catheter. The larger lumen measures the pressure in the pulmonary artery while the smaller lumen leads to a small balloon just proximal to the tip of the catheter. When inflated, the balloon serves to guide the catheter through the right atrium, right ventricle, and into proper position in the pulmonary artery. The catheter is inserted through an arm (antecubital) vein and advanced to the superior vena cava. After the catheter enters the vena cava, the balloon is fully inflated with air and allowed to float through the right atrium and right ventricle into the pulmonary artery. The balloon finally wedges in a small branch of the pulmonary artery; this is called the *pulmonary wedge position.* The course the catheter traverses in reaching the wedge position is illustrated in Figure 7.9. Continuous pressure recordings are made during passage of the catheter to verify its location. As shown in Figure 7.10 the pressure waves are distinctly different in the right ventricle, pulmonary artery, and pulmonary wedge position. The pressure recorded in the pulmonary wedge position is termed the *pulmonary capillary wedge pressure* (PCWP). It represents the pressure in the pulmonary capillary bed, which reflects the left ventricular end-diastolic pressure. PCWP cannot be measured continuously because the inflated balloon obstructs the flow of blood through a segment of the lung and can cause pulmonary embolism. Consequently, as soon as the PCWP is determined the balloon is deflated. Deflation of the balloon (with the catheter still in the wedge position) permits the pulmonary artery pressure (PAP) to be measured. In most instances there is a close correlation between pulmonary artery (diastolic) pressure and PCWP. Therefore by monitoring PAP (which can be performed continuously because the balloon is deflated), left ventricular performance may be evaluated constantly. These hemodynamic measurements are extremely important in determining a logical plan of treatment and should be utilized whenever possible.

Cardiac Output. Included in the overall hemodynamic assessment of cardiogenic shock is the measurement of cardiac output. This important study was seldom performed in patients with acute myocardial infarction until recent years because of the difficulty and complexity of the methods used; however after it was shown that cardiac output could be determined simply and quickly at the bedside with a modified Swan-Ganz catheter, this form of hemodynamic monitoring became a standard procedure in many coronary care units. The technique, called the thermodilution method, involves the use of a specially designed balloon-tipped catheter with a built-in electrode (thermister) to detect changes in temperature. The catheter is floated into the pulmonary artery and then cold saline solution is injected through one of the lumen of the catheter into the right atrium or vena cava. The resulting temperature change in the pulmonary artery is measured by the thermister electrode, and cardiac output is calculated according to the extent of the change. In effect, the greater the change in temperature in the pulmonary artery, the lower the cardiac output or, vice versa, the less the temperature change, the higher the cardiac output. Cardiac output measurements can be made repeatedly

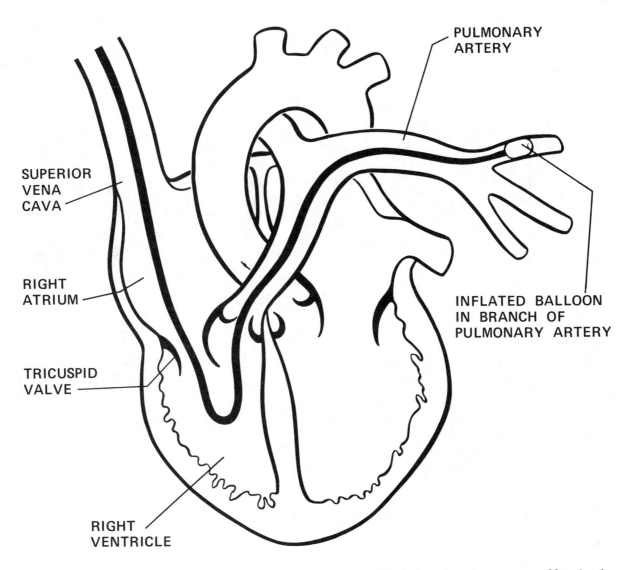

PULMONARY
ARTERY

SUPERIOR
VENA
CAVA

RIGHT
ATRIUM

TRICUSPID
VALVE

RIGHT
VENTRICLE

INFLATED BALLOON
IN BRANCH OF
PULMONARY ARTERY

Figure 7.9. The course of a Swan-Ganz catheter during passage through the heart to the pulmonary artery. Note that the inflated balloon is wedged in a branch of the pulmonary artery, which permits recording of the wedge pressure.

with no discomfort to the patient since the catheter remains in place; the information provided is valuable in evaluating the effects of treatment.

Central Venous Pressure. Although much less accurate than pulmonary artery pressure in assessing the extent of circulatory failure, measurement of central venous pressure (CVP) is still performed in many coronary care units under certain circumstances. Probably the main reason for measuring CVP rather than pulmonary artery pressure is inability, for one reason or other, to use the Swan-Ganz technique. Also, CVP determinations can be made almost immediately since, unlike the Swan-Ganz method, the equipment does not have to be standardized. The procedure involves no more than inserting a long polyethylene tube (catheter) into the superior vena cava by way of an arm, neck or subclavian vein.

The free end of the catheter is attached to a simple water manometer; the height of the water column in the manometer indicates the CVP. The normal CVP ranges between 5-10 cm H_2O. The disadvantage of measuring CVP is that it reflects the ability of the *right* ventricle to handle venous return, but offers much less information about left ventricular performance, which of course is the critical factor in cardiogenic shock. (As explained previously, when the left ventricle fails, a backward pressure develops throughout the pulmonary circulation; this increased pressure impedes right ventricular emptying and in turn causes a rise in pressure in the right atrium and vena cava.) Unfortunately, the relationship between the right heart and left heart pressures is not always consistent, and therefore the CVP is not a reliable index of left ventricular function. In fact, in some instances the CVP may be normal or only slightly elevated despite the presence of cardiogenic shock.

PRESSURE RECORDINGS DURING PASSAGE OF SWAN-GANZ CATHETER

Right Ventricle

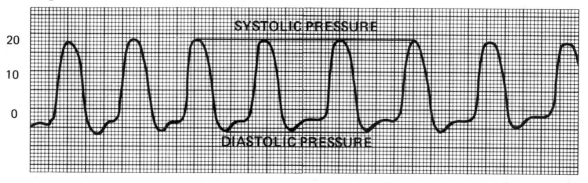

The catheter tip is in the right ventricle. The normal pressure in the right ventricle is 20 mm Hg systolic and 5 mm diastolic (20/5). In this example the pressure is 20/0 mm Hg.

Pulmonary Artery

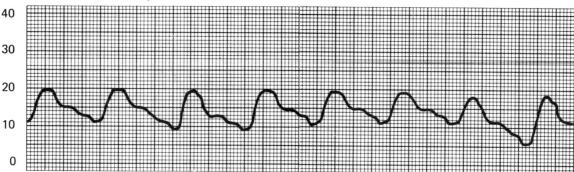

The catheter tip is in the pulmonary artery. The normal PAP is 25/10 mm Hg. In this case the systolic pressure is 20 mm Hg and the diastolic pressure between 10–12 mm Hg. The *diastolic* pulmonary artery pressure is used to assess left ventricular function; the pressure increases above 12 mm when the left ventricle begins to fail.

Pulmonary Capillary Wedge Pressure

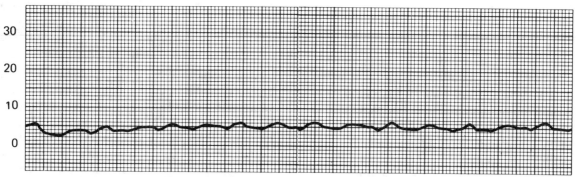

The catheter tip (with the balloon inflated) is in a small branch of the pulmonary artery. A PCWP of 5–12 mm Hg is considered normal. Levels above 12 mm Hg indicate reduced left ventricular emptying. The PCWP in this instance is about 5 mm Hg.

Figure 7.10.

However, in the vast majority of patients with cardiogenic shock the CVP is markedly elevated, usually to levels of 15-20 cm H_2O or more.

Urinary Output. Accurate measurement of urinary output is of such great importance in assessing the patient's physiological status that an indwelling (Foley) catheter should be placed into the bladder in the early stages of cardiogenic shock. The urinary volume is measured at 30-minute intervals.

Arterial Blood Gases. Cardiogenic shock, as noted, is accompanied by inadequate oxygenation and metabolic acidosis. The extent of these two disturbances is determined by arterial blood gas studies (pO_2 and pH). If an intraarterial catheter is used to monitor blood pressure, arterial blood samples can be collected through the tube; otherwise arterial puncture must be performed each time.

Supportive Therapy

With the appearance of the first signs of cardiogenic shock, several general measures are undertaken in an effort to preserve vital organ function until specific treatment can be instituted to improve cardiac performance (based on the results of hemodynamic studies). These initial steps, categorized as supportive therapy, include the following.

Administration of Oxygen. Oxygen is administered initially by means of a tight-fitting face mask. Arterial blood gas studies should be performed while the patient is receiving oxygen. If the results indicate inadequate arterial oxygenation (pO_2 levels of less than 75), assisted respiration may be necessary.

Relief of Pain. Patients with cardiogenic shock frequently develop ischemic chest pain because of reduced coronary blood flow and inadequate myocardial perfusion. Small doses of morphine (5-10 mg) should be administered intravenously to relieve this pain. (Intramuscular or subcutaneous injections are not advisable in this circumstance since drug absorption may be very slow in the presence of diminished circulation.)

Correction of Acidosis. As explained previously, inadequate tissue perfusion leads to lactic acidosis, a condition that even when of moderate severity adversely affects cardiac performance and contributes to the development of lethal arrhythmias. Consequently it is essential to detect and correct acidosis promptly. The presence of acidosis is determined by measurement of arterial blood pH. (The normal arterial blood pH is 7.35-7.45; levels lower than 7.35

indicate acidosis.) Lactic acidosis is treated with intravenous sodium bicarbonate (an alkali).

Specific Treatment (Drug Therapy)

Infusion of Fluids. Hypotension, oliguria, and other signs of cardiogenic shock sometimes develop in patients with acute myocardial infarction as the result of a reduction in the circulating blood (plasma) volume. The volume depletion, called *hypovolemia,* is usually caused by a combination of factors, including inadequate fluid intake, anorexia, vomiting, profuse sweating, and excessive fluid loss from vigorous diuretic therapy. This form of shock is characterized by *normal (or low)* pulmonary artery and central venous pressures (in contrast to the high levels that are expected with typical cardiogenic shock). The condition can be corrected by the administration of adequate amounts of intravenous fluids to expand the plasma volume. Consequently, if the PAP or CVP is not elevated, plasma volume expansion should be undertaken as the first step in treatment. Usually 200 cc of 5% dextrose solution is administered intravenously over a 10-minute period (20 cc/minute). If hypovolemia is a contributing factor to shock, this trial of fluid loading usually causes the blood pressure and urinary volume to increase promptly. Additional fluids are then infused according to clinical and hemodynamic responses. With marked volume depletion, albumin, whole blood, or low-molecular-weight dextran may be required to expand the intravascular volume sufficiently. As a general rule, patients who respond to volume expansion have a good chance for recovery.

Inotropic Drugs. Unless cardiogenic shock responds to plasma volume expansion (which happens in approximately 10% of cases), drug therapy is initiated in an attempt to increase the strength of myocardial contraction (and to raise the blood pressure). A variety of drugs are available for this purpose, but none is ideal. The main problem with these agents (categorized as inotropic drugs) is that in achieving their effect they increase myocardial oxygen consumption. An increase in myocardial oxygen consumption is especially dangerous in the presence of cardiogenic shock since additional oxygen deprivation may cause the area of infarction to enlarge, thus reducing pumping function even more. Despite this (and other) adverse physiologic effects, inotropic drugs must be used, at least temporarily, when the blood pressure is very low and perfusion of vital organs cannot be maintained. One or more of the following drugs may be administered in this circumstance: levarterenol (Levophed), dopamine (Inotropin), and dobutamide (Dobutrex). Although it is beyond the scope of this discussion to describe the precise pharmacologic actions and methods of administration of each of these agents, several general conclusions regarding inotropic therapy are pertinent. First, the results of treatment vary from patient to patient, and therefore trials with different drugs (or different dosages) may be necessary. Second, no attempt should be made to restore blood pressure to normal, preshock levels. As a general rule, the systolic pressure should be maintained in the range of 90-100 mm Hg; higher levels create an excessive myocardial oxygen demand. Third, inotropic drugs frequently induce serious arrhythmias; consequently, careful ECG monitoring is mandatory during the period of treatment. Fourth, inotropic drugs usually act promptly, and if definite improvement does not occur within an hour mechanical assistance of the circulation may be required.

Vasodilator Drugs. As noted previously, when cardiogenic shock develops the peripheral arterioles constrict (as a compensatory mechanism) to preserve adequate circulation to the vital organs. Although vasoconstriction is highly desirable at first, it may ultimately lead to a reduction in cardiac output because the left ventricle must pump against strong resistance in the arterial system (peripheral vascular resistance). In other words, increased peripheral vascular resistance can impede ventricular emptying and thereby diminish cardiac output. On this basis it has been proposed that *vasodilator* drugs be used to improve cardiac output if there is evidence of increased peripheral vascular resistance (as calculated from hemodynamic measurements). Unfortunately, this concept has limited application in the treatment of cardiogenic shock because vasodilator drugs tend to lower the blood pressure substantially. Occasionally, however, patients with cardiogenic shock exhibit systolic blood pressure above 100 mm Hg, in which case vasodilating agents may be administered cautiously. The two agents that appear most effective in increasing cardiac output in the presence of marked vasoconstriction are sodium nitroprusside and phentolamine. It must be emphasized that these vasodilating agents should *not* be used if the systolic blood pressure is less than 100 mm Hg.

Regulation of Heart Rate. An important measure in the treatment of cardiogenic shock is to maintain the heart rate above 60/minute but less than 120/minute, if possible. Heart rates beyond this range are ineffective and reduce the cardiac output. Therefore, in patients with abnormally slow or fast heart rates every effort must be made to control the rate as a means of improving cardiac output. This is achieved by the use of drugs or by electrical means (cardiac pacing or cardioversion), as described in subsequent chapters.

Mechanical Assistance of the Circulation

As apparent from the foregoing discussion drug therapy is designed primarily to increase cardiac output. However, for drugs to succeed in their purpose, the heart must receive an adequate amount of oxygen in order to preserve myocardial function; otherwise the infarcted area increases and treatment is to no avail. Thus the outcome of cardiogenic shock depends finally on the amount of oxygen available to the myocardium. Attempting to increase myocardial perfusion with inotropic drugs is often a lost cause because these agents also increase myocardial oxygen consumption. For this reason cardiologists now believe that if patients in cardiogenic shock do not respond promptly to drug therapy mechanical assistance of the circulation should be undertaken without delay. The object of mechanical assistance is to increase coronary blood flow and at the same time to decrease the workload of the heart. In this way myocardial function can be maintained, at least temporarily.

The best known and probably the most effective method of mechanical cardiac assistance involves the use of an *intraaortic balloon pump*. The principle of intraaortic balloon pumping (IABP) is as follows: When blood is ejected from the left ventricle into the aorta during systole, only a small amount of aortic blood flows through the coronary arteries. By far the greatest flow through the coronary circulation occurs during diastole (when the myocardium is in a resting state). The underlying purpose of IABP is to raise the diastolic pressure in the aorta momentarily after each contraction so that a larger volume of blood will flow through the coronary arteries. This is achieved by inserting a long, narrow balloon through a femoral artery into the thoracic aorta (Figure 7.11) and inflating it rapidly (with helium) at the onset of diastole. At the end of diastole (just before systole) the balloon is instantly deflated by a vacuum pump. The sudden decrease in aortic pressure lowers resistance to left ventricular pumping, thereby reducing the workload of the ventricle. The inflation-deflation system is automatically synchronized with the heartbeat, and IABP can be continued for many hours, if necessary. Drug therapy is used concomitantly with IABP, and if the patient's condition stabilizes, mechanical assistance is gradually decreased (weaned) and finally withdrawn.

Unfortunately, clinical experience has shown that relatively few patients with cardiogenic shock can in fact be weaned from the pump. In most cases as soon as IABP is diminished or stopped, signs of shock reappear. Thus, in its own right IABP has not signifi-

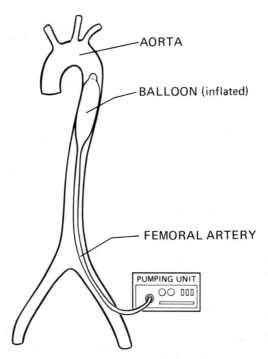

Figure 7.11. Position of an intra-aortic balloon pump.

cantly reduced mortality from cardiogenic shock. For example, reports from various medical centers, in which a total of more than 250 patients with cardiogenic shock were treated with IABP, indicate an overall mortality of 72%; only 28% of patients with shock survived the period of hospitalization. Nevertheless, IABP offers one major benefit: it provides time to search for potentially reversible causes of pump failure and to attempt emergency cardiac surgery in selected patients.

Acute Cardiac Surgery. Patients who do not respond to drugs or who cannot be weaned from IABP may be candidates for emergency cardiac surgery. The principle hope is that a coronary bypass operation, usually in conjunction with resection of a noncontractile portion of the myocardium (or other lesion), can restore adequate pumping performance. Toward this end, emergency cardiac catheterization and ventriculography are performed first, while cardiac function is being sustained with IABP. At present, this type of emergency surgery still has limited application except perhaps in large teaching centers.

Nursing Role in Cardiogenic Shock

Early Recognition of Cardiogenic Shock

The importance of early detection and treatment of cardiogenic shock cannot be overemphasized. Indeed the main hope for survival depends on improving tissue perfusion as soon as possible. To this end the nurse must be alert for any changes in the patient's clinical condition which suggest that cardiogenic shock is developing. *Early signs of cardiogenic shock can be recognized only by repeated, planned observation at the bedside.* In examining the patient it is essential to remember that inadequate cardiac output (and organ perfusion) produces multiple signs—all of which must be considered in evaluating the problem. Particular attention should be given to the following clinical findings:

1. A decrease in systolic blood pressure, especially if associated with narrowing of the pulse pressure
2. Mental confusion, apathy, anxiety, or lethargy
3. A reduction in urinary volume
4. Cool, moist skin.

Initial Treatment Program

When signs of cardiogenic shock appear (or if they are present on admission) the nurse should proceed promptly to initiate supportive therapy. The following measures are taken:

1. Notify the physician at once of the clinical findings.
2. Administer oxygen by means of a well-fitted face mask; the flow rate should be 8-10 liters/minute.
3. Inquire if the patient is experiencing chest pain. If so, intravenous morphine (5 mg) is usually ordered.

4. Adjust the flow rate of the intravenous infusion (5% dextrose in water) in accordance with the physician's instructions.
5. Insert an indwelling catheter into the urinary bladder. Measure and record the urinary volume every 20 minutes.
6. Measure the blood pressure every 15 minutes. By comparing serial readings, a continual fall in pressure can be distinguished from a stabilized level.
7. Observe the cardiac monitor carefully to identify changes in the heart rate and the development of arrhythmias. Because ventricular fibrillation is common in the presence of cardiogenic shock, a defibrillator should be at the bedside.
8. Place the patient in a supine position with a pillow under the head. The Trendelenburg position (used in hemorrhagic shock) is disadvantageous in cardiogenic shock.
9. Prepare for hemodynamic monitoring.
10. Record all clinical and laboratory findings sequentially (on a flow sheet) so that changes in the patient's condition can be readily observed.

Subsequent Treatment Program

The specific treatment program for cardiogenic shock is conducted jointly by physician and nurse members of the CCU team. The most important nursing duties include the following:

1. Mobilizing all necessary equipment, drugs, and materials at the onset so that efficient care can be provided uninterruptedly
2. Assisting the physician in performing hemodynamic studies (e.g., insertion of pulmonary artery and intraarterial catheters)
3. Measuring and recording blood pressure, pulmonary artery pressure, and urinary output at regular intervals in order to assess the effectiveness of treatment
4. Monitoring the heart rate and rhythm (cardiac monitoring)
5. Preparing and administering drug therapy in accordance with physicians' orders
6. Checking the patency of all intravenous and intraarterial lines, and adjusting the flow rate of intravenous fluids
7. Arranging for repeated laboratory studies (particularly arterial blood gases)
8. Preparing for assisted ventilation and endotracheal intubation if hypoxia cannot be controlled with nasal oxygen administration
9. Assembling and recording physiological and laboratory data in an organized way

10. Changing the patient's position at least every hour by tilting (slipping a pillow under one side) or elevating the head of the bed slightly
11. Staying with the patient to support him during this critical period.

THROMBOEMBOLISM

Patients with acute myocardial infarction are especially prone to develop intravascular clots (thrombi); the reason for this is uncertain, but several factors are thought to contribute to the problem. Venous stasis, which accompanies prolonged bed rest and muscular inactivity, probably plays an important role in promoting clot formation. However, recent studies (using radioactive isotopes to detect clots in the leg veins) indicate that thrombi often develop within the first 3 days after acute myocardial infarction, suggesting that immobilization itself is not the primary cause of intravascular clotting. There is suspicion that the increased clotting tendency may be inherent in patients with coronary disease and is related to certain blood factors which induce abnormal coagulation (hypercoagulability). Another cause for thrombus formation after acute myocardial infarction is injury to the endocardial lining of the heart by the infarction process. In this circumstance, circulating blood cells adhere to the damaged area and form clots within the chambers of the heart. These intracardiac clots are called mural thrombi. The majority of thrombi, however, arise in the deep veins of the lower extremities (peripheral thrombi). It is estimated that approximately 40% of all patients with acute myocardial infarction develop clots in the calf veins during the period of hospitalization. However, in only a small percentage of cases do these thrombi produce symptoms or affect the clinical course of myocardial infarction. The incidence of peripheral thrombosis is highest in elderly patients and in those with heart failure.

When a peripheral or mural thrombus breaks loose from its site of origin it migrates through the circulatory system as an *embolus*. Depending on where they ultimately lodge, emboli are classified as pulmonary, cerebral, or peripheral. These three types of embolization are discussed separately.

Pulmonary Embolism

Pulmonary emboli nearly always originate in the *deep veins of the legs.* When the thrombus is dislodged from the vein it travels through the inferior vena cava, right atrium, and right ventricle, and finally occludes a branch of the pulmonary artery. There is little chance of mural thrombi causing pulmonary embolism since these latter clots are confined almost exclusively to the *left* heart and consequently remain in the systemic rather than the pulmonary circulation. (In this sense, pulmonary embolism is not a direct result of acute myocardial infarction; the problem develops because of secondary factors.)

Of the three sites of thromboembolic complications, pulmonary embolism is by far the most common. Autopsy studies indicate that pulmonary embolism occurs in about 25% of patients with acute myocardial infarction. However, these embolic episodes are seldom death-producing; the total mortality from pulmonary embolism (in patients with acute myocardial infarction) is about 1-2% at most.

Clinical Manifestations of Pulmonary Embolism

The clinical response to pulmonary embolism depends on the size of the embolus and the degree of obstruction it produces in the pulmonary circulation. Most pulmonary emboli are small and do not produce distinct signs or symptoms; indeed the majority of embolic episodes go unnoticed. With a large pulmonary embolus (which occludes a major branch of the pulmonary artery) patients usually develop clinically recognizable findings. The typical features consist of sudden chest pain, dyspnea, cough (sometimes with hemoptysis), tachycardia, and marked anxiety. The chest pain, often described as crushing or oppressive in quality, may be located substernally or in the right or left side of the chest. The pain pattern frequently resembles that of acute myocardial infarction, but differs in that ordinarily it does not radiate to the arms or jaws and is usually increased by inspiration (pleuritic pain). Rapid respiration and tachycardia are observed in nearly all cases soon after the onset of the episode. Physical examination of the chest may reveal wheezing or rales, but these findings are inconstant. With a massive pulmonary embolus (obstructing more than 50% of the main pulmonary artery), hypotension and circulatory collapse develop; in this circumstance death usually occurs rapidly.

Several diagnostic tests are used to identify pulmonary embolism. X-ray examination of the chest, probably the most common method, is of minimal diagnostic help immediately after an embolic episode because the characteristic findings rarely appear at once. A normal chest x-ray offers no assurance that embolization has not occurred. A more reliable diagnostic procedure is the lung scan. By injecting a radioactive isotope intravenously and scanning the lung fields, the segment of the lung deprived of oxygen can be identified at an early stage. A comparison of a normal lung scan with one demonstrating a large pulmonary embolism is shown in Figure 7.12. The diagnosis of pulmonary embolism can sometimes be suspected from acute ECG changes that indicate an acute strain pattern of the right heart (which develops

from resistance in the pulmonary circulation created by the embolus). Arterial blood gas determinations may also be useful in establishing the diagnosis. Nearly all patients with large pulmonary emboli exhibit arterial oxygen undersaturation (while breathing room air).

The onset of pulmonary embolism is by no means constant or predictable; however, its sudden occurrence after straining during defecation or when the patient first gets out of bed after prolonged inactivity is common enough to merit special precautions.

Cerebral Embolism

Cerebral emboli, unlike pulmonary emboli, originate as *mural* thrombi. Clots from the injured wall of the left ventricle travel through the aorta and occlude arteries in the brain, producing cerebral infarction. In some instances the embolic episode occurs very soon after acute myocardial infarction so that it is not uncommon for patients to be admitted to a hospital with typical findings of a stroke when the underlying problem is in fact an acute myocardial infarction. In this situation the effects of the stroke usually dominate the clinical picture and obscure cardiac symptoms. (For this reason it is a wise practice to record an ECG routinely in all patients with sudden cerebrovascular events.)

Clinical Manifestations of Cerebral Embolism

The most characteristic feature of cerebral embolism is the *sudden* onset of the stroke. In contrast to customary (nonembolic) strokes, there are no premonitory warnings, and the neurologic findings appear abruptly. Therefore if a patient with acute myocardial infarction suddenly develops signs of a stroke, it can be assumed that cerebral embolism has developed as a complication of myocardial infarction. The clinical course after the attack depends on the location of the cerebral infarction and the extent of the neurologic deficit it produces. Motor weakness, paralysis, and speech disturbances are the most common findings; many patients develop loss of consciousness. Diagnostic studies are seldom necessary to confirm the diagnosis, but if uncertainty exists computerized axial tomography (CAT scan) may be utilized. The combination of an acute myocardial infarction and a stroke is usually overwhelming, particularly in elderly patients. Although as a rule death does not occur suddenly, the prognosis is extremely poor.

Peripheral Embolism

Like cerebral emboli, peripheral emboli arise from clots formed within the left heart. Although these

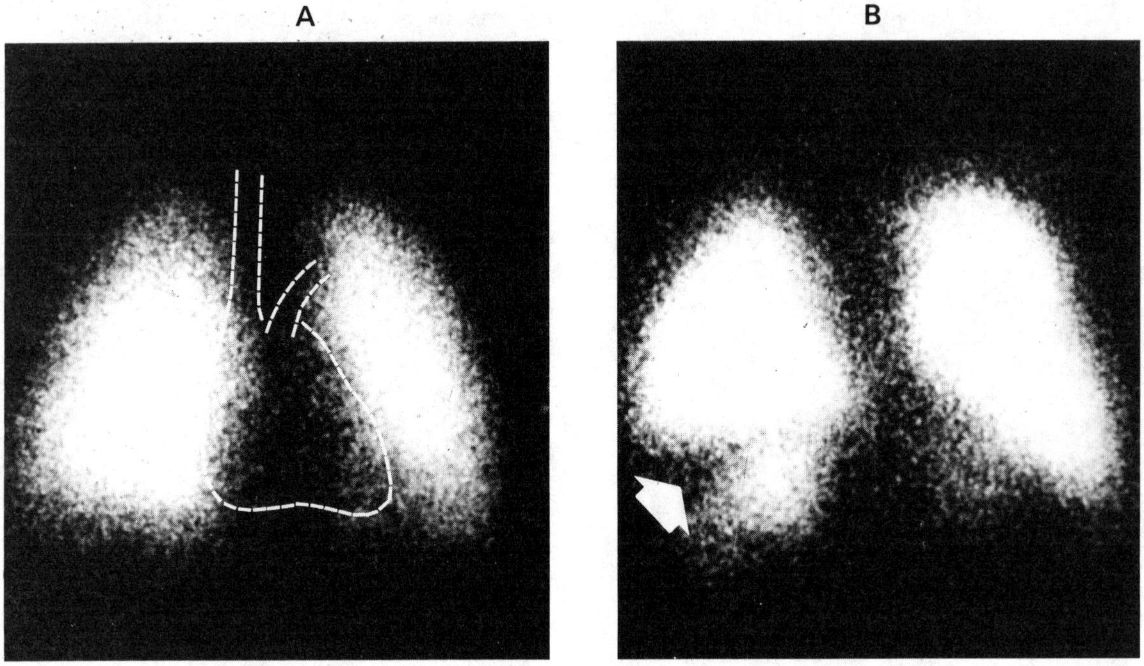

A

B

Figure 7.12. Lung scans: **A**–Normal; **B**–Large pulmonary embolism (arrow).

mural thrombi may lodge anywhere in the systemic arterial system, the most frequent site of peripheral embolism is in the femoral or iliac arteries supplying the lower extremities. The outcome of peripheral embolism depends on the artery involved and whether the embolus can be removed surgically (embolectomy).

**Clinical Manifestations of
Peripheral Embolism**

Embolic occlusion of the major arteries to the lower extremities produces a distinctive clinical picture. There is a sudden onset of pallor, coldness, and numbness of the involved extremity. Within minutes, the patient develops pain in the leg along with decreased sensation. Physical examination reveals an absence of arterial pulsations in conjunction with a cold, pale extremity. In some instances both extremities are involved simultaneously, indicating that the embolus is at the bifurcation of the aorta. Unless embolectomy can be performed promptly, gangrene develops.

Treatment of Thromboembolism

Because emboli originate as thrombi the ideal method of treatment for all forms of embolism is to *prevent* thrombus formation. Prevention can often be accomplished by means of prophylactic anticoagulant therapy; however, the value of this approach is a subject of controversy. Before the era of CCUs it was customary to administer anticoagulant drugs prophylactically to most patients with acute myocardial infarction. When it was demonstrated that thromboembolic complications accounted for only a small percentage of the total mortality, the routine use of anticoagulant therapy was all but abandoned by most physicians. At present, prophylactic anticoagulant treatment is reserved primarily for patients with the highest risk of developing thromboembolism (i.e., the elderly and those with circulatory failure). Even this practice is not fully endorsed since many clinicians believe that the danger of anticoagulant therapy—particularly uncontrolled bleeding—outweighs the benefit of attempting to prevent clot formation. A second method of reducing the incidence of thrombus formation is to avoid venous stasis whenever possible. This can often be achieved by exercising the extremities, changing the body position frequently, and minimizing the duration of complete bed rest. If embolism does occur, anticoagulant therapy is usually started immediately. In this situation the purpose of anticoagulants is not to treat the embolus but to prevent further clot formation at the site of origin and in turn to prevent additional emboli. Also, anticoagulant therapy may inhibit extension of the embolus. Heparin, which becomes active immediately after intravenous injection, is administered as soon as a thromboembolic complication is detected. This anticoagulant is continued for 5-7 days, after which oral agents are used.

Peripheral emboli involving the lower or upper extremities may be treated surgically. Although the operative risk is high in patients with acute myocardial infarction, embolectomy has been performed successfully in many instances.

Nursing Role in Thromboembolism

Prevention

The incidence of thrombus formation in the deep veins of the lower extremities can be reduced by thoughtful nursing care. The basic objective is to prevent venous stasis. Several measures are used for this purpose. During the period of bed rest after myocardial infarction the nurse should assist the patient in performing passive exercises at regular intervals. In addition, the patient should be encouraged to flex and extend his feet against a footboard. Elastic stockings may be applied to prevent venous pooling. If support stockings are used it is important to verify that they remain in proper position and do not produce a tourniquet effect. Placing pillows (or elevating the gatch of the bed) under the knees must be avoided, since they can obstruct venous flow in the extremities. The nurse should caution the patient about straining at defecation, and provide stool softeners or laxatives if needed.

Recognition of the Problem

Because pulmonary embolism often resembles acute myocardial infarction, the nurse must consider the possibility that recurrent chest pain may be due to an embolic complication. Whenever pulmonary embolism is suspected, the nurse should record a 12-lead ECG and prepare for arterial blood gas studies. Routine inspection of the legs for signs of thrombophlebitis (warmth, tenderness, or swelling) is important, particularly in high-risk patients.

Cerebral infarction can be recognized without difficulty. If the patient suddenly develops motor weakness, paralysis, or a speech disturbance, the physician should be notified at once.

Survival after peripheral embolism depends for the most part on the rapidity with which arterial blood flow can be surgically reestablished after occlusion has occurred; therefore the nursing role in detecting this complication at its onset is of crucial importance. Any delay in recognizing the problem increases the likelihood of irreversible tissue damage.

Treatment Program

With few exceptions, anticoagulant therapy is used in treating thromboembolic complications. The most rapid and effective method of anticoagulation is a constant intravenous infusion of heparin. This route of administration is preferable to intermittent dosages since it permits better anticoagulant control and reduces the risk of bleeding complications. A continuous intravenous drip containing 20,000 units of heparin in 500 cc dextrose solution is administered at a rate (usually 500-750 units per hour) that will achieve and maintain the activated partial thromboplastin time (APTT) at 2 to 2.5 the normal control value. The APTT level should be checked in 4-6 hours after heparin therapy is started and then once a day. Intravenous heparin may also be administered intermittently by way of a heparin lock positioned in a peripheral vein. The usual dosage with this method is 5000 to 10,000 units every 4-6 hours, depending on the APTT or clotting time.

During the course of anticoagulant therapy the nurse must observe the patient carefully for signs of bleeding. Excessive doses of anticoagulant drugs can cause hemorrhage anywhere in the body, but the most common bleeding sites are the skin, kidneys, and gastrointestinal tract. Careful examination of the body surface should be made during routine nursing care to detect evidence of ecchymosis. The urine and stools must be observed on each occasion. Any evidence of bleeding should be reported to the physician promptly. Anticoagulant therapy may have to be discontinued or anticoagulant antagonists (protamine sulfate or vitamin K_1) administered.

VENTRICULAR RUPTURE

Rupture of the ventricle is the least common of the major complications of acute myocardial infarction; however, it is the most lethal and probably accounts for 5% of all hospital deaths from myocardial infarction.

Ventricular rupture is nearly always associated with extensive transmural infarction involving through-and-through myocardial necrosis. The perforation, which develops suddenly, occurs in the center of the necrotic area (or at the junction of the infarcted area with healthy tissue) and is apparently due to softening and weakening of the muscle fibers. The rupture may involve either the outer wall of the left ventricle or the interventricular septal wall; the former site is about 10 times more common.

When the outer ventricular wall ruptures, blood rushes through the hole in the ventricle and instantly fills the surrounding pericardial sac. This extravasation of blood into the closed pericardium produces compression of the heart (*cardiac tamponade*) and prevents ventricular filling. Death usually occurs within minutes. When the rupture involves the interventricular septum (rather than the outer ventricular wall) the outcome is not necessarily fatal immediately, but the prognosis is very poor. In this situation blood from the left ventricle is forced into the right ventricle (because of the difference in pressures of the respective ventricles) and produces abrupt right ventricular overloading and, in turn, severe right heart failure.

For many years it was believed that physical activity during the early period after infarction was a major factor in causing ventricular rupture. It now appears that this concept is incorrect since many ruptures occur despite complete bed rest. Moreover, about one-third of cardiac ruptures develop within the first 2 days after hospitalization. Sustained hypertension and the use of anticoagulant therapy have also been incriminated as possible causes of ventricular rupture, but there is little evidence to substantiate either of these relationships. Perhaps the most significant factor in the development of ventricular rupture is the size and extent of the infarction and the degree of collateral circulation to the involved area. Curiously, ventricular rupture occurs more frequently in women than in men and is the only complication of acute myocardial infarction with a female preponderance; the reason for this is uncertain. The highest incidence of ventricular rupture is in the seventh decade of life.

Clinical Manifestations of Ventricular Rupture

Rupture of the outer ventricular wall is nearly always manifested by *sudden* death. Occasionally the patient may complain of recurrent chest pain just before the event, and a sudden fall in blood pressure and abrupt slowing of the heart rate is noted. Clinically, the picture is that of an arrhythmic death. Although the mechanical (pumping) action of the heart ceases immediately after cardiac rupture, the heart's electrical activity may persist for many minutes or longer (because electrical impulses continue to be generated even though the ventricles cannot contract). Thus during resuscitation attempts electrical activity may be noted on the cardiac monitor although the patient is dead.

When the interventricular septum perforates, the diagnosis can often be suspected by the sudden appearance of a loud systolic murmur which was not present previously. This finding, coupled with the abrupt development of *right* heart failure (due to the opening between the left and right ventricles), strongly suggests septal rupture. The diagnosis can be confirmed with the use of the Swan-Ganz catheter. A marked increase in oxygen saturation is found in the right heart (reflecting the passage of oxygenated blood from the left ventricle into the right ventricle).

Treatment of Ventricular Rupture

Rupture of the outer ventricular wall almost invariably produces death before any corrective measures can be attempted. Indeed the only hope for survival is immediate repair of the rupture site with excision of the infarcted area (infarctectomy). This procedure has been attempted very rarely, but with the growing availability of heart surgery teams it is conceivable that this form of emergency surgery may be used more often.

Unlike rupture of the ventricular wall, rupture of the septum does not necessarily result in immediate death, and there is an opportunity for surgical intervention in many cases.

Nursing Role in Ventricular Rupture

If sudden death occurs from ventricular rupture the nurse must make certain that the catastrophe is not in fact due to a treatable and reversible cause, specifically ventricular fibrillation or standstill. Cardiopulmonary resuscitation should be attempted immediately and continued until it is definitely ascertained that an arrhythmia is not responsible for the death-producing event.

Because of the potential ability to repair an interventricular septal rupture, the nurse should notify the physician immediately in the event a patient suddenly develops right heart failure associated with the appearance of a loud systolic precordial murmur. Preparation should be made promptly for the insertion of a Swan-Ganz catheter since the physician will confirm the diagnosis by measuring the pressure and arterial oxygen saturation in the right ventricle by means of this device.

CARDIAC ARRHYTHMIAS

Arrhythmias are by far the most frequent complication of acute myocardial infarction. At least 90% of all patients with acute infarction develop some disturbance in the rate, rhythm, or conduction of the heartbeat. Prior to the introduction of the system of intensive coronary care, nearly half of all myocardial infarction deaths were due to this single cause. Because of the extreme importance of arrhythmic complications, the remaining chapters of this book are dedicated to the identification and treatment of each of the common arrhythmias.

8

The Electrocardiographic Interpretation of Arrhythmias

Arrhythmias, by far the most frequent complication of acute myocardial infarction, can only be identified specifically by means of an electrocardiogram (ECG). Therefore it is absolutely essential that CCU nurses acquire a basic, usable knowledge of electrocardiography, at least as it pertains to the recognition of arrhythmias. The object of this and the following chapters is to describe the electrocardiographic basis of arrhythmia detection and interpretation.*

FUNDAMENTALS OF ELECTROCARDIOGRAPHY

Impulse Formation

Each normal heartbeat is the result of an electrical impulse that originates in a specialized area in the wall of the right atrium called the *sinoatrial (SA)*

---

*When we conceived the nurse-centered system of intensive coronary care it was our impression that nurses required a comprehensive course in electrocardiography not unlike that offered to house officers. Experience has shown, however, that an overly detailed training program is unnecessary and that nurses can fulfill their roles successfully with considerably less instruction than anticipated. The following discussion therefore focuses only on those aspects of electrocardiography that permit the nurse to assume clinical responsibilities in the CCU.

node. This island of tissue serves as a "battery" for the heart and normally discharges an electrical force 60 to 100 times a minute in rhythmic fashion. Because the SA node controls the heart rate it is designated the *pacemaker.* However, most other areas of the heart also have the potential ability to initiate impulses (an inherent property of cardiac muscle), but they assume this role only under abnormal circumstances. Whenever the SA node is displaced as the pacemaker the new site of impulse formation is called an *ectopic* pacemaker.

Conduction of Impulse

The original impulse is transmitted from the atria to the ventricles along a network of specialized cells called the *conduction system.* When the impulse reaches and stimulates the ventricular muscles, myocardial contraction occurs.

The electrical conduction from the SA node to the contractile cells of the ventricle is seen in Figure 8.1.

The Cardiac Cycle

When an impulse from the SA node (or an ectopic pacemaker) stimulates the Purkinje-myocardial cells, it causes a discharge of electrical forces that have been stored within the cell membrane. This electrical process is called *depolarization;* it results in myocardial contraction. After depolarization occurs, the

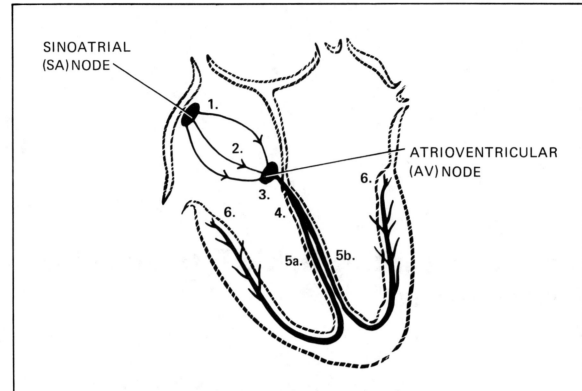

A. The impulse originates in the *SA node* (1).

B. It spreads through the atrial muscles along three bands of tissue known as the *internodal tracts* (2), causing atrial contraction.

C. It reaches the *AV node* (3) where it is momentarily slowed before passing on to the *bundle of His* (4).

D. The impulse descends through the bundle of His and down the *right and left bundle branches* (5A and 5B).

E. Reaching the terminal *Purkinje fibers* (6) the impulse stimulates the ventricular myocardial cells at the Purkinje-myocardial junction.

F. Ventricular contraction then occurs.

Figure 8.1. The conduction system of the heart.

muscle cells recover and restore electrical charges. This recovery process is called *repolarization*. Under normal circumstances the next impulse from the SA node arrives when repolarization has been completed, after which activation can occur again. The combined periods of stimulation (depolarization) and recovery (repolarization) constitute the electrical events of the cardiac cycle.*

---

*The discharge and the storage of electrical forces within the myocardial cells during depolarization and repolarization are associated with a chemical process involving the exchange of sodium and potassium ions across the myocardial cell membrane. This subject is discussed in Chapter 16.

THE ELECTROCARDIOGRAM

The electrical activity associated with depolarization and repolarization of cardiac muscle can be recorded and analyzed by means of electrocardiography. The basis of the technique is as follows: electrical currents emanating from the heart are transmitted through surrounding tissues to the body surface where they can be detected by electrodes placed on the extremities (or the chest wall). These electrical forces are then directed through a sensitive galvonometer (the basic component of an electrocardiographic machine), which produces a series of upward and downward deflections according to changes in the heart's electrical activity. The resulting waves are then amplified (for greater visibility) before being inscribed on a moving strip of graph paper; the graphic recording is called an electrocardiogram.* Analysis of the wave forms permits the identification of cardiac arrhythmias and the diagnosis of acute myocardial infarction (among many other conditions).

Electrocardiographic Leads

Because the electrical forces generated by the heart travel in multiple directions simultaneously, it is necessary to record the flow of current in several different planes if a comprehensive view of the heart's electrical activity is to be obtained. There are three major planes for detecting electrical activity, called lead I, lead II, and lead III, which are recorded by placing electrodes on the right arm, left arm, and left leg. (In practice, a fourth electrode is placed on the right leg; it serves as a ground electrode and is not a part of an electrical lead.) Each of the three leads records the difference in electrical forces between two electrode sites. As shown in Figure 8.2, lead I is derived from electrodes on the right arm and left arm; lead II from electrodes on the right arm and left leg; and lead III from electrodes on the left arm and left leg. From an electrical standpoint, a hypothetical triangle (called the Einthoven triangle) is formed by these three leads with the heart in the center. In other words, each lead is electrically equidistant from the heart.

Since these leads record electrical forces in three different planes, it is understandable that an ECG obtained from each of the leads will have a different appearance. An example of the variation of electrocardiographic patterns in leads I, II, and III (recorded simultaneously) is depicted in Figure 8.3.

To understand why the electrocardiographic deflections (waves) differ in the three leads it is necessary to consider briefly a fundamental principle of electricity: electrical current flows between two poles (or electrodes), one of which is positive (+) and the other negative (−).

When the current flows *toward* the positive pole, the electrocardiograph will record an upward (positive) deflection:

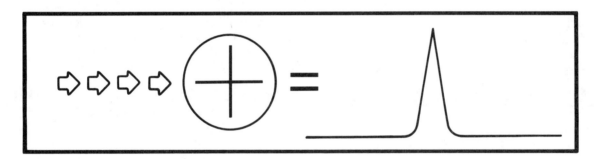

Conversely, when the current flows *away* from the positive electrode, the electrocardiograph will record a downward (negative) deflection:

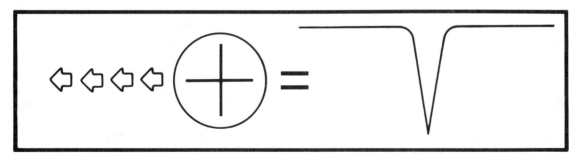

The respective positions of the positive (+) and negative (−) electrodes in leads I, II, and III are shown in Figure 8.4. Thus the deflection (waves) observed on an ECG depend on which lead is recorded.

A complete electrocardiograph consists of 12 separate leads: the 3 standard leads (I, II, and III), 3

---

*The instrument which receives electrical impulses from the heart and transforms them into a graphic record is called an *electrocardiograph*. The printed record obtained from the electrocardiograph is an electrocardiogram.

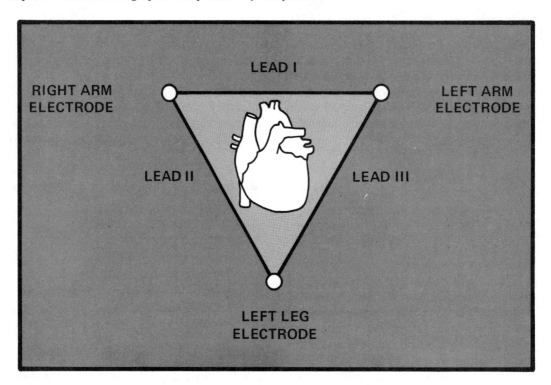

Figure 8.2. Standard electrocardiographic leads.

modified (augmented) leads (aVR, aVL, and aVF), and 6 leads positioned across the chest wall (V1, V2, V3, V4, V5, and V6). A full 12-lead electrocardiogram is reproduced in Figure 8.5. Note that each lead produces a different electrocardiographic pattern because of the variation of the electrode positions.

Monitoring Leads

Cardiac monitors depict only a single lead, which is determined by the position of the positive and negative electrodes attached to the chest wall. Using the conventional electrode position the resultant lead is similar to standard lead II. With a modified chest electrode position the lead is equivalent to lead V1. While these two chest leads are the most useful for detecting the majority of arrhythmias, by no means can they identify all rhythm disturbances. It is important to recognize this limitation of cardiac monitoring and when the interpretation of an arrhythmia is in doubt the chest leads may have to be repositioned (to obtain a more distinctive lead), or a 12-lead electrocardiogram recorded.

It must also be understood that the ECG seen on the monitor will depend on which particular lead is being used; therefore attempting simply to memorize certain patterns as a means of identifying arrhythmias is of no avail. For example, the ECGs shown in Figure 8.6 were recorded simultaneously from a conventional (lead II) monitoring lead and from a modified (V1) lead. The difference in the appearance of the wave forms in the two leads makes it readily apparent that memorizing patterns is not a useful way to learn the interpretation of arrhythmias.

ELECTROCARDIOGRAPHIC WAVE FORMS

The electrical activity during the cardiac cycle is characterized by five separate waves or deflections which are designated as P, Q, R, S, and T; these letters were arbitrarily selected and have no additional meaning. Before considering the meaning of each of these deflections it is necessary to discuss two key features of electrocardiographic waves: their amplitude (or voltage) and their duration.

Amplitude (voltage) is measured by a series of horizontal lines on the ECG. Each horizontal line is 1 millimeter apart and represents one-tenth of a millivolt (the basic unit of intensity of the heart's electrical activity). Thus in Figure 8.7 we see that the deflection extends nine lines (9 millimeters) above the baseline; this indicates that the voltage of the wave is 0.9 millivolt. The amplitude of the wave reflects only its electrical force and has no relation to the muscular strength of ventricular contraction.

Duration of a wave is measured by a series of vertical lines, also 1 millimeter apart. The time interval between each vertical line is 0.04 second. Accordingly, the width of the deflection shown in Figure 8.7 extends for 3 millimeters and represents 0.12 second (0.04 × 3).

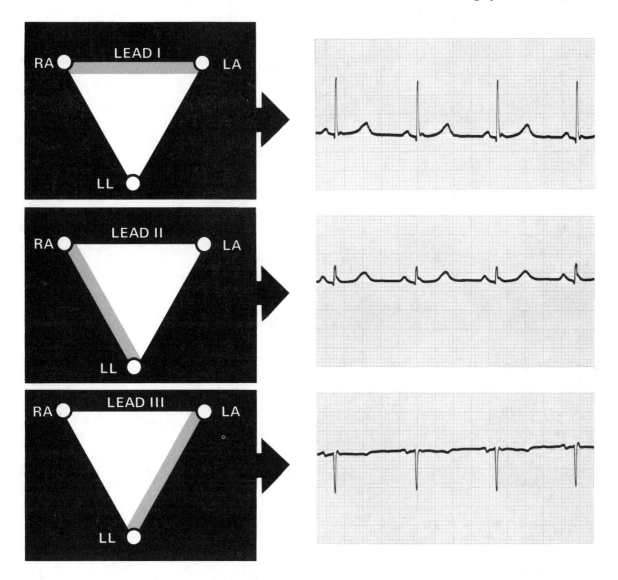

Figure 8.3. Electrocardiographic patterns as recorded from leads, I, II, and III.

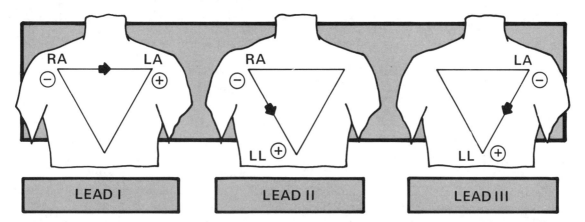

Figure 8.4. Positions of positive (+) and negative (−) electrodes for lead I, lead II, and lead III. RA = right arm, LA = left arm, LL = left leg.

The relationship between voltage and time is demonstrated in the ECG in Figure 8.8.

To simplify the measurement of the wave forms, every *fifth* line, both horizontally and vertically, is inscribed boldly, producing a series of larger squares. These large squares then represent 0.5 millivolt vertically and 0.20 second horizontally, as shown in Figure 8.9.

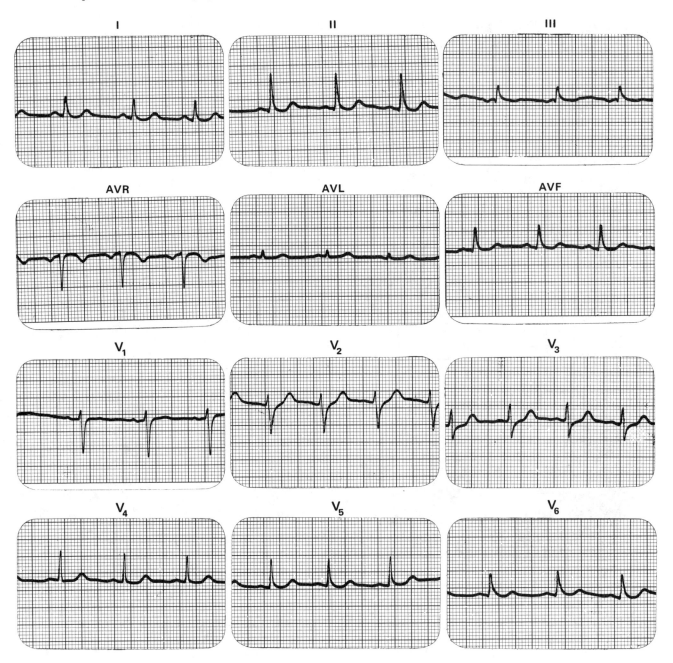

Figure 8.5. A 12-lead electrocardiogram.

The Normal Electrocardiogram

A normal electrocardiogram consists of a series of five successive waves designated by the letters P, Q, R, S, T. The significance of each of these waves is described below but, in brief, the P wave represents electrical activation (depolarization) of the atria; and the QRS complex of the ventricles; the T wave is produced by ventricular recovery (repolarization). The distances between the waves are called intervals or segments. The configuration of one complete ECG complex demonstrating the waves and intervals is seen in Figure 8.10.

P Wave

This wave represents the electrical activity associated with the original impulse from the SA node and its passage through the atria.

If P waves are present and are of normal size and shape it can be assumed that the stimulus began in the SA node. If these waves are absent or abnormally positioned, it implies the impulse originated outside the SA node. Therefore the identification of P waves is of critical importance in differentiating normal sinus rhythm from *ectopic* rhythms.

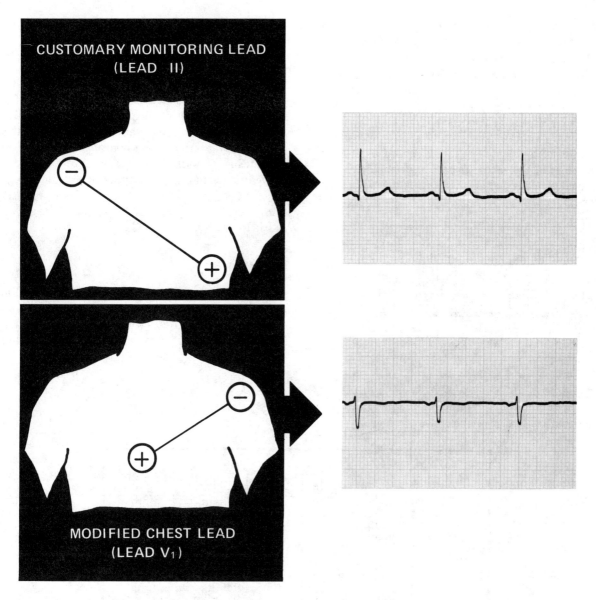

Figure 8.6. Electrocardiograms recorded simultaneously from conventional and modified chest leads.

P-R Interval

The period from the beginning of the P wave to the beginning of the QRS complex is designated the P-R interval. It represents the time taken for the original impulse to pass from the SA node, through the atria and AV node, to the ventricles.

With normal conduction the duration of this interval is no more than 0.20 second. If the duration of the P-R interval exceeds 0.20 second it can be reasoned that a conduction delay (block) exists in the area of the AV node (or less likely, below the AV node). In some instances the P-R interval is unusually short (less than 0.10 second), which indicates that the impulse reached the ventricle through a shorter-than-normal (accessory) pathway. Abnormally short P-R intervals are observed in the Wolff-Parkinson-White syndrome and the Lown-Ganong-Levine syndrome

(as described in the chapters on conduction disorders).

QRS Complex

These waves represent depolarization of the ventricular muscle. The depolarization process starts at the endocardium of the ventricle and progresses outward to the epicardial surface. This results in a complex consisting of an initial downward deflection (Q wave), a tall upward deflection (R wave), and a second downward deflection (S wave). These three deflections comprising the QRS complex vary in size according to the lead being recorded. For example, there may be a tall R wave and a small S wave (Figure 8.11A) or a small R wave and a deep S wave (Figure 8.11B). In many instances, again depending on lead placement, one or more of the three components in the

QRS complex may not be seen. For instance, in Figure 8.11C the complex does not include a Q wave.

The QRS interval is measured from the beginning of the Q wave to the end of the S wave. (If a Q wave, R wave, or S wave is absent the QRS complex is measured from the beginning to the end of the remaining waves.) The normal duration of the QRS complex is always *less* than 0.12 sedond. When the duration of the complex is 0.12 second or more it indicates that the ventricles have been stimulated in a delayed or abnormal manner (e.g., a bundle branch block).

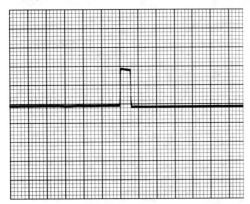

Figure 8.7. Measurement of wave amplitude (voltage).

ST Segment

This interval describes the time period between the completion of depolarization and the beginning of repolarization (recovery) of the ventricular muscles. Normally this segment is *isoelectric*, meaning it is neither elevated nor depressed because the positive and negative forces are equally balanced during this period. Elevation or depression of the ST segment indicates an abnormality in the onset of recovery of the ventricular muscle, usually because of injury (e.g., acute myocardial infarction). Examples of isoelectric, depressed, and elevated ST segments are shown in Figure 8.12.

T Wave

This wave represents the major portion of the recovery phase after ventricular contraction. Any condition which interferes with normal repolarization (e.g., myocardial ischemia) may cause the T waves to

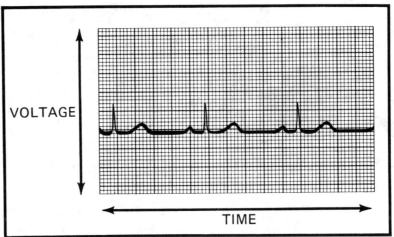

Figure 8.8. Relationship between voltage and time.

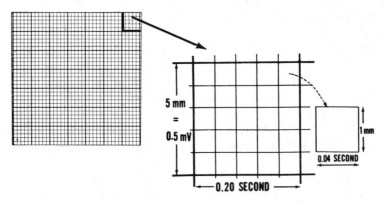

Figure 8.9. Electrocardiographic measurements.

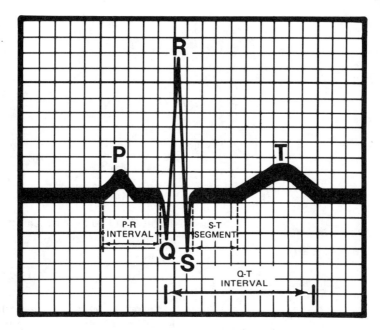

Figure 8.10. Normal electrocardiogram.

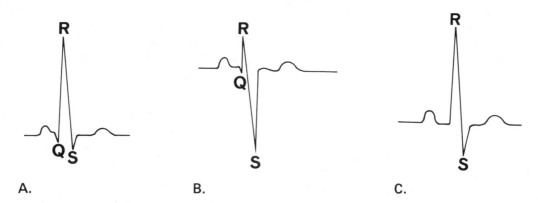

A.   B.   C.

Figure 8.11. Various configurations of QRS complex.

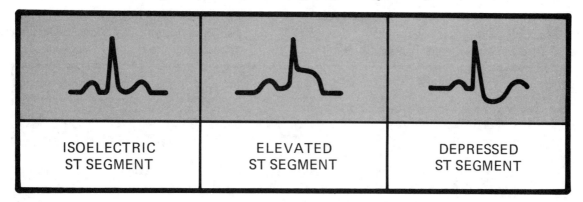

| ISOELECTRIC ST SEGMENT | ELEVATED ST SEGMENT | DEPRESSED ST SEGMENT |

Figure 8.12. ST segments.

invert. Examples of inverted T waves are depicted in Figure 8.13.

QT Interval

This interval defines the total duration of the combined phases of depolarization and repolarization of the ventricular muscle. In other words, it represents the total period of ventricular stimulation and recovery (see Figure 8.10).

The QT interval is measured from the *beginning* of the QRS complex to the *end* of the T wave. The interval varies with heart rate, but with normal sinus rhythm the duration seldom exceeds 0.40 second.

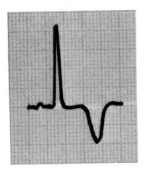 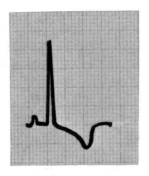 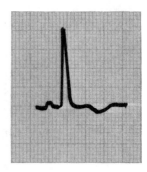

Figure 8.13. Illustrations of inverted T waves.

Significance of the Electrocardiogram

By analyzing the wave forms and intervals just described, certain deductions can be made which offer indirect information about the heart. It is important to realize that the ECG does not depict the actual physical condition of the heart or its function; it simply reveals the electrical activity of the heart. Thus an ECG may be normal in the presence of heart disease unless the pathologic process actually disturbs the electrical forces. For example, a patient may have coronary atherosclerosis which has not produced myocardial ischemia or injury and, consequently, no abnormality will be seen on the ECG.

The ECG, however, can be correlated with the systolic and diastolic phases of ventricular action as shown in Figure 8.14. Note that ventricular contraction (systole) begins at the peak of the QRS complex, after electrical stimulation has occurred, and ends near the completion of the T wave. Diastole commences at this time and continues until the next R wave.

Electrocardiography has many valuable uses in medical practice, but its major importance is in the diagnosis of acute myocardial infarction and the identification of abnormal cardiac rhythms.

ARRHYTHMIAS

A normal cardiac mechanism is characterized by normal sinus rhythm and normal conduction of impulses. *Normal sinus rhythm* means that the SA node controls the heart beat, discharging impulses regularly at a rate of 60-100 per minute. *Normal conduction* indicates there is no obstruction or delay in the passage of impulses from the SA node through the AV node and ventricles. Therefore, among the main features of a normal electrocardiogram are:

1. a heart rate within the normal range of 60-100 per minute
2. regularity of the cardiac rhythm
3. normal P waves, each of which is followed by a ventricular (QRS) complex
4. a P-R interval between 0.10 and 0.20 second in duration
5. a QRS complex ranging from 0.04 to 0.12 second, indicating that sinus node impulses reached both ventricles on schedule.

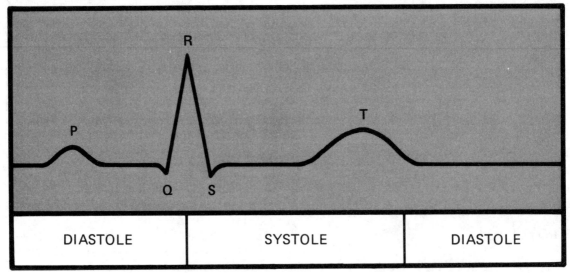

Figure 8.14. Relationship of electrocardiogram to diastole and systole.

Examples of normal electrocardiograms are shown in Figure 8.15.

When either rate, rhythm or conduction fails to conform to normal standards, the resulting disorder is called an *arrhythmia.**

Classification of Arrhythmias

Arrhythmias can be categorized into two main groups, according to their underlying mechanism:

1. disturbances in impulse formation
2. disturbances in conduction of impulses.

Disturbances in Impulse Formation

We know that under normal conditions the SA node serves as the pacemaker for the heart, and that it generates impulses regularly at a rate of 60-100/minute. If for some reason normal sinus rhythm is disrupted either because the SA node discharges abnormally, or because a pacemaker from another site (an ectopic pacemaker) gains control of the heartbeat, the resulting disorder is called a *disturbance in impulse formation.*

Arrhythmias in this category are divided according to the site of the impulse formation as follows:

a) disturbances arising in the SA node (sinus rhythms)
b) disturbances arising in the atria (atrial arrhythmias)
c) disturbances arising in the AV nodal area (nodal or junctional arrhythmias)
d) disturbances arising in the ventricle (ventricular arrhythmias).

These disorders of impulse formation may be further subdivided according to the mechanism of the arrhythmia. There are 6 major arrhythmic mechanisms:

a) tachycardia (heart rate greater than 100/minute)
b) bradycardia (heart rate less than 60/minute)
c) premature (ectopic) beats
d) escape beats
e) flutter
f) fibrillation.

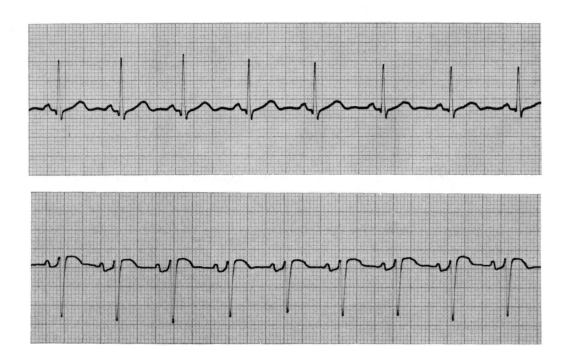

Figure 8.15. Normal electrocardiograms.

---

*In a strict sense the term arrhythmia indicates an absence of normal rhythm and, therefore, might be restricted to this one type of disorder. In practice, however, the term has been used collectively for many years to describe all clinical disorders of the heart beat, including disturbances in rate, rhythm and conduction. Despite its long-established usage, the term arrhythmia has been challenged in recent years by some linguists who feel that the broader word *dysrrhythmia* is more appropriate and should be used instead. It seems to us that a change in terminology at this late date for the sake of linguistic purism serves no purpose and can only lead to confusion. Therefore, as in previous editions of this book, we have retained the term arrhythmia.

Table 8.1. Arrhythmias Due to Disturbances in Impulse Formation

A. *Sinoatrial (SA) Node Arrhythmias*
  Sinus Tachycardia
  Sinus Bradycardia
  Sinus Arrhythmias
  Wandering Pacemaker
  Sinoatrial Arrest

B. *Atrial Arrhythmias*
  Premature Atrial Contractions
  Atrial Tachycardia
  Atrial Flutter
  Atrial Fibrillation
  Atrial Standstill

C. *AV Nodal Area (Junctional) Arrhythmias*
  Premature Junctional Contractions
  Passive Junctional Rhythm (escape beats)
  Paroxysmal Junctional Tachycardia
  Nonparoxysmal Junctional Tachycardia

D. *Ventricular Arrhythmias*
  Premature Ventricular Contractions
  Ventricular Tachycardia
  Ventricular Fibrillation

On the basis of this combined classification (involving site of impulse formation and mechanism of arrhythmia), the term *sinus tachycardia* indicates that the impulse originates in the SA node but that the heart rate is faster than 100/minute (tachycardia). By contrast, *ventricular tachycardia* means that impulses originate in the ventricles (rather than the SA node) at a rate, again, above 100/minute. Similarly, the term *atrial tachycardia* describes an arrhythmia originating in the atria, which produces a heart rate greater than 100/minute. The classification of common arrhythmias due to disturbances in impulse formation is shown in Table 8.1. Each of these arrhythmias is considered separately in the following chapters.

Disturbances of Conduction

A conduction disturbance refers to a block or abnormal delay in the passage of cardiac impulses from the SA node, through the atrioventricular (AV) node, through the left and right bundle branches, to the Purkinje system in the ventricles. Blocks may occur at any point along the course of the conduction system, but it is customary to classify these disorders according to three main anatomic sites with the following subdivisions:

1. **Blocks within the SA node or atria**
   (Sinoatrial Blocks)

2. **Blocks between the atria and ventricles**
   (Atrioventricular (AV) Blocks)
     First-degree AV Block
     Second-degree AV Block
     Third-degree (complete) AV Block

3. **Blocks within the ventricles**
   (Intraventricular Blocks)
     Left Bundle Branch Blocks
     Right Bundle Branch Blocks
     Bilateral Bundle Branch Blocks
     Ventricular Standstill

Classification of Arrhythmias by Prognosis

In addition to the method just described, arrhythmias can also be classified in a general way (but not categorically) according to their seriousness or prognosis. This division of arrhythmias is useful to nurses caring for patients with acute myocardial infarction since it considers the relative importance of various arrhythmias from a clinical standpoint. It is essential to realize, however, that this classification is only a broad index and is not truly dependable in assessing the actual prognosis of an individual arrhythmia. Using this classification three prognostic categories of arrhythmias can be established:

Minor Arrhythmias. These disorders are not of *immediate* concern because they usually do not affect the circulation, nor do they warn of the development of more serious arrhythmias.

Major Arrhythmias. These disturbances either reduce the pumping efficiency of the heart or herald the onset of lethal arrhythmias. They require prompt treatment.

Death-Producing Arrhythmias. These are lethal arrhythmias and require immediate resuscitation in order to prevent death.

The classification of arrhythmias according to seriousness or prognosis is shown in Table 8.2.

Table 8.2. Classification of Arrhythmias According to Prognosis

Minor Arrhythmias	*Major Arrhythmias (cont'd.)*
Sinus Tachycardia	Atrial Fibrillation
Sinus Bradycardia	Passive Junctional Rhythm
Sinus Arrhythmia	Paroxysmal Junctional Tachycardia
Wandering Pacemaker	Nonparoxysmal Junctional Tachycardia
Premature Atrial Contractions	Premature Ventricular Contractions (when frequent or in pairs)
Premature Junctional Contractions	Ventricular Tachycardia
Premature Ventricular Contractions (when infrequent)	First-Degree AV Heart Block
	Second-Degree AV Heart Block
Major Arrhythmias	Third-Degree (Complete) Heart Block
Sinus Tachycardia (when persistent)	Bundle Branch Block
Sinus Bradycardia (when rate is 50 or less per minute)	
Sinoatrial Arrest or Block	*Death-Producing Arrhythmias*
Atrial Tachycardia	Ventricular Fibrillation
Atrial Flutter	Ventricular Standstill

Interpretation of Arrhythmias from the Electrocardiogram

Electrocardiographic interpretation of specific arrhythmias involves a deliberate analysis of cardiac rate, rhythm and conduction. Most arrhythmias can be identified correctly by following the five basic steps described below. Attempting to interpret arrhythmias without adhering to this type of orderly process can only lead to confusion and error.

Step 1. Calculate the heart rate. Four methods may be used to determine the heart rate from the electrocardiogram:

a. Count the number of R waves in a 6-second strip of the ECG tracing. Multiply this sum by 10 to get the heart rate per minute. Since the electrocardiographic paper is marked at 3-second intervals (at the top margin), the approximate heart rate can be estimated very quickly with this simple method, as shown below:

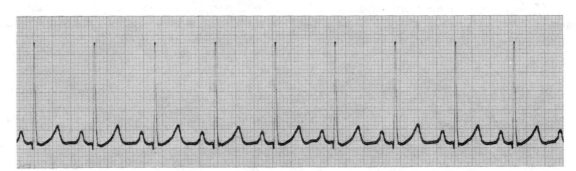

Note that there are 9 R waves in the 6-second ECG strip. Therefore the heart rate is approximately 90/minute (9 × 10).

b. Commercially available rate calculators, which measure the distance between R waves, may be placed on the ECG and the heart rate read directly from the rate scale.

c. Count the number of large squares between two R waves and divide this sum into 300 to obtain the rate per minute. For example, in the ECG shown below there are 4 large squares between two consecutive R waves. Dividing 300 by 4 indicates that the heart rate is 75/minute.

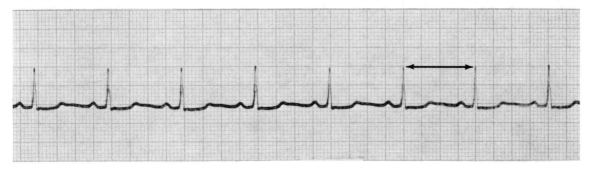

d. Count the number of small squares between two R waves (an R-R interval) and convert this sum into heart rate by using a rate conversion table. (A rate conversion table is found on the inner side of the back cover of this book.) In the ECG depicted below each R-R interval consists of 12 small squares. Thus the heart rate, as determined from the rate conversion table, is 125/minute. This method of rate calculation is more accurate than those described above, but it can be used if the heart rhythm is regular.

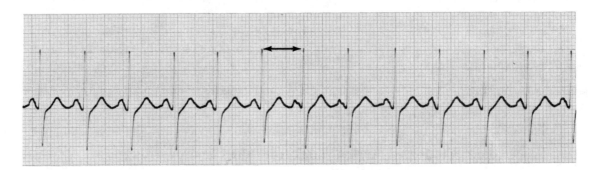

On the basis of heart rate determination alone, arrhythmias can be classified as: a) slow rate (*brady-arrhythmias*), where there are less than 60 beats/minute; b) normal rate arrhythmias, where the rate is between 60-100 beats/minute; and c) fast rate (*tachy-arrhythmias*), where there are more than 100 beats/minute. Since many arrhythmias are characterized only by rate changes, rate calculation is essential in interpreting any ECG.

Step 2. Determine the regularity (rhythm) of the R waves. The regularity of the heart beat can often be determined by simply looking at the ECG: If the R-R intervals are equal, without any obvious variation in their length, it can be concluded that the rhythm is regular. In many instances, however, scanning is unreliable and it is necessary to measure the R-R intervals precisely with ECG calipers to ascertain if the R waves are in fact regular. When the difference between R-R intervals is more than 0.12 second, the ventricular rhythm is described as abnormal or irregular. Many arrhythmias are characterized by either regular or irregular rhythms and therefore this single finding is an important step in the process of arrhythmia interpretation. An example of a regular ventricular rhythm is shown below. Note that there are 19 small squares between each R wave.

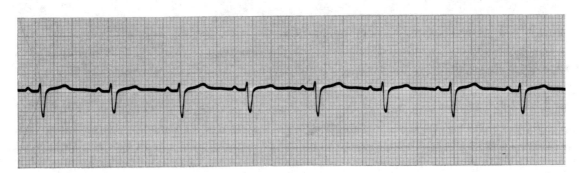

An example of an irregular ventricular rhythm is depicted in the following ECG. The R-R intervals vary from 1.02 second to 1.40 second.

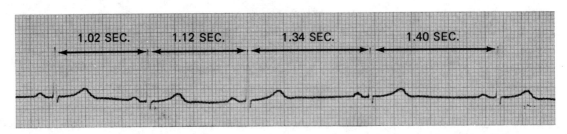

Step 3. Identify and examine the P waves. Although usually less conspicuous than the other waves of the cardiac cycle, P waves often provide more information about the type and mechanism of a cardiac arrhythmia than any of the other wave forms. For this reason it is mandatory to search for P waves and to examine their size, shape, and position. A normal P wave (as seen in the standard monitoring lead) is upright, smoothly rounded, and precedes each QRS complex. If these findings exist, it means that the heart beat originates in the SA node and sinus rhythm is present. In contrast, the absence of P waves or an abnormality in configuration or position indicates that impulses arise outside the SA node and that an ectopic pacemaker is in control. In the following ECG P waves cannot be identified, reflecting an ectopic pacemaker below the SA node.

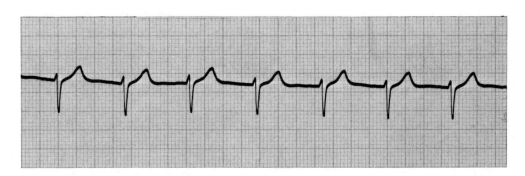

Step 4. Measure the P-R interval. Normally the duration of this interval should be between 0.10 and 0.20 second. Prolongation of the P-R interval beyond 0.20 second indicates a delay in the passage of impulses from the SA node to the ventricle. Conversely, a P-R interval of less than 0.10 second indicates that sinus impulses reach the ventricles sooner than expected through an abnormal pathway (called an accessory pathway). The P-R interval of the ECG shown below is within normal limits (0.16 second).

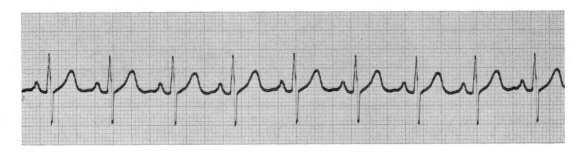

Step 5. Measure the duration of the QRS complexes. The width of the QRS complex represents the time required for a stimulus to activate both ventricles. The normal duration of the QRS complex is no more than 0.12 second. If there is an obstruction in one of the bundle branches, activation of the ventricles will be delayed, as manifested electrocardiographically, by widening of the QRS complex beyond 0.10 second. Two examples of abnormally widened QRS complexes (greater than 0.12 second) are depicted.

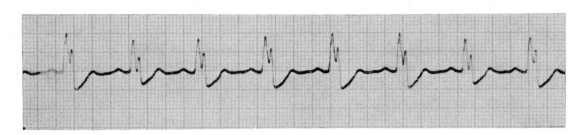

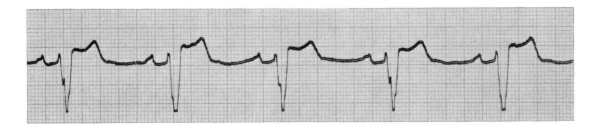

Interpretation of Specific Arrhythmias

The application of the five-step orderly process just described in identifying and interpreting specific arrhythmias is considered in the following paragraphs, using the ECG shown in Figure 8.16 as the first example.

5. QRS Complexes. These complexes of ventricular activation measure 0.06 second, indicating that there is no conduction disorder in the bundle branches or the Purkinje network.

Interpretation: Analyzing these facts, we can conclude that the only abnormality detected in the ECG is a rate of about 40/minute, which is distinctly

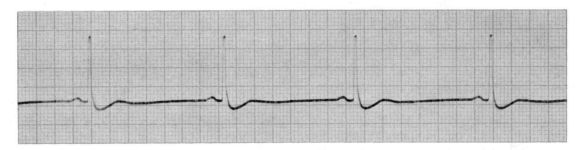

Figure 8.16.

Analysis of ECG

1. Heart Rate. There are 4 R waves in the 6 second ECG strip. This means that the heart rate is approximately 40/minute. (Since the R-R intervals consist of 37 small squares, the heart rate, according to the rate conversion table, is actually 41/minute.)

2. Rhythm. The R-R intervals are essentially equal (varying by only one small square, a normal finding). We know therefore that this arrhythmia is characterized by a regular rhythm.

3. P Waves. A P wave occurs before each QRS complex and is normal in configuration. This indicates that the impulses originated in the SA node.

4. P-R Interval. This interval measures 0.16 second (4 small squares), which is within normal limits (0.10 to 0.20 second). Consequently, we can infer that conduction from the SA node to the ventricles is not disturbed.

below the lower limits of normal (60/minute). Since there are no disturbances in conduction (both the P-R interval and the QRS complexes are normal) we know that the slow heart rate is due to a *disturbance in impulse formation.* The presence of a normal P wave before each QRS complex tells us that the site of impulse formation is in the SA node itself. However the SA node is discharging too slowly, which accounts for the heart rate of 40/minute. Thus the interpretation of this arrhythmia is *sinus bradycardia.*

Another demonstration of the five basic steps used in arrhythmia interpretation is presented in Figure 8.17.

Analysis of ECG

1. Heart rate. That there are 7 R waves in 6 seconds indicates that the heart rate is approximately 70/minute. (Since the R-R intervals are comprised of 21 small squares, the precise heart rate is 72/minute.)

2. Rhythm. The R waves occur at very regular intervals and therefore the rhythm can be categorized as regular.

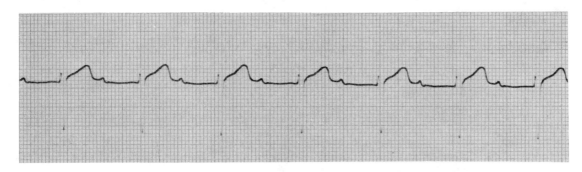

Figure 8.17.

3. P waves. A normal P wave precedes each QRS complex, indicating a sinus rhythm.

4. P-R interval. The time from the beginning of a P wave to the onset of a QRS complex is 0.44 second (11 small squares). This interval is markedly prolonged, far exceeding the top normal P-R interval (0.20 second).

5. QRS complexes. These complexes are 0.06 second in duration and show no abnormalities.

Interpretation: Based on the information obtained from the ECG it can be concluded that impulse formation is normal: the impulses originate in the SA node at a rate of 70/minute with a regular rhythm—the criteria of normal sinus rhythm. However, conduction is not normal: the P-R interval is distinctly prolonged (0.44 second), indicating a delay in the passage of impulses somewhere between the SA node and the ventricles. Since the QRS complexes are of normal duration (0.06 second) we know that once the delayed impulse reached the bundle branches it proceeded normally thereafter and stimulated the ventricles. The delay is at the level of the atrioventricular (AV) node. This particular *disturbance in conduction* is called a *first-degree atrioventricular (AV) block,* the details of which are described in later chapters.

9

Arrhythmias Originating in the Sinoatrial (SA) Node

SINUS TACHYCARDIA
SINUS BRADYCARDIA
SINUS ARRHYTHMIA
WANDERING PACEMAKER
SINOATRIAL ARREST (AND SA BLOCK)

This group of arrhythmias results from disturbances of impulse formation in the SA node.

The SA node retains its normal role as pacemaker, but instead of discharging impulses at regular intervals 60-100 times/minute the rate either exceeds 100/minute (sinus tachycardia) or is less than 60/minute (sinus bradycardia), or the node does not discharge rhythmically (sinus arrhythmia). In some instances the pacemaker site wanders from the SA node to nearby areas (wandering pacemaker). If the SA node fails to discharge an impulse at the expected time, the arrhythmia is called sinus arrest.

Impulse formation in the SA mode is under the control of the sympathetic and parasympathetic nervous systems. Overactivity of one of these normally balanced forces leads to disturbances in rate, rhythm, or site of impulse formation. When the sympathetic system is dominant the heart rate speeds, and when the parasympathetic system (vagal influence) is in control the rate slows. The node itself is seldom the source of these arrhythmic disturbances, but ischemic damage to the SA node can occur from myocardial infarction.

As a general rule, sinus node disorders are not dangerous and can be considered as minor arrhythmias. However, if the heart rate is very slow (less than 50/minute) or very fast (greater than 130/minute) the risk is significantly increased, in which case the arrhythmia would be classified as a major arrhythmia.

SINUS TACHYCARDIA

Mechanism

The SA node is the pacemaker and discharges impulses regularly at a rate faster than 100/minute. This acceleration in heart rate often reflects overactivity of the sympathetic nervous system resulting from fever, anxiety, or physical activity. Of greater importance, sinus tachycardia may be a manifestation of heart failure. In this situation the heart rate increases through reflex mechanisms to compensate for reduced stroke volume.

Danger in Acute Myocardial Infarction

1. Tachycardia tends to increase the work of the heart and its oxygen consumption. This expenditure may lead to heart failure, myocardial ischemia (angina), or possibly an increase in the size of an infarction, particularly if the rapid rate is persistent.
2. *RISK:* The danger depends primarily on the etiology of the fast heart rate. When sinus tachycardia is due to anxiety, fever, or physical activity, the risk is usually not great. On the other hand, if sinus tachycardia develops as a consequence of heart failure, the danger is distinctly increased and the prognosis then varies with the cardiac reserve and the duration of the tachycardia.

Clinical Features

1. In most instances, sinus tachycardia does not produce any symptoms. However, if the tachycardia is very rapid or sustained, patients may develop angina or dyspnea.
2. The only pertinent physical finding is a fast, regular heart rate, usually 100-150/minute. An ECG is required to distinguish sinus tachycardia from other tachyarrhythmias.
3. Sinus tachycardia terminates gradually, unlike other tachycardias (e.g., paroxysmal atrial tachycardia) which cease abruptly.

Treatment

1. The first step in treatment is to identify the underlying cause of the arrhythmia rather than attempt to slow the rate. Always to be considered is the possibility that sinus tachycardia represents a sign of early left ventricular failure.
2. Once the cause of sinus tachycardia is recognized, treatment is directed at correction of the basic problem. For example, when the rapid rate is due to temperature elevation, aspirin may be effective; or if the tachycardia is secondary to anxiety, tranquilizers or sedatives may be helpful in reducing the rate.
3. If sinus tachycardia produces ischemic pain, opiates may be indicated.
4. When sinus tachycardia is due to left ventricular failure, administration of digitalis is usually effective in controlling the heart rate (as well as in increasing the force of myocardial contraction).
5. Drug therapy aimed solely at reducing the heart rate, without consideration of the underlying cause of sinus tachycardia, is ill advised.

Nursing Role

1. Identify the rapid-rate arrhythmia as sinus tachycardia and document it with a rhythm strip.
2. Examine the patient at regular intervals, always seeking possible causes for the arrhythmia (e.g., elevated temperature, apprehension).
3. When the source of sinus tachycardia cannot be readily identified, be suspicious that left ventricular failure exists and attempt to elicit other evidence of early heart failure (e.g., orthopnea, cough, restlessness).
4. If the patient develops symptoms secondary to the arrhythmia or if the clinical signs change, the physician should be notified.
5. Discuss the use of sedatives, tranquilizers, aspirin, and digitalis with the physician.
6. If anxiety seems to be the cause of sinus tachycardia, attempt to alleviate the emotional stress through nursing intervention.

SINUS TACHYCARDIA—IDENTIFYING ECG FEATURES

1. Rate:	Usually 100-150 beats/minute.
2. Rhythm:	Regular.
3. P waves:	Normal, and precede each QRS complex.
4. P-R interval:	Normal, indicating that conduction from the SA node through the ventricles is not disturbed.
5. QRS:	Normal.

Sinus Tachycardia (Figure 9.1)

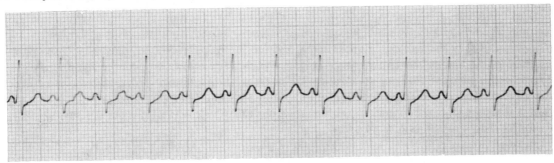

Rate:	About 130/minute (Actual rate: 125/minute).
Rhythm:	Regular.
P waves:	Normal, and precede each QRS complex.
P-R interval:	Normal (0.12 second).
QRS:	Normal (duration 0.08 second).
Comment:	Other than the rapid heart rate no other abnormalities are present.

Sinus Tachycardia (Figure 9.2)

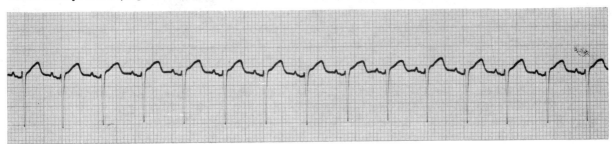

Rate:	About 140/minute (136/minute).
Rhythm:	Regular.
P waves:	Normal.
P-R interval:	Normal (0.12 second).
QRS:	Normal (0.04 second).
Comment:	Note the difference in the configuration of the QRS complexes in the two examples shown. Figure 9.1 was recorded with a conventional monitoring lead (lead II) while Figure 9.2 was recorded with a modified chest lead (MCL).

CASE HISTORY

A 42-year-old male has been in the CCU for 2 days with a stable pulse rate ranging from 75-90/minute. An ECG showed an acute anterior infarction with normal sinus rhythm. While his wife was visiting, the patient became obviously upset and the monitor showed sinus tachycardia at a rate of 130/minute. The nurse assessed the clinical condition of the patient and could find no change other than the rapid heart rate. She calmed the patient by talking with him and continued to assess the heart rate. In addition she administered an ordered sedative. One hour later the pulse rate was 90/minute.

SINUS BRADYCARDIA

Mechanism

Sinus bradycardia exists when the SA node discharges regularly at a rate slower than 60 beats/minute. The underlying cause of the slow rate is parasympathetic (vagal) dominance of the SA node, resulting from either pain, drugs, myocardial ischemia, or other factors (including sleep). Sinus bradycardia occurs more frequently with acute inferior myocardial infarction than acute anterior infarction (because of ischemia of the SA node).

Danger in Acute Myocardial Infarction

1. The main threat of sinus bradycardia is that it may allow a faster ectopic focus to take over as pacemaker. Ventricular rates below 50/minute predispose to serious ventricular and atrial arrhythmias.
2. The slow rate may also reduce cardiac output, particularly in elderly patients, thus reducing coronary and cerebral blood flow. In this circumstance, angina, syncope or heart failure may develop.
3. *RISK:* Sinus bradycardia with heart rates of less than 50/minute can lead to several arrhythmic and hemodynamic complications (particularly in the first hours after infarction) and for this reason must be regarded as a *warning* arrhythmia. When the rate is more than 50/minute, sinus bradycardia is usually well tolerated and classified as a minor arrhythmia.

Clinical Features

1. Sinus bradycardia seldom produces symptoms unless the rate is slow enough to reduce cardiac output.
2. The only physical sign is a slow, regular heart rate, usually 40-60 beats/minute.

Treatment

1. Sinus bradycardia should be treated only under the following circumstances:
   a. if there are any signs or symptoms indicating a reduction in cardiac output (syncope, hypotension, angina, or heart failure)
   b. if premature ventricular contractions develop during the period of bradycardia
   c. if the rate is persistently less than 50/minute, particularly in elderly patients or those with previous myocardial damage.
2. Atropine, which blocks the vagal effect on the SA node, is usually effective in accelerating the heart rate and should be the initial therapy. The drug is given intravenously in a dosage of 0.5-1.0 mg.
3. If atropine is unsuccessful, isoproterenol (Isuprel) will often increase the heart rate. This agent is administered by a slow intravenous infusion containing 1 mg isoproterenol in 500 cc glucose solution.
4. If drug therapy fails, or if its effect is short-lived, temporary transvenous pacing may be required to maintain a normal heart rate, particularly if heart failure is present.
5. Drugs with known bradycardic effects such as digitalis, reserpine, morphine, or beta-blocking agents should be avoided or discontinued in the presence of sinus bradycardia.

Nursing Role

1. Carefully review the ECG to ascertain that the slow rate is due to sinus bradycardia rather than another cause, such as heart block or nodal (junctional) rhythm. Document the arrhythmia.
2. Record the heart rate at frequent intervals for comparative purposes; this is particularly important when drug therapy is used in an attempt to increase the rate.
3. Assess the patient's clinical course regularly to determine if there are signs or symptoms of decreased left ventricular performance.
4. Observe the ECG pattern repeatedly for evidence of premature ventricular contractions. If these occur, notify the physician.
5. If the heart rate falls below 50/minute, advise the physician.

SINUS BRADYCARDIA—IDENTIFYING ECG FEATURES

1. Rate:		Usually 40-60/minute, but may be slower.
2. Rhythm:		Regular.
3. P waves:		Normal, and precede each QRS complex.
4. P-R interval:		Normal.
5. QRS:		Normal.

Sinus Bradycardia (Figure 9.3)

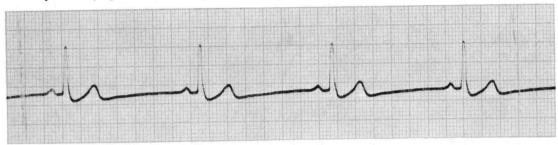

Rate:	About 40/minute (43/minute).
Rhythm:	Regular.
P waves:	Normal.
P-R interval:	Normal (0.16 second).
QRS:	Normal (0.08 second).
Comment:	Sinus bradycardia differs from normal sinus rhythm only in that the rate is less than 60/minute.

Sinus Bradycardia (Figure 9.4)

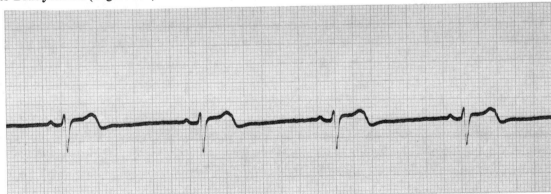

Rate:	About 40/minute.
Rhythm:	Regular.
P waves:	Normal; each P wave is followed by a QRS complex.
P-R interval:	Normal (0.12 second).
QRS:	Normal (0.08 second).
Comment:	The usual cause of sinus bradycardia is increased vagal tone, which slows discharges from the SA node.

CASE HISTORY

A 78-year-old man was brought to the CCU 1 hour after an episode of severe chest pain. On admission the blood pressure was 90/60 and the pulse rate 48/minute. On the monitor frequent premature ventricular beats were noted. The nurse notified the physician of these findings. Atropine (0.6 mg) was administered intravenously and within 5 minutes the blood pressure rose to 114/76, the heart rate increased to 76/minute, and the premature ventricular contractions lessened.

SINUS ARRHYTHMIA

Mechanism

In sinus arrhythmia impulses arise from the SA node but not with a completely regular rhythm. The irregularity of discharge is due to variation of vagal influence on the SA node, resulting in *alternating* periods of slow and fast rates. In most instances this effect is related to the phases of respiration with the rate increasing during inspiration and slowing during expiration.

Danger in Acute Myocardial Infarction

1. Sinus arrhythmia causes no hemodynamic effects nor does it warn of more serious arrhythmias. Consequently it can be regarded as an unimportant and nondangerous arrhythmia.
2. *RISK:* None.

Clinical Features

1. The pulse is irregular, but the patient is unaware of this minor disturbance in rhythm.
2. The diagnosis of sinus arrhythmia can be verified with an ECG but it may be suspected clinically if a change in heart rate occurs with deliberate breath-holding.

Treatment

No treatment is indicated.

Nursing Role

1. Ascertain that the irregular rhythm is due to sinus arrhythmia and document with an ECG strip.
2. Make certain that the irregularity is not a manifestation of a more serious arrhythmia (e.g., atrial fibrillation).

CASE HISTORY

A 70-year-old woman was admitted to the unit with a typical history of acute myocardial infarction. While taking the patient's pulse the nurse noted an irregular rhythm. From the monitor she recognized that the problem was sinus arrhythmia and recorded this finding on the admission sheet. The arrhythmia persisted all during the patient's stay in the CCU. No treatment was given for this minor arrhythmia.

SINUS ARRHYTHMIA—IDENTIFYING ECG FEATURES

1. Rate:		The heart rate per minute is usually normal (60-100); however the rate increases during inspiration and then slows during expiration.
2. Rhythm:		Irregular. There is a variation of at least 0.12 second between the longest and shortest R-R intervals.
3. P waves:		Normal, and precede each QRS complex.
4. P-R interval:		Normal.
5. QRS:		Normal.

Sinus Arrhythmia (Figure 9.5)

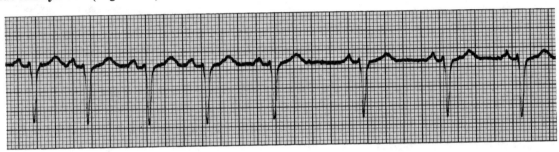

Rate:	About 80/minute.
Rhythm:	Irregular. There is a variation of at least 0.12 second between the longest and shortest R-R intervals.
P waves:	Normal. Each P wave is followed by a QRS complex.
P-R interval:	Normal (0.16 second).
QRS:	Normal (0.08 second).
Comment:	The rate increases during inspiration and slows during expiration.

Sinus Arrhythmia (Figure 9.6)

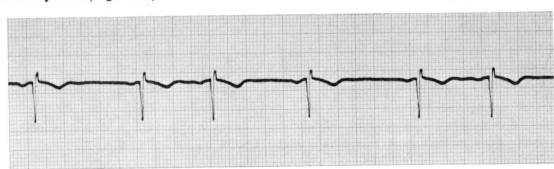

Rate:	About 60/minute.
Rhythm:	Irregular. The R-R intervals vary by more than 0.12 second.
P waves:	Normal but inverted (because of the particular monitoring lead being used).
P-R interval:	Normal (0.20 second).
QRS:	Normal (0.08 second).
Comment:	The key feature of sinus arrhythmia is the irregularity of the rhythm with otherwise normal wave forms.

WANDERING PACEMAKER

Mechanism

With a wandering pacemaker, impulses arise in a normal manner in the SA node, but occasionally the pacemaker wanders from the SA node to the atria or the AV nodal areas. This shifting of the pacemaker from the SA node to adjacent tissues is manifested electrocardiographically by transient changes in the size, shape, and direction of P waves. A wandering pacemaker is usually caused by varying vagal tone (just as the case with sinus arrhythmia). With increased vagal tone the SA node slows, allowing a pacemaker in the atria or AV nodal area, which may become slightly faster than the SA node under these conditions to take over briefly as pacemaker. As soon as vagal tone decreases the SA node speeds up and regains control of the heartbeat again.

Danger in Acute Myocardial Infarction

1. There is no particular danger from a wandering pacemaker. The arrhythmia usually reflects fluctuating depression of the SA node by vagal influence.
2. *RISK:* None.

Treatment

1. No treatment is needed in most instances.
2. If depression of the SA node permits the AV nodal area to dominate the pacemaker role, atropine can be used to block the vagal influence.
3. If a wandering pacemaker develops during digitalis therapy, the drug may be withheld temporarily to see if the arrhythmia is drug-related and will disappear with cessation of digitalis.

Nursing Role

1. When a wandering pacemaker is noted on the monitor, document the arrhythmia with a rhythm strip.
2. Observe the ECG subsequently to verify that the SA node has not relinquished complete control to the atria or AV nodal area.

CASE HISTORY

On the second day after admission to the CCU a 56-year-old man with an acute inferior wall infarction developed ECG evidence of a wandering pacemaker. The nurse noted that the configuration of the P waves varied at different times and realized that the pacemaker site was changing during these periods. Because these episodes were infrequent and since the SA node remained the dominant pacemaker, the nurse concluded that the problem was not serious and no treatment was given.

WANDERING PACEMAKER—IDENTIFYING ECG FEATURES

1. **Rate:**   Usually normal but may be slow (because of vagal dominance).
2. **Rhythm:**   Essentially regular, but the R-R intervals may vary as the pacemaker site shifts.
3. **P waves:**   As the pacemaker wanders to the atria or AV nodal area, the shape, position or direction of the P waves change, reflecting the different sites of origin of the impulse. However, a P wave precedes every QRS complex.
4. **P-R interval:**   The conduction time to the ventricle depends on the actual site of impulse formation. On this basis the P-R interval may vary slightly depending on the changing pacemaker location.
5. **QRS:**   Normal. Conduction from the AV node to the ventricle is unaffected, so there is a normal QRS complex regardless of the size, shape or position of the P waves.

Wandering Pacemaker (Figure 9.7)

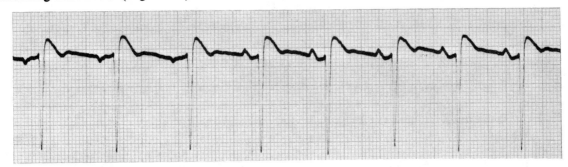

Rate:	About 80/minute.
Rhythm:	Nearly regular.
P waves:	In the first 3 complexes the P waves are inverted (indicating an atrial pacemaker). When the pacemaker shifts back to the SA node (the last 5 complexes) the P waves return to normal.
P-R interval:	Normal (0.16 second).
QRS:	Normal (0.08 second).
Comment:	The pacemaker shifts from the SA node to the atria.

Wandering Pacemaker (Figure 9.8)

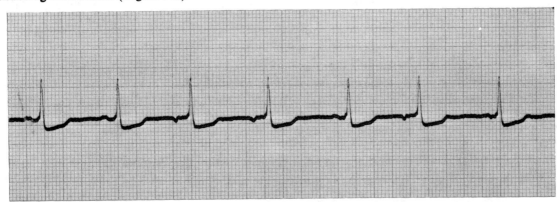

Rate:	About 70/minute.
Rhythm:	Regular.
P waves:	The size, shape and direction of the P waves vary as the pacemaker changes position.
P-R interval:	Normal (0.20 second).
QRS:	Normal (0.06 second).
Comment:	The pacemaker moves back and forth between the SA node and the atria.

SINOATRIAL ARREST (AND SA BLOCK)

Mechanism

Under certain circumstances, the SA node fails to initiate an impulse at the expected time in the cardiac cycle. In the absence of an impulse from the SA node neither the atria or the ventricles are stimulated and therefore an entire PQRST complex drops out for one beat (or more). This is called *sinoatrial (SA) arrest.* In other instances the impulse is initiated normally but is blocked *within* the SA node and never reaches the atria or ventricles. Again, the PQRST sequence is absent. This condition is designated *SA block* or, more specifically, SA exit block. Although SA arrest is a disturbance of impulse formation and SA exit block a disturbance of conduction, it is often impossible to determine from an ECG which of the two mechanisms is responsible for the dropped beat. For this reason the terms SA arrest and SA block are used interchangeably, or grouped together and called *sinus pauses.* Sinoatrial arrest (or block) may result from excessive vagal dominance of the SA node or from digitalis or quinidine toxicity; however neither of these factors is probably as important as ischemic injury of the SA node secondary to acute myocardial infarction.

Danger in Acute Myocardial Infarction

1. When infrequent, SA arrest (or block) is not of great importance and usually reflects excessive vagal activity.
2. Repeated episodes of SA arrest or very prolonged pauses between beats suggests ischemic damage to the SA node, a condition that is potentially dangerous.
3. When related to overdosages of digitalis (or quinidine), the arrhythmia assumes special significance since the drug may lead to further depression of SA node activity and result in atrial standstill.
4. *RISK:* SA arrest is usually not serious, but is potentially dangerous when the episodes are repetitive or prolonged as the result of ischemic damage or drug overdoses.

Clinical Features

1. Patient may notice pauses in the heartbeat and describe this sensation; however, most are unaware of the arrhythmia.
2. The only physical finding is a pause detected while taking the pulse or listening to the heartbeat.
3. If the missed beats occur frequently or consecutively, cerebral insufficiency manifested as syncope or vertigo may develop.

Treatment

1. If SA arrest occurs only occasionally, the condition is usually self-limiting and requires no treatment.
2. If the periods of SA arrest are frequent or prolonged, atropine (0.5-1.0 mg intravenously) will frequently restore normal SA impulse formation or conduction by inhibiting vagal effect on the SA node. Isoproterenol can also be used for this purpose.
3. If SA arrest does not subside spontaneously or fails to respond to drug therapy, a transvenous pacemaker may be required.
4. If SA arrest occurs in patients receiving digitalis or quinidine, the drugs should be discontinued promptly.

Nursing Role

1. When SA arrest is noted, document the arrhythmia with a rhythm strip.
2. If SA arrest occurs frequently or if more than two consecutive beats are missed, notify the physician promptly.
3. If SA arrest develops in patients receiving digitalis or quinidine, further dosages of these drugs should be withheld until reordered by the physician.

SINOATRIAL ARREST (AND SA BLOCK)—IDENTIFYING ECG FEATURES

1. **Rate:**	Usually slow (40-70/minute) but may be normal.
2. **Rhythm:**	Basic rhythm is normal except for the missing beats.
3. **P waves:**	The P wave is absent with the missed beat since the SA node either did not discharge or the impulse failed to reach the atrium.
4. **P-R interval:**	The entire PQRST complex is missing for one or more beats; thus no P-R interval during sinus arrest.
5. **QRS:**	No QRS complex is produced when the SA node impulse is absent or blocked.

Sinoatrial Arrest (or block) (Figure 9.9)

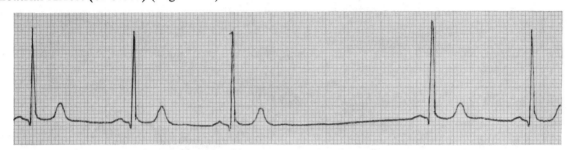

Rate:	About 50/minute.
Rhythm:	Regular except for sinus pause between third and fourth QRS complexes.
P waves:	The P wave anticipated after the third complex is absent.
P-R interval:	No P-R interval during SA arrest; other P-R intervals are normal.
QRS:	No QRS complex for one beat; other QRS complexes normal.
Comment:	The duration of the pause is exactly twice the R-R interval of the two previous beats, suggesting that the SA node continued to discharge normally but that one impulse was blocked in the node (SA block).

Sinoatrial (SA) Arrest (Figure 9.10)

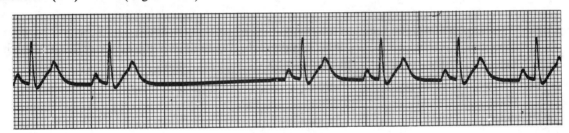

Rate:	About 60/minute.
Rhythm:	Regular except for one period of sinus arrest.
P waves:	Absent with missed beat; otherwise normal.
P-R interval:	Absent with missed beat; otherwise normal (0.16 second).
QRS:	Absent when SA node failed to discharge; otherwise normal (0.08 second).
Comment:	The duration of the pause is not an exact multiple of the other R-R intervals. This implies that the SA node failed to discharge during this period (SA arrest) and then started again suddenly.

CASE HISTORY

A 61-year-old man was admitted to the CCU with an acute inferior infarction. On examining the patient the nurse noted that the pulse was 50/minute and occasionally irregular. The ECG revealed sinus bradycardia with episodes of SA arrest. In some instances there were as many as three missed beats in a row. The physician ordered atropine (1 mg intravenously), which promptly accelerated the heart rate and restored normal sinus function.

OTHER EXAMPLES OF ARRHYTHMIAS ORIGINATING IN THE SINOATRIAL (SA) NODE

Note:

The following ECG strips are meant to fulfill four basic purposes:

1) to provide additional examples of the arrhythmias discussed in the preceding pages
2) to demonstrate certain variations of the ECG patterns of these arrhythmias
3) to illustrate that more than one arrhythmic disorder may be present at the same time
4) to introduce other details of arrhythmia interpretation.

Normal Sinus Rhythm with Inverted T Waves (Figure 9.11)

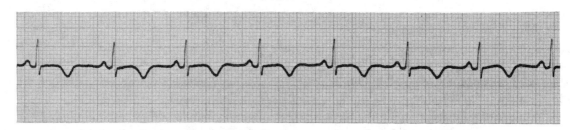

Rate:	About 80/minute (Actual rate: 75/minute)
Rhythm:	Regular.
P waves:	Normal.
P-R interval:	Normal (0.12 second).
QRS:	Normal (0.04 second).
Comment:	The T waves are inverted, a common manifestation of myocardial ischemia. However, abnormalities of T waves or ST segments do not affect arrhythmia interpretation, and this ECG shows normal sinus rhythm (NSR).

Sinus Tachycardia (Figure 9.12)

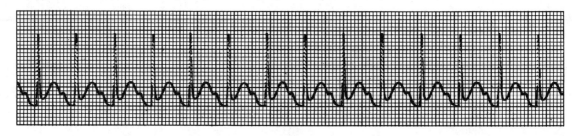

Rate:	About 140/minute.
Rhythm:	Regular.
P waves:	Because of the rapid rate, the P waves encroach on the preceding T waves.
P-R interval:	Normal (less than 0.20 second, but not clearly measurable).
QRS:	Normal (0.06 second).
Comment:	A careful search for P waves, often hiding in the preceding T waves, is an essential step in interpreting arrhythmias.

Sinus Bradycardia with Prominent U Waves (Figure 9.13)

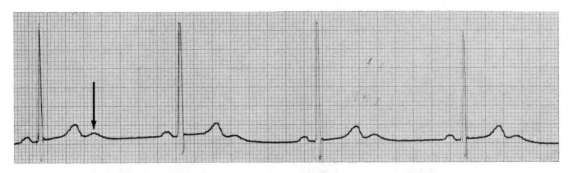

Rate:	About 40/minute.
Rhythm:	Regular.
P waves:	Normal. A P wave precedes each QRS complex.
P-R interval:	Normal (0.16 second).
QRS:	Normal (0.06 second).
Comment:	Immediately after each T wave is another wave called a U wave (see arrow). U waves, particularly when they are prominent, often reflect low serum potassium levels.

Sinus Bradycardia with Conduction Disorder (Figure 9.14)

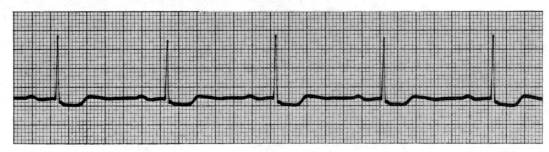

Rate:	About 50/minute.
Rhythm:	Regular.
P waves:	Normal.
P-R interval:	Prolonged (0.32 second), indicating a first-degree AV heart block.
QRS:	Normal (0.04 second).
Comment:	This ECG shows both a disturbance in impulse formation (sinus bradycardia) and a disturbance in conduction (first-degree AV block).

Sinus Arrhythmia and Sinus Bradycardia (Figure 9.15)

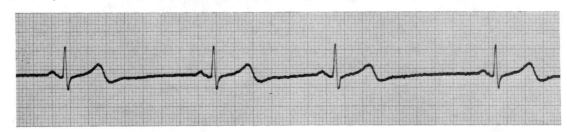

Rate:	About 40/minute.
Rhythm:	Irregular.
P waves:	Normal.
P-R interval:	Normal (0.16 second).
QRS:	Normal (0.08 second).
Comment:	Sinus bradycardia and sinus arrhythmia often occur together, both resulting from increased vagal tone.

Wandering Pacemaker (Figure 9.16)

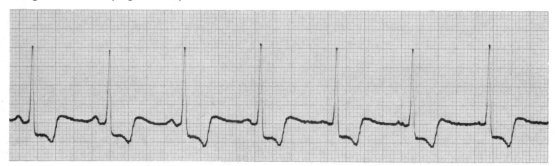

Rate:	About 70/minute.
Rhythm:	Regular.
P waves:	The P waves are normal with the first 4 beats, but then their size and shape change as the pacemaker wanders to the atria.
P-R interval:	Normal (0.20 second) during normal sinus rhythm.
QRS:	Normal duration (0.08 second).
Comment:	Marked (4mm) ST segment depression and T wave inversion, as seen in this tracing, reflect myocardial disease.

Sinoatrial (SA) Arrest (Figure 9.17)

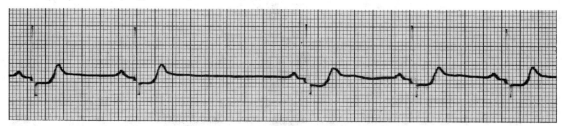

Rate:	About 50/minute.
Rhythm:	Regular except for one missed beat.
P waves:	Normal.
P-R interval:	Normal (0.16 second).
QRS:	Normal (0.06 second).
Comment:	This sinus pause, manifested by the absence of one PQRST complex, is not a multiple of the other R-R intervals and, therefore, represents SA arrest (rather than SA block).

Sinoatrial Pause with Sinus Arrhythmia (Figure 9.18)

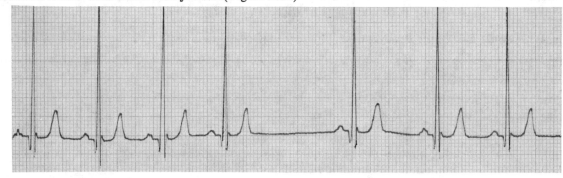

Rate:	About 70/minute.
Rhythm:	Irregular as the result of the sinoatrial pause and sinus arrhythmia.
P waves:	Normal.
P-R interval:	Normal (0.16 second).
QRS:	Normal (0.10 second).
Comment:	After 4 normal beats the SA node fails to discharge (or the impulse is blocked in the node), creating a pause before the sinus node discharges again. Sinus arrhythmia is evident after the SA pause, suggesting that both arrhythmias were the result of increased vagal tone.

10

Arrhythmias Originating in the Atria

PREMATURE ATRIAL CONTRACTIONS
PAROXYSMAL ATRIAL TACHYCARDIA
ATRIAL FLUTTER
ATRIAL FIBRILLATION
ATRIAL STANDSTILL

As noted previously, the atria, the AV nodal area, and the ventricles all have the *potential* capacity to serve as pacemaker, but the SA node retains control because it normally discharges impulses at an inherently faster rate than the other sites. If for some reason a focus in the atrial walls initiates impulses more rapidly than those arising from the SA node, the ectopic site in the atria replaces the SA node as pacemaker. This may occur for only one beat (premature atrial contraction) or continuously (atrial tachycardia, atrial flutter, or atrial fibrillation), depending on the degree and persistence of irritability of the abnormal focus.

When impulses originate in the atria, outside the SA node, at rates of *less than 200/minute,* P waves are usually visible but are distorted in shape, indicating that the SA node is not in command. In this situation each impulse reaches the AV node and passes through to the ventricles without difficulty. Consequently, a normal QRS complex follows each P wave (atrial tachycardia).

When the atria are stimulated *200-400 times/minute,* the AV node is unable to accept each impulse and blocks every second, third, or fourth atrial beat. The impulses that do pass the AV node are conducted normally thereafter to the ventricles. For example, in atrial flutter the atrial rate is two, three, or four times greater than the ventricular response and there are two, three, or four P waves between each normal QRS complex.

If the atria are stimulated at extremely fast rates (*400-1000 times/minute*), the atrial muscles are no longer capable of responding to these repetitive impulses, and the individual fibers comprising the atrial muscle merely twitch, or *fibrillate.* The atria do not actually contract in this circumstance, and P waves are not seen. Because of this chaotic atrial activity, impulses reach the AV node at a rapid, irregular rate. The AV node blocks most of these rapid impulses, and those that pass to the ventricles do so at irregular intervals. Consequently, the ventricular rhythm is irregular (atrial fibrillation).

Atrial arrhythmias result primarily from irritability of the atrial muscle usually caused by ischemic damage or by overdistention (stretching) of the atrial wall. Atrial rhythm disturbances associated with a rapid ventricular rate are categorized as major arrhythmias because they increase myocardial oxygen demand and also reduce pumping efficiency of the heart. These latter arrhythmias must not be allowed to persist.

147

PREMATURE ATRIAL CONTRACTIONS

Mechanism

When an ectopic focus in the atrium discharges before the SA node, a *premature atrial contraction* (PAC) results. Because the impulse arises outside the SA node, the P wave of the ectopic beat is abnormally shaped or inverted. Conduction from the AV node to the ventricles is not affected and therefore the QRS complex is normal. Following the premature beat there is a slight pause before the next normal sinus impulse arises. This pause—called an incomplete compensatory pause—occurs because the ectopic impulse discharges the nearby SA node and the node must recover before it can discharge again. (The compensatory pause is discussed in more detail in the discussion of premature ventricular contractions.)

Premature atrial contractions usually reflect irritability of the atrial musculature and may be provoked by atrial distention or various drugs.

Danger in Acute Myocardial Infarction

1. By themselves PACs have no particular significance; however they indicate atrial irritability and may forewarn of impending serious atrial arrhythmias, e.g., paroxysmal atrial tachycardia or atrial fibrillation. When PACs increase beyond 6/minute, the arrhythmia assumes more importance in this regard.
2. *RISK:* PACs pose no immediate danger but may herald the onset of atrial fibrillation or other sustained atrial arrhythmias, particularly when they occur frequently.

Clinical Features

1. Normally the patient is unaware of PACs; however, a beat that occurs sooner than expected may be heard with a stethoscope.
2. Positive identification can be made only by ECG.

Treatment

1. If PACs occur rarely and do not increase in frequency, treatment is usually unnecessary.
2. If the number of PACs increases during a period of observation, it is advisable to use antiarrhythmic drugs to control these ectopic beats. Digitalis alone or in combination with quinidine is usually effective in this circumstance.

Nursing Role

1. Distinguish PACs from other causes of irregular heart rhythm and document their presence on an ECG.
2. Carefully observe the frequency of these premature beats for comparative purposes and advise the physician of any significant increase in the number of these beats.
3. Be aware that atrial fibrillation or other serious atrial arrhythmias may develop abruptly in the presence of frequent premature atrial beats.

CASE HISTORY

A 69-year-old man exhibited occasional PACs during the first day after admission. These ectopic beats occurred at a rate of 2-4/minute, and were duly noted by the nurse and recorded on hourly rhythm strips. On the second hospital day, the frequency of PACs increased to 10-20/minute; and some of them occurred consecutively for 2-3 beats. The nurse advised the physician of these changes and digoxin was started to suppress this increasing atrial ectopic activity. Within 8 hours the number of PACs diminished greatly and by 24 hours the arrhythmia was almost completely suppressed.

PREMATURE ATRIAL CONTRACTIONS—IDENTIFYING ECG FEATURES

1.	**Rate:**	Usually normal.
2.	**Rhythm:**	After a PAC there is a slight delay (incomplete compensatory pause) before the next normal beat. This pause creates a mild irregularity in the cardiac rhythm.
3.	**P waves:**	Either abnormally shaped or inverted, and differ from normal P waves originating in the SA node.
4.	**P-R interval:**	Usually normal, but may be short or prolonged.
5.	**QRS:**	Usually normal, indicating that there is no disturbance in conduction from the AV node to the ventricles.

Premature Atrial Contractions (Figure 10.1)

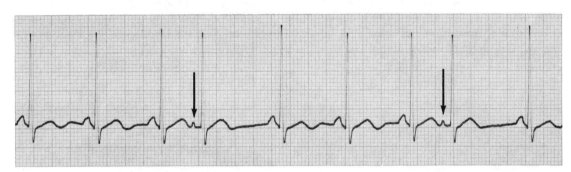

Rate:	About 90/minute.
Rhythm:	The two premature atrial contractions (PACs) and the pauses that follow them create an irregular rhythm.
P waves:	The size and shape of the P waves of the PACs (see arrow) are different than the P waves of normal beats. However, a P wave precedes each QRS.
P-R interval:	Normal (0.16 second).
QRS:	Normal (0.08 second).
Comment:	The most distinguishing feature of an ectopic beat arising in the atria (a PAC) is that the configuration of the P wave differs from the other P waves.

Premature Atrial Contraction (Figure 10.2)

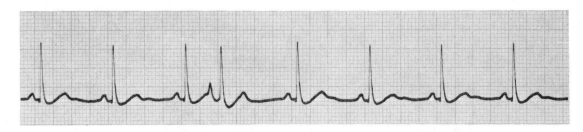

Rate:	About 70/minute.
Rhythm:	Irregular.
P waves:	The P wave of the PAC is hidden in the T wave of the preceding complex, producing a sharp pointed wave, differing from the other P or T waves.
P-R interval:	Normal (0.12 second).
QRS:	Normal (0.08 second).
Comment:	P waves are often obscured by the preceding T waves, particularly if the PAC occurs soon after the previous beat.

PAROXYSMAL ATRIAL TACHYCARDIA

Mechanism

Paroxysmal atrial tachycardia (PAT) is caused by the rapid discharge on an ectopic focus in the atria, occurring at a regular rate of 150-250/minute, which replaces the SA node as pacemaker. In this sense, PAT is a consecutive series of rapidly occurring premature atrial contractions. The ventricles respond to each atrial impulse and therefore the atrial and ventricular rates are identical. When PAT is associated with acute myocardial infarction it often reflects atrial distention secondary to heart failure.

Danger in Acute Myocardial Infarction

1. The rapid heart rate tends to reduce cardiac output because the volume of blood ejected with each contraction (stroke volume) is decreased as a result of the very short ventricular filling time between beats. The decrease in cardiac output may lead to left ventricular failure, particularly if the tachycardia is sustained. Cerebral circulation can also be affected, resulting in syncope.
2. The fast ventricular rate increases the demand for and consumption of oxygen by the myocardium. Consequently, additional myocardial ischemia or angina may result. The longer that PAT persists, the greater the threat of further myocardial injury.
3. *RISK:* PAT is a dangerous arrhythmia with acute myocardial infarction but not a direct cause of death. The risk is directly proportional to the duration of the arrhythmia.

Clinical Features

1. Characteristically, paroxysmal atrial tachycardia (PAT) occurs *suddenly,* sometimes without warning, but is usually preceded by premature atrial contractions.
2. Most patients are immediately aware of the rapid heart action and frequently describe a fluttering sensation in the chest, lightheadedness, angina, or dyspnea.
3. The arrhythmia is usually transient and ends *abruptly,* even without treatment.

Treatment

1. Initially an attempt should be made to terminate the arrhythmia by reflex vagal stimulation (e.g., carotid sinus massage). This technique is frequently effective.
2. If PAT cannot be terminated by vagal stimulation and the patient describes angina or symptoms of left ventricular failure, elective precordial shock (cardioversion) should be used promptly; this method seldom fails to restore sinus rhythm.
3. If the rapid rate does *not* produce obvious symptoms, drug therapy can be attempted. Although several different drugs can be used for this purpose, the calcium-blocking agent, verapamil, appears to be the most effective in terminating PAT (see Chapter 16). Among other drugs that may be used in this situation are: morphine, given intravenously, rapid-acting digitalis preparations or propranolol (Inderal).
4. If PAT occurs repetitively, prophylactic antiarrhythmia therapy is advisable. Quinidine, administered orally, is probably the most effective agent in this circumstance.

Nursing Role

1. The onset of PAT will trigger the high-rate alarm system of the monitor.
2. Examine the patient and verify the rapid pulse rate.
3. Document the arrhythmia with a rhythm strip.
4. Notify the physician immediately.
5. Assess the patient's clinical signs with particular reference to the presence of angina or signs of left ventricular failure. Record the blood pressure.
6. If the patient has signs or symptoms related to the rapid rate, prepare for precordial shock (elective cardioversion).
7. Have appropriate drugs ready for use at the bedside.

PAROXYSMAL ATRIAL TACHYCARDIA—IDENTIFYING ECG FEATURES

1. **Rate:**   150-250/minute.
2. **Rhythm:**   Regular.
3. **P waves:**   An abnormal P wave precedes each QRS complex. However, the P waves can seldom be identified because they are buried in the preceding T waves.
4. **P-R interval:** In most instances the P-R interval cannot be measured because the P waves are obscured.
5. **QRS:**   Usually normal.

Paroxysmal Atrial Tachycardia (Figure 10.3)

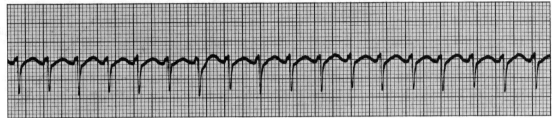

Rate: About 180/minute.
Rhythm: Regular.
P waves: Not identifiable; probably buried in preceding T waves.
P-R interval: Not measurable since P waves cannot be identified specifically.
QRS: Normal, indicating that all atrial impulses are conducted to the ventricles normally.
Comment: Atrial tachycardia increases the work of the heart substantially but, fortunately, it often terminates spontaneously after a few minutes.

Paroxysmal Atrial Tachycardia (Figure 10.4)

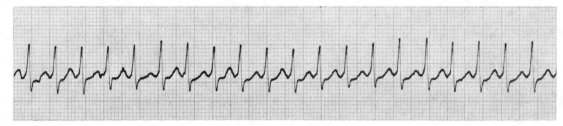

Rate: About 200/minute.
Rhythm: Regular.
P waves: Cannot be identified specifically, probably superimposed on preceding T waves.
P-R interval: Not measurable since P waves cannot be delineated.
QRS: Normal (0.08 second), indicating that all atrial impulses are conducted normally through the ventricles.
Comment: In this typical example of paroxysmal atrial tachycardia (PAT), the ventricles respond regularly to each atrial impulse; i.e., a QRS complex follows every P wave on a 1:1 basis. However, under certain conditions (especially digitalis toxicity), some atrial impulses are blocked in the AV node and not conducted to the ventricles. As a result, every P wave is not followed by a QRS complex, and the 1:1 relationship no longer exists. This latter arrhythmia is called *PAT with block*.

CASE HISTORY

A 55-year-old woman with an acute infarction had been in normal sinus rhythm for 48 hours after admission. At 4 PM the pulse rate was 82 and regular, and an hourly ECG strip taken by the nurse showed a normal sinus rhythm. At 4:10 PM the tachycardia alarm sounded and the monitor showed a heart rate of 160. At the bedside the nurse confirmed the rapid rate. The patient complained of chest pain and was obviously frightened. The nurse ran a rhythm strip and recognized PAT. She called the physician immediately and prepared for precordial shock. By the time the physician arrived several minutes later, the arrhythmia had stopped abruptly. In reviewing the rhythm strip it was apparent that the patient had a run of PAT which lasted for less than 3 minutes.

ATRIAL FLUTTER

Mechanism

Atrial flutter, like paroxysmal atrial tachycardia, is a manifestation of a rapid ectopic atrial pacemaker. The atrial rate is 250-400/minute. The AV node is unable to conduct all of these impulses but usually allows every second, third, or fourth impulse to reach the ventricles and cause contraction. The ventricular rate is therefore determined by the extent of the block in the AV node. For example, if the atrial rate is 300/minute and the AV node blocks every second impulse (2:1 block), the ventricular rate will be 150/minute. The atrial flutter may result from heart failure, increased catecholamine secretion, injury to the SA node, and other causes.

Danger in Acute Myocardial Infarction

1. When atrial flutter is associated with a rapid ventricular rate, cardiac output usually decreases and the myocardial oxygen consumption increases (as with other rapid-rate arrhythmias, e.g., PAT). This impairment predisposes to left ventricular failure and myocardial ischemia.
2. If the ventricular rate is not increased, left ventricular performance may not be affected significantly.
3. *RISK:* Atrial flutter is a serious arrhythmia because of its potential hemodynamic consequences. It is usually more persistent than PAT and therefore a greater threat.

Clinical Features

1. The occurrence of symptoms depends fundamentally on the ventricular rate. If the ventricular response is rapid (e.g., 150/minute) the patient may describe palpitations, angina, or dyspnea. If the ventricular rate is normal (e.g., with a 4:1 block) the arrhythmia may produce no signs or symptoms.
2. Atrial flutter can be identified only by means of an ECG.

Treatment

1. Atrial flutter can be instantly terminated by precordial shock (cardioversion) with very low discharge energies (less than 50 watt-seconds). Because of its predictable effectiveness, cardioversion should be the initial treatment, especially when the ventricular rate is rapid.
2. Drug therapy is seldom successful in restoring normal sinus rhythm. However, digitalis preparations, beta-blockers, or calcium blocking agents (verapamil) are often used to control the ventricular rate (by increasing the degree of AV block). Other pharmacologic means for terminating atrial flutter (quinidine, for example) are rarely effective.

Nursing Role

1. When atrial flutter develops, the high-rate alarm may or may not sound, depending on the *ventricular* rate.
2. Identify the arrhythmia on the monitor and document with a rhythm strip.
3. Assess the patient's clinical status. Determine if the patient has angina or dyspnea. Record the blood pressure and pulse rate.
4. Notify the physician promptly after this arrhythmia is identified.
5. If the patient complains of angina or if there is evidence of left ventricular failure, prepare for elective cardioversion (see Chapter 14).
6. If digitalis or other drugs are used to treat atrial flutter, carefully record the heart rate and rhythm response.

CASE HISTORY

Six hours after admission to the unit, a 71-year-old man developed atrial flutter. This was noted by the nurse when the high-rate alarm sounded. The ventricular rate was 150/minute. The nurse went to the bedside and noted that the patient was apprehensive and dyspneic. She immediately notified the physician, and then recorded the blood pressure and pulse rate, and documented the arrhythmia. Anticipating that precordial shock would be used because of the circulatory impairment induced by the arrhythmia, the nurse prepared for the procedure. Cardioversion was accomplished as soon as the physician arrived, and normal sinus rhythm was restored. The patient's symptoms disappeared promptly.

ATRIAL FLUTTER—IDENTIFYING ECG FEATURES

1. Rate:	The ventricular rate may range from 60-160/minute, depending on the number of atrial impulses passing through the AV node. The atrial rate is 250-400/ minute.
2. Rhythm:	The ventricular rhythm is most often regular. However, as a result of varying degrees of block in the AV node from time to time, the ventricular rhythm may become slightly irregular.
3. P waves:	There are characteristic atrial oscillations described as sawtooth waves which are easily identifiable. These waves (called F waves or flutter waves) occur regularly at a rate of 250-400/minute.
4. P-R interval:	The P-R interval (actually the F-R interval) has no meaning and is not measured.
5. QRS:	The QRS complex is normal, indicating that conduction beyond the AV node is not disturbed. However, only one-half, one-third, or one-fourth of the atrial impulses are conducted through the AV node and reach the ventricle. The resulting disparity between atrial and ventricular rates is described as atrial flutter with 2:1, 3:1, or 4:1 block.

Atrial Flutter (Figure 10.5)

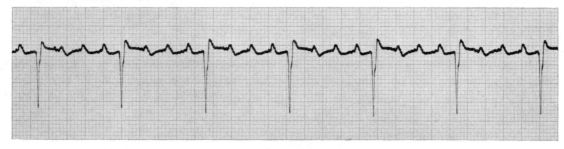

Rate:	The ventricular rate is about 70/minute (65/minute) while the atrial rate is 260/minute.
Rhythm:	Regular.
P waves:	There are 4 F waves between each R wave. Note the typical sawtooth appearance of these atrial waves.
P-R interval:	In the absence of P waves there is no P-R interval. The F-R interval has no significance.
QRS:	Normal (0.06 second). Every fourth atrial impulse is conducted to the ventricle producing a QRS complex.
Comment:	Note that there are 4 flutter waves for each QRS complex. This is called *atrial flutter with 4:1 block.*

Atrial Flutter (Figure 10.6)

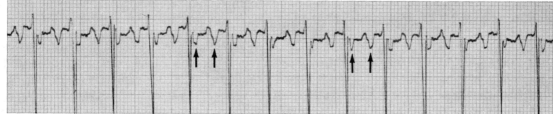

Rate:	The *ventricular* rate is about 140/minute. The *atrial* rate is about 280/minute.
Rhythm:	Regular.
P waves:	There are two F waves between ventricular complexes. These waves, which are inverted in the lead (see arrows), have a sawtooth appearance, but not as distinctively as in atrial flutter with 4:1 block (as in Figure 10.5 above).
P-R interval:	Not determinable.
QRS:	Every second atrial impulse is conducted to the ventricle. This is called atrial flutter with 2:1 block. The QRS complexes are normal.
Comment:	Atrial flutter with 2:1 block should always be suspected when there is a regular ventricular rate of 140-160/minute. A careful search for F waves should be made in this circumstance.

ATRIAL FIBRILLATION

Mechanism

In atrial fibrillation, ectopic foci in the atria discharge impulses at a rate of 400-500/minute. The atrial muscles cannot respond uniformly to this very rapid, irregular stimulation. Instead, the individual muscle fibers respond on their own in a wholly disorganized way. The net effect is a mere twitching of the atrial walls rather than true atrial contraction. In a sense the atria are no more than quivering tubes connecting the great veins to the ventricles, and they provide no assistance in filling the ventricles.

The extremely rapid, irregular impulses from the atria bombard the AV node but the node can conduct only a small percentage of them to the ventricles; the rest are blocked. The impulses that pass through the AV node do so at irregular intervals, creating an irregular ventricular rhythm.

The ventricular rate during atrial fibrillation can vary from 40-160/minute, depending on the number of impulses conducted to the ventricles and the degree of AV block. When the ventricular response (rate) is more than 100/minute, atrial fibrillation is classified as rapid and when less than 60/minute as slow.

Danger in Acute Myocardial Infarction

1. The major danger of atrial fibrillation is a reduction in the pumping efficiency of the heart (decreased cardiac output). This inefficiency results not only from the rapid, irregular ventricular response but also from the loss of effective atrial contraction. (Normally the atrium serves as a booster pump for ventricular filling, and the loss of atrial contraction can cause a 20% reduction in cardiac output). The resulting hemodynamic deficit may lead to left ventricular failure and additional myocardial ischemia.
2. With atrial fibrillation there is a propensity for clots to form within the noncontracting atria. Mural thrombi, with subsequent embolization in the circulatory system, may develop on this basis.
3. *RISK:* Atrial fibrillation is a dangerous arrhythmia from a hemodynamic standpoint, especially when the ventricular rate is rapid.

Clinical Features

1. Most patients with atrial fibrillation are aware of the irregular heart action and describe palpitations or "skipping" of the heartbeat. This disturbing sensation is usually more pronounced when the ventricular rate is rapid.
2. The grossly *irregular* rhythm is so characteristic of atrial fibrillation that this physical sign by itself is almost diagnostic of the arrhythmia.
3. In most instances the peripheral pulse rate is slower than the heart (apical) rate. This *pulse deficit* results from variations in the volume of blood ejected with each ventricular contraction; at times the stroke volume is inadequate to produce a peripheral pulse.
4. If the ventricular rate is persistently rapid, evidence of left ventricular failure may be anticipated.

Treatment

1. Atrial fibrillation can be treated with either drug therapy or by electrical means (elective precordial shock). The choice depends on several factors: the ventricular rate, the duration of the arrhythmia, and above all the presence or absence of circulatory insufficiency as manifested by left ventricular failure or angina.
2. If a patient develops left ventricular failure or angina as a direct consequence of rapid atrial fibrillation, the arrhythmia should be terminated without delay by means of synchronized precordial shock (cardioversion) to restore normal sinus rhythm.
3. If atrial fibrillation is *not* accompanied by signs of impaired circulation, then drug therapy should be the primary method of treatment. Digitalis is the cornerstone of this program. The drug controls the rapid ventricular rate by increasing the degree of block at the AV node, but it usually does not restore normal sinus rhythm.
4. If digitalis fails to slow the ventricular rate, verapamil (a calcium blocking agent) is usually very effective. In fact, many cardiologists prefer verapamil to digitalis because of its lower incidence of side effects in this particular situation.
5. When atrial fibrillation is of longstanding duration (existing before the acute infarction) and is not associated with a rapid ventricular rate, attempts to restore normal sinus rhythm are not usually indicated.

ATRIAL FIBRILLATION—IDENTIFYING ECG FEATURES

1. **Rate:** The ventricular rate may be normal (60-100/minute), rapid (greater than 100/minute), or slow (less than 60/minute), depending on the number of atrial impulses conducted to the ventricles.

2. **Rhythm:** The ventricular rhythm is totally irregular. This irregularity is the most typical finding of atrial fibrillation.

3. **P waves:** P waves are not present because of chaotic atrial activity. They are replaced by small, irregular, rapid oscillations called f (fibrillatory) waves.

4. **P-R interval:** There is no P-R interval.

5. **QRS:** Normal, but occur at irregular intervals. Most of the atrial impulses that bombard the AV node are blocked, but those that do pass through are conducted normally through the ventricles. Thus the conduction pattern of atrial fibrillation is manifested by the absence of P waves and the presence of normal QRS complexes, occurring at totally irregular intervals.

Atrial Fibrillation (Figure 10.7)

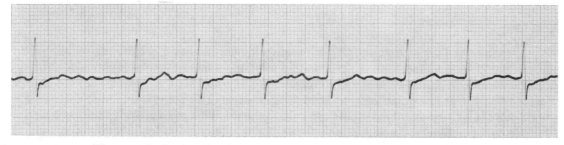

Rate: The ventricular rate is about 80/minute.
Rhythm: Irregular.
P waves: Absent. Fibrillatory (f) waves of different sizes and shapes are present instead.
P-R interval: Not determinable.
QRS: Of normal duration (0.08 second), but complexes occur irregularly.
Comment: The most characteristic feature of atrial fibrillation is the irregular ventricular rhythm. This finding, in conjunction with absent P waves, confirms the diagnosis of atrial fibrillation.

Rapid Atrial Fibrillation (Figure 10.8)

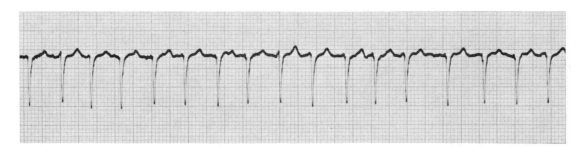

Rate: The average ventricular response is about 170/minute.
Rhythm: Irregular.
P waves: Absent. (Note the variation in the shape and size of the T waves resulting from superimposed fibrillatory (f) waves.)
P-R interval: Not measurable because of absence of P waves.
QRS: Normal duration (0.06 second).
Comment: Rapid atrial fibrillation reduces cardiac output substantially, and the ventricular rate must be slowed promptly.

Nursing Role

1. *If atrial fibrillation develops abruptly or is present and rapid at the time of admission:*
   a. Document the arrhythmia with a rhythm strip and notify the physician.
   b. Ascertain if the arrhythmia is compromising circulatory efficiency and inquire specifically if the patient has chest pain or dyspnea.
   c. Record the pulse rate, the extent of the pulse deficit, and the blood pressure.
   d. Prepare for elective cardioversion and have intravenous digitalis preparations at bedside.
2. *If atrial fibrillation is not rapid or if it existed before the present infarction:*
   a. Observe the patient's clinical status in a planned manner, always seeking evidence of left ventricular failure. Carefully record pulse rate, apical rate, and blood pressure.
   b. Obtain serial rhythm strips at regular intervals for comparative purposes.
   c. Advise the physician of any significant increase or decrease of the ventricular rate, or of the development of signs or symptoms which suggest left ventricular failure.
3. If digitalis or quinidine is used to treat atrial fibrillation, observe the ECG for signs of drug overdosages (see Chapter 16). If the ventricular rate falls below 60/minute, further administration of these drugs should be discussed with the physician.
4. Because of the possibility of embolization secondary to atrial fibrillation, this potential complication should always be considered during careful clinical assessment.

CASE HISTORY

A 72-year-old man was admitted to the CCU with acute pulmonary edema. The nurse initiated a planned treatment program which included morphine (15 mg intravenously), the administration of oxygen, and an intravenous injection of furosemide. Although there was improvement within the next hour, the patient was still very dyspneic. The pulse rate was 136 and irregular, and rales were heard throughout the entire chest. The ECG revealed rapid atrial fibrillation. It was felt that the decrease in cardiac output (which produced left ventricular failure) was related in part to the inefficient pumping action associated with the rapid ventricular rate. Accordingly, digoxin was administered intravenously (0.5 mg) in an attempt to slow the ventricular response. After two additional doses of digoxin within the next 12 hours, the ventricular response decreased to 70-80/minute. Clinical improvement was clearly evident during this period.

Atrial Fibrillation with Normal Ventricular Rate (Figure 10.9)

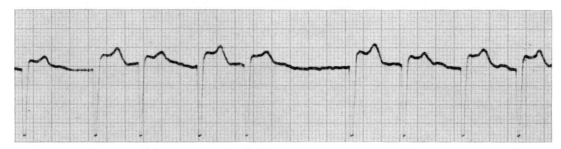

Rate:	The ventricular rate is about 90/minute.
Rhythm:	Grossly irregular.
P waves:	Absent. Fibrillatory waves are shallow in this particular lead.
P-R interval:	Not measurable.
QRS:	Normal (0.08 second).
Comment:	The ST segments are distinctly elevated (2-3 mm) and there are no R waves. These are signs of acute myocardial infarction (as described in Chapter 2).

Slow Atrial Fibrillation (Figure 10.10)

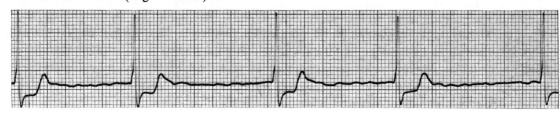

Rate:	The ventricular rate averages about 50/minute.
Rhythm:	Irregular.
P waves:	Shallow, fibrillatory waves are present.
P-R interval:	Not measurable.
QRS:	Normal (0.10 second).
Comment:	The slow ventricular response is caused by advanced AV block, allowing only a few atrial impulses to pass through to the ventricles. Atrioventricular block may be due to damage to the AV node or to digitalis toxicity. In either case digitalis should not be administered since it increases the degree of AV block and may slow the rate even further.

Atrial Fibrillation/Flutter (Figure 10.11)

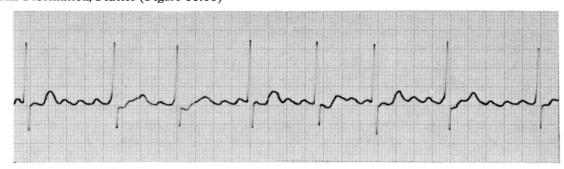

Rate:	Ventricular rate is about 80/minute.
Rhythm:	Irregular.
P waves:	Absent, being replaced by sawtooth F waves of atrial flutter and irregular f waves of atrial fibrillation.
P-R interval:	Not determinable.
QRS:	Normal (0.08 second), indicating conduction below AV node is normal.
Comment:	The irregular ventricular rhythm indicates atrial fibrillation; but the sawtooth F waves suggest atrial flutter. In this sense the arrhythmia represents a combination of both arrhythmias and is often called atrial fibrillation/flutter.

ATRIAL STANDSTILL

Mechanism

Atrial standstill denotes that the SA node and the atria have lost their ability to generate any electrical impulses. As a result, atrial contractions cease (atrial standstill) and the ventricles are stimulated by a lower pacemaker in either the AV nodal area or the ventricles. Usually the pacemaker descends progressively: first the SA node, then the atria, and then the AV nodal area fail, leaving only an undependable ventricular pacemaker to sustain the heart beat. This sequence is called *downward displacement of the pacemaker.* In most cases it is a terminal arrhythmia associated with severe left ventricular failure or cardiogenic shock. In patients with acute myocardial infarction atrial standstill is seldom reversible, indicating extensive damage or severe ischemia of the higher pacemaking centers. Rarely, however, does atrial standstill develop from overdosages of digitalis or quinidine. Atrial standstill may also occur in the presence of hyperkalemia and is described as atrial paralysis, a reversible condition.

Danger in Acute Myocardial Infarction

1. Failure of the SA node and the atria to initiate impulses leaves the AV nodal area and the ventricles as the only remaining pacemakers. These latter centers are far less dependable than higher pacemakers and *ventricular standstill* may occur at any time.
2. Downward displacement of the pacemaker usually indicates irreversible damage of the higher pacing centers in the heart and often heralds death.
3. *RISK:* Atrial standstill is an extremely ominous arrhythmia and is usually a forerunner of death due to advanced left ventricular failure.

Clinical Features

1. Atrial standstill with downward displacement of the pacemaker is seen most often in patients with severe circulatory failure. The arrhythmia itself does not produce specific signs or symptoms.
2. The disappearance of P waves, particularly in patients with advanced circulatory failure, suggests that downward displacement of the pacemaker is occurring because of damage to the SA node and atria.
3. When the pacemaker has descended to the AV nodal area, the ECG has the same characteristics of an arrhythmia originating in the AV nodal area (as described in the next chapter). However, the differences in clinical circumstances and in prognosis between the two arrhythmias make it important to consider atrial standstill and AV nodal arrhythmias as separate entities.

Treatment

1. When atrial standstill occurs with advanced heart failure or cardiogenic shock, survival is very unlikely. The only hope is to improve left ventricular function and tissue oxygenation with intraaortic balloon pumping and vigorous drug therapy.
2. A transvenous pacing catheter should be inserted as soon as there is suspicion that the SA node or atria are failing as pacemakers, and the ventricular pacing should be carried out during the course of treatment for left ventricular failure.
3. If atrial standstill is a result of digitalis toxicity or hyperkalemia (rather than a reflection of progressive ischemia), measures to correct these disorders should be initiated immediately.

Nursing Role

1. The P waves should be examined repeatedly in all patients with advanced left ventricular failure. The abrupt disappearance of the P waves in this situation suggests the onset of atrial standstill.
2. Notify the physician immediately and document the changing P wave pattern with a rhythm strip.
3. Verify the patient's clinical status. Death may occur during downward displacement of the pacemaker even though ventricular complexes are observed on the monitor. In other words, although electrical activity may still be present, the severely ischemic myocardium is unable to respond and its pumping action ceases (a condition called electromechanical dissociation).
4. At the first suggestion of atrial standstill, prepare for the insertion of a transvenous pacemaker.

ATRIAL STANDSTILL—IDENTIFYING ECG FEATURES

1. **Rate:**	Usually slow (40-60/minute), but depends on the site of the pacemaker.
2. **Rhythm:**	The ventricular rhythm is generally regular, except in the dying heart where ventricular ectopic beats may be interspersed.
3. **P waves:**	P waves are absent and there is essentially a straight line between the QRS complexes.
4. **P-R interval:**	Absent. There is no electrical activity in the SA node or atria.
5. **QRS:**	The configuration of the QRS complex depends on the site of the pacemaker. If the ventricle is stimulated from the AV nodal area the QRS complex may be normal. However, if the impulse originates within the ventricle itself the QRS will be widened and distorted.

Atrial Standstill (Figure 10.12)

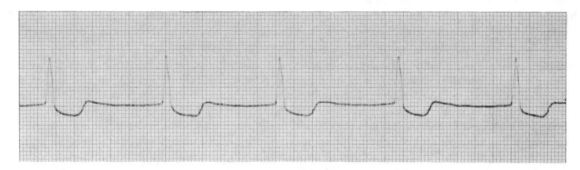

Rate:	About 50/minute.
Rhythm:	Regular.
P waves:	Absent (no atrial activity).
P-R interval:	Not determinable.
QRS:	Normal (0.10 second).
Comment:	The absence of P waves indicates that all atrial activity has ceased and that the pacemaker is now in the AV nodal area.

CASE HISTORY

A 69-year-old man with an acute anteroseptal infarction was admitted to the CCU with obvious signs of left ventricular failure. The response to treatment was poor and the patient remained in heart failure. The ECG showed normal sinus rhythm with a heart rate of 84/minute. About 8 hours after admission, the nurse noted that the heart rate suddenly slowed to 50/minute and that the P waves had disappeared. The physician was notified immediately. Although a temporary pacemaker was inserted, the patient died several hours later. Death was due to power failure with downward displacement of the pacemaker. The ECG change from normal sinus rhythm to atrial standstill is shown in the following examples (Figures 10.13A and Figure 10.13B).

Figure 10.13A. Normal sinus rhythm.

Figure 10.13B. Atrial standstill.

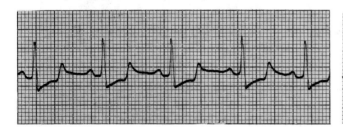

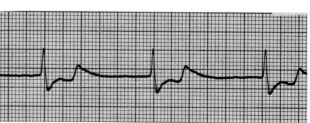

OTHER EXAMPLES OF
ARRHYTHMIAS ORIGINATING IN THE ATRIA

Premature Atrial Contraction with Aberrant Conduction (Figure 10.14)

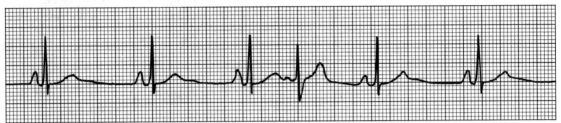

Rate:	About 60/minute.
Rhythm:	The otherwise regular rhythm is interrupted by the PAC.
P waves:	The P wave of the atrial premature beat differs in size and shape from the normal P waves of the other beats.
P-R interval:	Normal (0.12 second).
QRS:	The QRS complex of the PAC is wider and of a somewhat different configuration than the other ventricular complexes. This variation is due to abnormal conduction of the premature atrial impulse through the ventricles (aberrant conduction).
Comment:	In this example the degree of aberration is only moderate. However, in other instances aberrant conduction may be far more pronounced, resulting in a wide, distorted QRS complex that can resemble a premature *ventricular* contraction (PVC).

Paroxysmal Atrial Tachycardia (Figure 10.15)

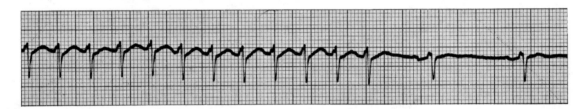

Rate:	185/minute during PAT.
Rhythm:	Regular.
P waves:	Not identified specifically during PAT.
P-R interval:	Not measurable.
QRS:	Normal (0.08 second).
Comment:	This example demonstrates the sudden cessation of paroxysmal atrial tachycardia and the resumption of normal sinus rhythm.

Paroxysmal Atrial Tachycardia with Block (Figure 10.16)

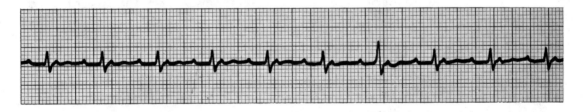

Rate:	The ventricular rate is 100/minute while the atrial rate is 200/minute.
Rhythm:	Regular.
P waves:	There are *two* P waves between each QRS complex. (One P wave occurs immediately after the QRS complex and below the T wave.)
P-R interval:	The atrial impulses that are conducted to the ventricles have a top normal P-R interval (0.20 second).
QRS:	Normal (0.08 second).

Comment: The atrial rate is 200/minute, typical of atrial tachycardia. The ventricular rate, however, is only 100/minute, indicating that every other atrial impulse is blocked. This arrhythmia, called PAT with block, is a common manifestation of *digitalis toxicity*. (The possibility that the arrhythmia is atrial flutter with 2:1 block can be excluded on the basis of the atrial rate, which would be 300 or more/minute with atrial flutter.)

Atrial Flutter with 4:1 Block (Figure 10.17)

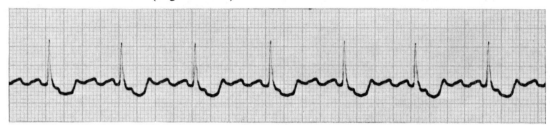

Rate:	Ventricular: 75/minute. Atrial: 300/minute.
Rhythm:	Regular.
P waves:	Four F waves occur during each R-R interval (4:1).
P-R interval:	Not determinable.
QRS:	Normal (0.08 second).
Comment:	Three of the four flutter waves between each QRS complex are clearly evident. The fourth occurs immediately after the R wave and produces a notch in the ST segment.

Atrial Flutter with 2:1 Block (Figure 10.18)

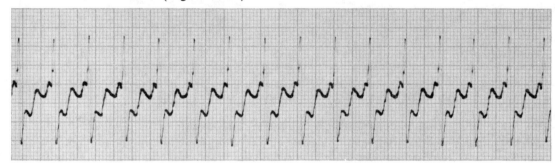

Rate:	Ventricular rate about 150/minute. Atrial rate about 300/minute.
Rhythm:	Regular.
P waves:	There are two flutter waves between QRS complexes, creating a sawtooth appearance.
P-R interval:	Not determinable.
QRS:	Normal.
Comment:	In general, atrial flutter with 2:1 block is more difficult to recognize than atrial flutter with 4:1 block. The reason is that flutter waves are often superimposed on other waves when the ventricular rate is fast (as in 2:1 block).

Atrial Fibrillation (Figure 10.19)

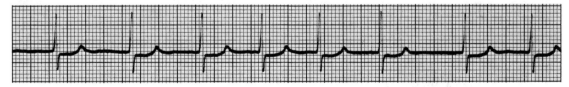

Rate:	About 80/minute.
Rhythm:	Irregular.
P waves:	No identifiable P waves or fibrillatory (f) waves.
P-R interval:	Not measurable.
QRS:	Normal (0.08 second).
Comment:	The diagnosis of atrial fibrillation is evident from 1) the absence of P waves and 2) the irregular ventricular rhythm. Although fibrillatory (f) waves can often be identified in atrial fibrillation, none are visible in this particular recording lead.

Atrial Flutter with Varying AV Block (Figure 10.20)

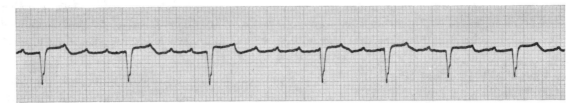

Rate:	Ventricular rate is about 70/minute.
Rhythm:	Irregular.
P waves:	Flutter waves occur regularly at a rate of about 250/minute. Some of the flutter waves are buried in the QRS complexes.
P-R interval:	Not significant.
QRS:	Normal (0.08 second).
Comment:	Unlike typical atrial flutter, which is characterized by a regular ventricular rate, this recording shows atrial flutter with a varying degree of AV block (3:1, 4:1, 5:1), which produces an irregular rhythm. Varying AV block is usally a manifestation of disturbed AV function.

Atrial Fibrillation with High Degree AV Block (Figure 10.21)

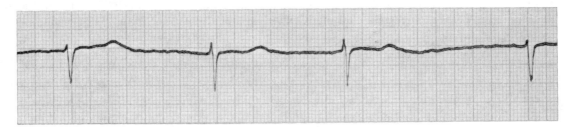

Rate:	Ventricular response is about 80/minute.
Rhythm:	Irregular.
P waves:	None. Very shallow fibrillatory waves are seen occasionally.
P-R interval:	None (since there are no P waves).
QRS:	Normal (0.09 second).
Comment:	Although the atria discharges impulses very rapidly (atrial fibrillation), only a few of these impulses are conducted to the ventricles. The very slow ventricular response (about 40/minute) indicates a high degree of block at the AV node, resulting from either digitalis or AV nodal disease. In any event, a ventricular rate of only 40/minute is usually hemodynamically ineffective and cannot be tolerated for long.

Atrial Standstill (Figure 10.22)

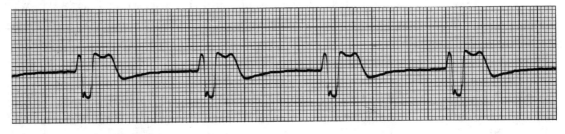

Rate:	About 40/minute.
Rhythm:	Regular.
P waves:	None.
P-R interval:	None.
QRS:	Wide (0.20 second) and distorted, indicating their ventricular origin.
Comment:	There is no evidence of atrial activity (atrial standstill) because the higher centers have been knocked out. A ventricular pacemaker has assumed control. This pattern, in which there is no longer any atrial or junctional activity, and only a ventricular pacemaker remains, occurs in the latter stages of downward displacement of the pacemaker.

11

Arrhythmias Originating in the AV Nodal Area (Junctional Arrhythmias)

PREMATURE JUNCTIONAL CONTRACTIONS
JUNCTIONAL RHYTHM
PAROXYSMAL JUNCTIONAL TACHYCARDIA
NONPAROXYSMAL JUNCTIONAL TACHYCARDIA
(Accelerated Junctional Rhythm)

Recent studies have shown that the AV node itself does not initiate impulses and that the site of origin of what had been called nodal rhythms is actually in the junctional tissue surrounding the AV node. In deference to this anatomic fact, disturbances previously classified as nodal arrhythmias are now properly termed *junctional arrhythmias.*

Normally the AV junction discharges impulses only when its inherent rate is faster than the SA node or atria. This usually occurs because the higher centers are suppressed temporarily (for one reason or other), allowing the normally slower AV junction to take over as pacemaker, at a rate of 40-60/minute. When this happens, the resulting arrhythmia is described as a junctional rhythm or a junctional escape rhythm (meaning that the pacemaker has "escaped" from the SA node to the AV junction).

On some occasions junctional arrhythmias are caused to accelerate impulse formation in the AV junction which exceeds the discharge rate of the SA node, even though the SA node is not depressed. Two arrhythmias may result from this increased activity in the AV junction: paroxysmal junctional tachycardia and nonparoxysmal junctional tachycardia (often called accelerated junctional rhythm).

Like the atria and the ventricles, the AV junction can also produce premature beats (premature junctional contractions).

Junctional arrhythmias (except for premature junctional contractions) must be regarded as major arrhythmias; they demand prompt attention.

PREMATURE JUNCTIONAL CONTRACTIONS

Mechanism

A premature junctional contraction (PJC) is similar to a premature atrial contraction except that the impulse arises from an ectopic focus in the *AV junctional area* rather than the atria. The impulse is transmitted downward through the His-Purkinje system and produces a normal QRS complex, which occurs earlier than expected in the rhythm cycle. The junctional impulse is also transmitted upward to the atria (retrograde conduction), causing atrial stimulation. Retrograde atrial activation usually results in an *inverted* P wave which occurs just before or just after (or during) the QRS complex, depending on the site of the ectopic focus in the junctional area and the speed of retrograde conduction. After a premature junctional beat there is an incomplete compensatory pause until the next sinus impulse arises. PJCs probably reflect irritability of the junctional tissues.

Danger in Acute Myocardial Infarction

1. Although it has been speculated that PJCs may give rise to junctional tachycardia in the same sense that atrial premature beats may trigger atrial fibrillation, this sequence has not been proven. Consequently, PJCs cannot be regarded as a distinct forerunner of junctional tachycardia.
2. Infrequent or isolated PJCs have no significant effect on circulatory efficiency.
3. PJCs probably represent a sign of irritability of the junctional tissue, and an increase in the frequency of these ectopic beats may reflect ischemic injury to the nodal or His bundle areas.
4. *RISK:* Premature junctional contractions are not serious in their own right and can be classified as a minor arrhythmia.

Clinical Features

1. Although PJCs produce some irregularity of the heart beat, patients seldom experience any symptoms.
2. PJCs cannot be distinguished from other premature beats by clinical examination; the arrhythmia can be identified only by ECG.

Treatment

1. If PJCs occur infrequently, treatment is unnecessary.
2. If their frequency increases, these ectopic beats can usually be terminated by administering lidocaine or procainamide intravenously.

Nursing Role

1. Identify premature *junctional* contractions and distinguish them from more serious premature *ventricular* contractions.
2. If the relative frequency of PJCs increases, notify the physician.
3. If PJCs are treated with an intravenous infusion of lidocaine or procainamide, adjust the rate of flow to control these ectopic beats.

CASE HISTORY

A 58-year-old man with an acute inferior myocardial infarction developed infrequent ectopic beats during the second day of hospitalization. From the monitor lead alone, the nurse was unable to decide whether these beats were premature junctional contractions or premature ventricular contractions. When the frequency of these ectopic beats increased gradually over the next 3 hours, a 12-lead ECG was taken to identify their specific origin. Premature junctional contractions were evident. The physician was notified, and it was decided that no therapy was necessary.

PREMATURE JUNCTIONAL CONTRACTIONS
IDENTIFYING ECG FEATURES

1. **Rate:**   Normal.
2. **Rhythm:**   Regular except for the premature beat and the pause that follows.
3. **P waves:**   Because the atria are stimulated in a *retrograde* manner by impulses originating in the junctional tissue, the shape and position of the P waves vary with the conduction time to the atria. Usually the P waves are *inverted* and occur either immediately before or after the QRS complex. In many instances P waves cannot be identified at all, being buried in the QRS complexes.
4. **P-R interval:** When a P wave precedes the QRS complex, the P-R interval is usually shortened (less than 0.12 second).
5. **QRS:**   Normal because conduction from the AV junctional area to the Purkinje network is not disturbed. (Occasionally, however, the impulse may be transmitted abnormally, producing a wide QRS complex. This is called aberrant conduction.)

Premature Junctional Contraction (Figure 11.1)

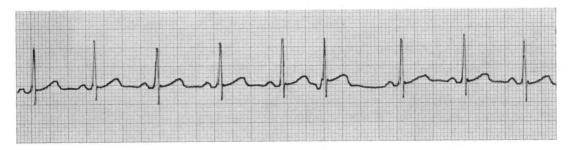

Rate:	About 90/minute.
Rhythm:	Regular except for one PJC.
P waves:	The P wave of the PJC is inverted and occurs immediately before the QRS complex.
P-R interval:	Shortened (0.08 second) in PJC; other P-R intervals are normal.
QRS:	Normal (0.06 second).
Comment:	An inverted P wave with a very short P-R interval indicates retrograde conduction from AV junction to atria.

Premature Junctional Contraction (PJC) (Figure 11.2)

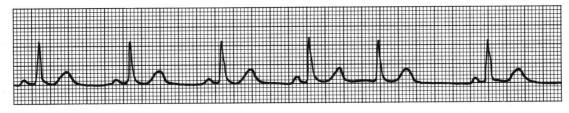

Rate:	About 60/minute.
Rhythm:	A regular rhythm is interrupted by one premature beat and the pause that follows it.
P waves:	The P wave of the PJC is not visible, hidden in the QRS complex.
P-R interval:	Not measurable.
QRS:	Normal (0.09 second).
Comment:	The P wave of the PJC is hidden in the QRS complex because the atria and ventricles are depolarized simultaneously (i.e., retrograde conduction speed equals anterograde conduction speed). If the atria were depolarized first, the P wave would precede the QRS complex. If depolarized after the ventricles, the P waves would follow the QRS complex.

JUNCTIONAL RHYTHM

Mechanism

If for any reason the SA node fails to initiate impulses or discharges too slowly, the AV junction may assume control of the cardiac rhythm, replacing the SA node as pacemaker. When this occurs a *junctional rhythm* exists. In other words, a junctional rhythm develops because of default of the primary (SA node) pacemaker and serves as a safety mechanism to sustain the heartbeat. Because the pacemaker has "escaped" from the SA node to the AV junction, the rhythm is also described as a *junctional escape rhythm.*

In this circumstance the AV junction discharges impulses at its own intrinsic rate of 40-60/minute. The impulses travel *upward* to activate the atria and *downward* to stimulate the ventricles. Depending on the relative speed of retrograde and anterograde conduction, the P waves may precede, follow, or be hidden within the QRS complexes. Since ventricular stimulation is not disturbed, the QRS complexes are normal.

The suppression of the SA node, which permits a junctional rhythm to develop, is often the result of excessive vagal activity. Other causative factors are ischemic damage to the SA node, and digitalis or quinidine toxicity.

Danger in Acute Myocardial Infarction

1. Because of the inherently slow rate of junctional impulses (40-60/minute), ectopic foci with more rapid rates may take over the pacemaking function. Such foci may cause either junctional or ventricular tachycardia, especially in the presence of myocardial ischemia.
2. A junctional pacemaker is not dependable and there is a danger of downward displacement of the pacemaker to the ventricle.
3. As with other slow-rate arrhythmias, cardiac output may decrease significantly, leading to myocardial ischemia or heart failure.
4. *RISK:* Although most patients can tolerate a junctional rhythm without difficulty, the arrhythmia is nevertheless dangerous because it indicates a less dependable pacemaker than the SA node is in command. Also, there is a potential threat of other ectopic rhythms developing as well as the adverse hemodynamic consequences resulting from the slow rate.

Clinical Features

1. A junctional rhythm seldom produces symptoms, unless the rate is very slow (about 40/minute).
2. At the bedside, a junctional rhythm resembles sinus bradycardia. Both arrhythmias are characterized by a slow regular rate of 40-60/minute. An ECG is necessary to distinguish the two arrhythmias.
3. A junctional rhythm is often transient (lasting for only a few beats) after which the SA node regains control.

Treatment

1. There is no specific drug therapy for a junctional rhythm, but atropine is sometimes successful in increasing the discharge rate of the SA node, allowing it to regain control.
2. If the slow heart rate compromises the circulation, a transvenous pacemaker should be used to increase the ventricular rate (and, in turn, the cardiac output).
3. If ventricular ectopic beats develop in the presence of a junctional rhythm, they are best controlled by rate acceleration (cardiac pacing or atropine). For some reason lidocaine is less effective in terminating ventricular ectopic beats that develop during slow heart rates than it is in controlling premature ventricular beats that occur during normal or fast heart rates.
4. If the arrhythmia is secondary to digitalis or quinidine overdosages, the offending drug should be withdrawn.

Nursing Role

1. Identify the arrhythmia as a junctional rhythm. Rule out the possibility that the slow heart rate is due to sinus bradycardia or advanced heart block. A 12-lead ECG may be necessary.
2. Observe the monitor carefully for premature ventricular beats, which are likely to develop in the presence of a slow rate. Notify the physician if such ectopic activity is noted.
3. Be alert for symptoms of heart failure or myocardial ischemia, particularly when the rate is below 50/min.
4. If a junctional rhythm develops *suddenly*, notify the physician.
5. If the patient is receiving digitalis or quinidine, discuss the further use of these drugs with the physician before administering the next dose.

JUNCTIONAL RHYTHM—IDENTIFYING ECG FEATURES

1. **Rate:**   Slow, usually 40-60/minute.
2. **Rhythm:**   Regular.
3. **P waves:**   The P waves may occur a) before the QRS, b) after the QRS, or c) may not be visible, being buried with the QRS complex. When present, the P waves are usually inverted.
4. **P-R interval:** When the P waves precede the QRS complexes the P-R interval is shortened (less than 0.12 second), reflecting retrograde stimulation of the atria by a pacemaker in the AV junction.
5. **QRS:**   Normal, indicating that conduction downward through the ventricular pathways is not disturbed.

Junctional Rhythm (Figure 11.3)

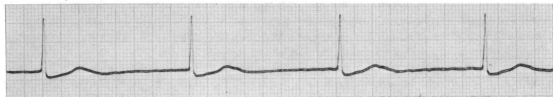

Rate:	About 40/minute.
Rhythm:	Regular.
P waves:	None visible.
P-R interval:	Not measurable.
QRS:	Normal (0.06 second)
Comment:	The presence of this junctional rhythm (at a rate of about 40/minute) indicates that the SA node is no longer discharging or is firing at a rate of less than 40/minute. A junctional rhythm is a safety mechanism that preserves the heartbeat if higher pacemakers fail, as in this example.

AV Junctional Rhythm (Figure 11.4)

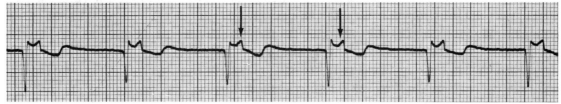

Rate:	About 60/minute (54/minute).
Rhythm:	Regular.
P waves:	Occur after QRS complexes, as evident by the notch in the ST segment (see arrows).
P-R interval:	Indeterminate.
QRS:	Normal (0.06 second).
Comment:	That the P wave follows the QRS complex indicates that the ventricles were activated by the junctional impulses before the atria. Put differently, anterograde conduction to the ventricles was faster than retrograde conduction to the atria.

CASE HISTORY

A 56-year-old man was admitted to the CCU with a heart rate of 48/minute. He was in no distress, and there was no evidence of left ventricular failure. On a rhythm strip the nurse noted that the P waves were inverted and followed the QRS complexes, from which she concluded that the bradycardia was due to a junctional rhythm. Two hours later the patient developed premature ventricular contractions (PVCs) at a rate of 4-6/minute. When 4 PVCs occurred consecutively (ventricular tachycardia) lidocaine was administered. It was not effective in suppressing the ectopic beats. After an unsuccessful attempt at increasing the heart rate with intravenous atropine, a transvenous pacemaker was inserted and the ventricle paced at a rate of 80/minute. The ectopic beats disappeared promptly.

PAROXYSMAL JUNCTIONAL TACHYCARDIA

Mechanism

Paroxysmal junctional tachycardia (PJT) is similar in most respects to paroxysmal atrial tachycardia except that the ectopic focus is in the AV junction rather than the atria. Both arrhythmias begin and end *suddenly* and both are characterized by a regular, rapid rate of 140-250/minute.

Impulses from the AV junction are conducted normally to the ventricles and retrogradely to the atria. As with other junctional arrhythmias the P waves occur before, after, or during the QRS complexes, depending on the speed of retrograde conduction.

PJT may develop secondary to ischemia to the AV junction, but increased catecholamine secretion and metabolic disturbances are probably more common causes. Digitalis toxicity is occasionally the underlying mechanism of PJT.

Danger in Acute Myocardial Infarction

1. The rapid ventricular rate usually results in a decrease in cardiac output and predisposes to left ventricular failure. This threat is directly related to the duration of the tachycardia.
2. PJT increases myocardial oxygen demand and may produce angina or additional ischemic damage.
3. *RISK:* PJT is a dangerous arrhythmia from a hemodynamic standpoint, particularly if the episode is prolonged.

Clinical Features

1. The clinical presentation of PJT closely resembles paroxysmal atrial tachycardia with the *sudden* onset and termination of a rapid, regular rhythm (140-250/minute).
2. The symptoms are those anticipated with a very fast ventricular rate: dyspnea, apprehension, and angina are common, especially if the tachycardia is sustained.
3. It is often difficult and sometimes impossible to distinguish PJT from PAT electrocardiographically. The rapid rate frequently obscures the position of the P waves and in this circumstance the two arrhythmias are collectively called *paroxysmal supraventricular tachycardia* (PSVT), indicating that the location of the ectopic focus may be either atrial or junctional.

Treatment

1. Vagal stimulation by means of carotid sinus massage may terminate PJT and is usually the first step in treatment.
2. If PJT is *sustained* and results in angina or signs of left ventricular failure, the arrhythmia should be terminated *immediately* with synchronized precordial shock (cardioversion).
3. If the arrhythmia produces no obvious symptoms and the patient is not in distress, drug therapy can be attempted initially. Digitalis or propranolol given intravenously are often effective in this situation.
4. Even if the paroxysm of junctional tachycardia is of short duration and subsides spontaneously without treatment, antiarrhythmic therapy should nevertheless be instituted in an attempt to prevent recurrent episodes. The choice of drugs for this purpose includes propranolol, quinidine, digitalis, and calcium blocking agents.

Nursing Role

1. PJT will trigger the high-rate alarm system. Document the arrhythmia with a rhythm strip. (If P waves cannot be identified from the monitor lead, recordings from other leads should be made.)
2. Go to the bedside and examine the patient. Inquire about angina and dyspnea and assess the clinical status.
3. Notify the physician promptly.
4. If the patient describes angina, record a 12-lead ECG to identify ischemic changes.
5. If the arrhythmia persists or signs of left ventricular failure are present, prepare for elective precordial shock.

PAROXYSMAL JUNCTIONAL TACHYCARDIA
IDENTIFYING ECG FEATURES

1. **Rate:** Usually 140-250/minute.
2. **Rhythm:** Regular.
3. **P waves:** May precede, follow, or be hidden in QRS complexes, depending on speed of retrograde conduction to the atria.
4. **P-R interval:** If P waves precede the QRS complexes, the P-R interval is usually less than 0.12 second.
5. **QRS:** Normal, since conduction to the ventricles is not disturbed.

Paroxysmal Junctional Tachycardia (Figure 11.5)

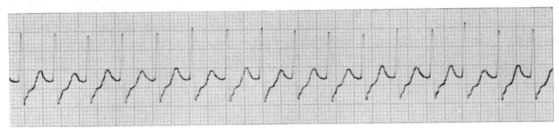

Rate:	160/minute.
Rhythm:	Regular.
P waves:	Follow the QRS complexes, being visible on the ST segments.
P-R interval:	Not determinable.
QRS:	Near normal. (Although widened, the QRS complexes appear to be 0.10 second in duration.)
Comment:	It is often difficult to distinguish PJT from PAT by a monitor lead alone. A 12-lead ECG may be necessary to identify the position of the P waves.

Paroxysmal Junctional Tachycardia (Figure 11.6)

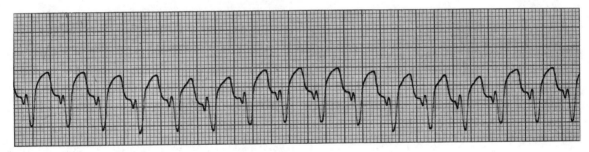

Rate:	About 160/minute.
Rhythm:	Regular.
P waves:	Inverted, and immediately precede the QRS complexes.
P-R interval:	Shortened (0.06 second).
QRS:	Normal (0.08 second).
Comment:	This arrhythmia began abruptly and terminated spontaneously 3 minutes later in typical paroxysmal fashion.

CASE HISTORY

A 72-year-old man with an acute anterior infarction experienced no complications during the first 8 hours after admission to the CCU. Then, suddenly the high-rate alarm sounded. The nurse noted a rate of 200/minute. The monitor revealed normal QRS complexes followed by inverted P waves. The patient was apprehensive and described "chest fullness." The blood pressure was 86/52. Oxygen and nitroglycerin were administered and the physician was notified. Two minutes later, before any other treatment was given, the arrhythmia stopped spontaneously and the patient's symptoms cleared promptly. Prophylactic therapy was instituted to prevent recurrent episodes of PJT.

NONPAROXYSMAL JUNCTIONAL TACHYCARDIA
(Accelerated Junctional Rhythm)

Mechanism

In nonparoxysmal junctional tachycardia (NPJT) an irritable focus in the AV junction replaces the SA node as pacemaker and discharges at a rate of 70-130/minute (in contrast to paroxysmal junctional tachycardia in which the rate is 140-250/minute). Even though the heart rate during NPJT may be less than 100/minute, as is often the case, the arrhythmia is nevertheless described as a tachycardia. The reason for this seemingly contradictory terminology is that the inherent rate of impulse formation in the AV junction is only 40-60/minute (junctional rhythm) and therefore any rate above 60/minute is, in effect, a tachycardia for the AV junction. In the same sense, NPJT can be described as an *accelerated junctional rhythm.*

NPJT often develops during the course of advanced heart failure or cardiogenic shock and in this circumstance probably represents a stage of downward displacement of the pacemaker in a severely damaged heart (see Atrial Standstill). However, NPJT may occur independently of circulatory failure. In this situation the most common cause is digitalis toxicity.

Danger in Acute Myocardial Infarction

1. When NPJT develops in association with heart failure or cardiogenic shock it usually indicates that extensive myocardial damage is present and that further downward displacement of the pacemaker (to the ventricles) may occur.
2. In its own right, NPJT may contribute to a reduction in cardiac output because the atrial component of ventricular filling is lost with a junctional pacemaker.
3. When NPJT is due to excessive digitalis, further administration of the drug can produce advanced heart block or ventricular standstill.
4. *RISK:* NPJT is a serious arrhythmia in patients with acute myocardial infarction and is usually associated with a high mortality. Death, however, is not due to the arrhythmia itself but to underlying myocardial damage. When digitalis is the causative factor and the problem is recognized, the prognosis is good.

Clinical Features

1. Unlike paroxysmal junctional tachycardia, NPJT develops and terminates *gradually,* rather than abruptly. This gradual rate change is the most distinctive feature of the arrhythmia.
2. When the arrhythmia accompanies advanced left ventricular failure the signs and symptoms of heart failure dominate the clinical picture.
3. In the absence of circulatory failure, NPJT seldom produces symptoms or physical findings.
4. NPJT can be identified only by ECG.

Treatment

1. There is no specific treatment for NPJT. When circulatory failure is present the treatment program is aimed at improving left ventricular function, after which the arrhythmia may disappear.
2. Because of the threat of further downward displacement of the pacemaker to the ventricles, a transvenous pacemaker may be inserted.
3. If there is any possibility that NPJT is the result of digitalis toxicity, the drug should be stopped immediately and potassium administered intravenously.

NONPAROXYSMAL JUNCTIONAL TACHYCARDIA
IDENTIFYING ECG FEATURES

1. Rate:	Usually 70-130/minute. Rates below 60/minute indicate a junctional escape rhythm and rates about 140/minute suggest paroxysmal junctional tachycardia.
2. Rhythm:	Regular.
3. P waves:	May occur before or after the QRS complex or may not be present.
4. P-R interval:	Retrograde conduction to the atria may or may not occur. When a P-R interval is identifiable the interval is usually less than 0.12 second.
5. QRS:	Normal, because conduction from the AV junction to the ventricles is not affected.

Nonparoxysmal Junctional Tachycardia (Accelerated Junctional Rhythm) (Figure 11.7)

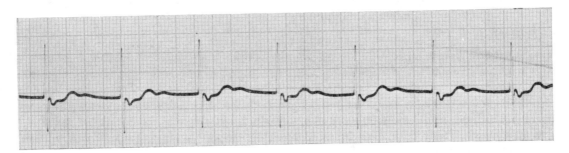

Rate:	About 70/minute.
Rhythm:	Regular.
P waves:	Inverted and occur immediately after QRS complexes.
P-R interval:	Not determinable.
QRS:	Normal (0.06 second).
Comment:	This arrhythmia is often called *accelerated junctional rhythm* because its rate is faster than the inherent rate of junctional tissue (40-60/minute) and, yet, it is much slower than paroxysmal junctional tachycardia (140-220/minute). Since the arrhythmia is not actually a tachycardia (rate more than 100/minute), it seems appropriate to adopt the new term "accelerated junctional rhythm."

Nursing Role

1. Because the arrhythmia develops gradually and its rate is between 70 and 130/minute, the monitor alarm system will *not* be activated and therefore the identification depends on careful monitor observation.

2. Ascertain that the arrhythmia is NPJT and document it with a rhythm strip.

3. Be especially alert for this arrhythmia among patients with advanced circulatory failure or cardiogenic shock and notify the physician immediately once identification has been made.

4. Prepare for the insertion of a transvenous pacemaker, which may be utilized in the treatment program.

5. Always consider the possibility of digitalis intoxication when NPJT develops in the absence of circulatory failure. Consult the physician before administering the next dose.

Nonparoxysmal Junctional Tachycardia (Accelerated Junctional Rhythm) (Figure 11.8)

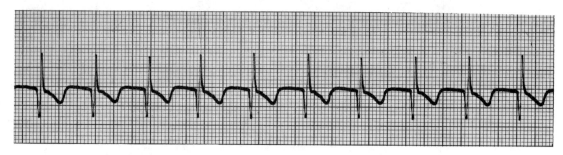

Rate:	About 100/minute.
Rhythm:	Regular.
P waves:	Not visible, probably buried in QRS complexes.
P-R interval:	Not measurable in the absence of P waves.
QRS:	Normal (0.10 second).
Comment:	In contrast to paroxysmal junctional tachycardia, which develops abruptly, the arrhythmia shown here developed gradually and its rate never exceeded 100/minute.

CASE HISTORY

A 74-year-old man was admitted to CCU with severe chest pain and signs of marked left ventricular failure. The ECG revealed an acute anterior wall myocardial infarction and the presence of sinus tachycardia. The patient was treated with furosemide and digoxin but showed little improvement during the next 2 hours. The nurse noted that the heart rate gradually decreased from 130 to 80/minute. She suspected at first that the rate slowing was due only to digitalis, but on examining a rhythm strip she noted a change in the P waves, which were now inverted and followed the QRS complexes. It was apparent that the patient had developed NPJT, and the physician was notified immediately.

OTHER EXAMPLES OF ARRHYTHMIAS ORIGINATING IN THE AV JUNCTION

Supraventricular Ectopic Beats: Either PJCs or PACs (Figure 11.9)

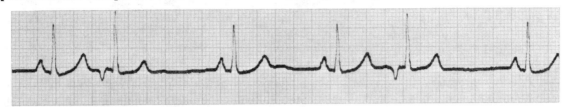

Rate:	About 70/minute.
Rhythm:	Regular except for premature ectopic beat.
P waves:	The fourth P wave occurs prematurely and is inverted.
P-R interval:	The P-R interval of the premature beat is 0.12 second.
QRS:	Normal (0.06 second).
Comment:	Although the P waves of the two ectopic beats are inverted, this does not indicate that they are PJCs. The P waves of atrial ectopic beats may also be inverted. However, the P-R intervals of PJCs should be less than 0.12 seconds, while they can be longer with PACs. In this example (where the P-R interval is 0.12 second) the ectopic beats are best classified as *supraventricular ectopic beats,* meaning that they are either atrial or junctional in origin.

Junctional Rhythm (to Normal Sinus Rhythm) (Figure 11.10)

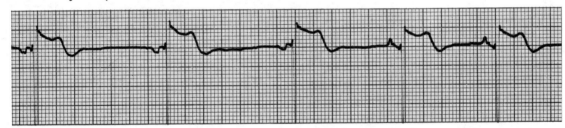

Rate:	During junctional rhythm: 45/minute. During normal sinus rhythm: 64/minute.
Rhythm:	Regular (but at different rates).
P waves:	Inverted with junctional rhythm; upright with normal sinus rhythm.
P-R interval:	Normal (0.12 second during junctional rhythm).
QRS:	Normal (0.08 second).
Comment:	The first three beats originate in the AV junction at a rate of 45/minute. The SA node, which apparently had been suppressed, suddenly regains control as the pacemaker starting with the fourth beat. Note the faster heart rate during sinus rhythm, which explains why the SA node resumed its control.

Junctional Rhythm (Figure 11.11)

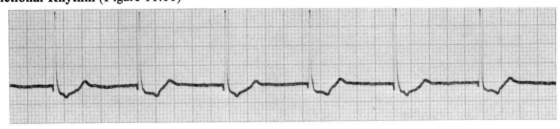

Rate:	About 60/minute.
Rhythm:	Regular.
P waves:	Occur after QRS complexes and appear as downward notches in ST segments.
P-R interval:	Not determinable.
QRS:	Normal (0.06 second).
Comment:	A junctional rhythm is a protective or escape mechanism which develops when the SA node or atria are suppressed.

Junctional Escape Beat (Figure 11.12)

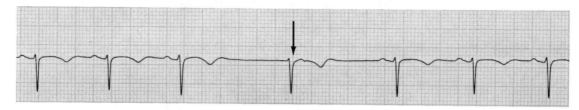

Rate:	About 70/minute.
Rhythm:	Irregular.
P waves:	About 3 beats, the next anticipated P wave is not visible (junctional escape beat). The P waves occur regularly thereafter.
P-R interval:	Normal except with junctional escape beat, where indeterminate.
QRS:	Normal (0.06 second), including junctional escape beat.
Comment:	After three beats there is a pause (due, perhaps, to sinus arrest or block or marked sinus bradycardia). In any event, after 1.2 seconds no sinus or atrial beat has occurred. As a protective mechanism, the AV junction—the next downward pacemaker—discharges an impulse to stimulate the ventricles and prevent cessation of the heartbeat. This junctional beat is called a *junctional escape beat.* Note that the escape beat does not occur unless the heart rate slows and the R-R interval is prolonged, even if just for one beat.

Paroxysmal Junctional Tachycardia (Figure 11.13)

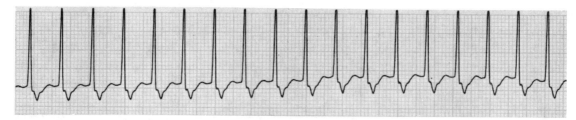

Rate:	About 180/minute.
Rhythm:	Regular.
P waves:	Occur after QRS complexes, producing spiked appearance of T waves.
P-R interval:	Not determinable.
QRS:	Normal (0.04 second).
Comment:	Sharp, spiked T waves usually indicate that a P wave is superimposed. Hidden P waves, as in this example, can often be located through this T wave sign.

Supraventricular Tachycardia (Figure 11.14)

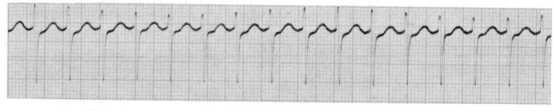

Rate:	160/minute.
Rhythm:	Regular.
P waves:	Not identifiable.
P-R interval:	Not determinable.
QRS:	Normal (0.06 second).
Comment:	This rapid tachycardia is characterized by a regular rhythm with QRS complexes of normal duration. The normal QRS complexes indicate that the arrhythmia originated *above* the ventricles. However, since P waves cannot be identified, the tachycardia may be either atrial tachycardia (PAT) or junctional tachycardia (PJT) or atrial flutter with 2:1 block. For this reason arrhythmias of this type (without identifiable P waves) are often categorized as *supraventricular tachycardias.* Only by using additional leads can a definite interpretation be made.

Accelerated Junctional Rhythm (Figure 11.15)

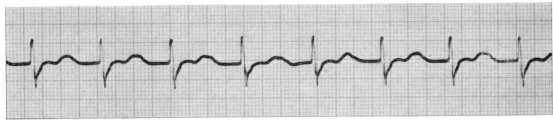

Rate:	About 80/minute.
Rhythm:	Regular.
P waves:	Not identified, probably buried in QRS complexes.
P-R interval:	Not measurable.
QRS:	Normal (just less than 0.12 second).
Comment:	This arrhythmia is often called an *accelerated junctional rhythm* because its rate is faster than the inherent rate of junctional tissue (40-60/minute). On the other hand, it is much slower than paroxysmal junctional tachycardia (140-220/minute).

Accelerated Junctional Rhythm (Figure 11.16)

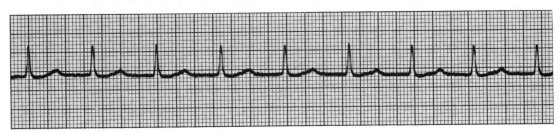

Rate:	About 90/minute.
Rhythm:	Regular.
P waves:	None visible.
P-R interval:	Not determinable.
QRS:	Normal (0.08 second).
Comment:	Since the normal discharge rate of the AV junction is 40-60/minute, the arrhythmia represents an accelerated junctional rhythm. Unlike an escape junctional rhythm, which occurs by default and is a protective mechanism, accelerated junctional rhythms (or nonparoxysmal junctional tachycardia as it is still called) are active rhythms; they may be caused by various drugs.

12

Arrhythmias Originating in the Ventricles

PREMATURE VENTRICULAR CONTRACTIONS
VENTRICULAR TACHYCARDIA
ACCELERATED IDIOVENTRICULAR RHYTHM
VENTRICULAR FIBRILLATION

Disturbances in the heartbeat that originate in the SA node, the atria, or the AV junction areas are jointly classified as *supraventricular* arrhythmias. If the impulse begins in the ventricles, below the level of the AV nodal area, the resulting disorder is termed a *ventricular* arrhythmia.

The most common ventricular arrhythmia (in fact, the most common of all arrhythmias) is the premature ventricular contraction (PVC). Practically all patients with acute myocardial infarction exhibit PVCs during the first few days after the attack. Premature ventricular beats result from the discharge of an ectopic focus within the ventricular walls (or the conduction pathway) before the expected arrival of the next impulse from a supraventricular center. These ectopic beats usually represent a sign of myocardial irritability secondary to ischemia, and the frequency and type of PVCs is probably a fair index of the degree of ischemic irritation.

There is good evidence that ventricular fibrillation, the most frequent cause of sudden death, is a direct consequence of myocardial irritability, and that this lethal arrhythmia usually begins with a premature ventricular contraction. The scale of myocardial irritability leading to ventricular fibrillation can be viewed as follows:

1. isolated premature ventricular contractions
2. complex premature ventricular contractions (occurring more than 6 times/minute), or originating from more than one ventricular focus (multifocal premature beats), or occurring in pairs (couplets)
3. a series of three or more *consecutive* premature contractions occurring at a rapid rate (ventricular tachycardia)
4. ventricular fibrillation.

Although the relationship between PVCs and ventricular fibrillation is clearly established, it should not be assumed that all ventricular ectopic beats are potentially dangerous. *It is only in the presence of myocardial ischemia that PVCs are likely to provoke ventricular fibrillation.* Many normal individuals without evidence of heart disease display premature ventricular beats which pose no threat at all.

Ventricular tachycardia is an immediate forerunner of ventricular fibrillation in many instances. In addition to this extreme threat, ventricular tachycardia, when sustained, seriously endangers the circulation by markedly reducing cardiac output. For these reasons this ventricular arrhythmia must never be allowed to persist.

Accelerated idioventricular rhythm, like ventricular tachycardia, represents a series of consecutive ventricular ectopic beats. However, these beats occur at a rate of only 50-100/minute, compared to the much faster rate of ventricular tachycardia (140-250/minute). Furthermore, accelerated idioventricular rhythm does not lead to ventricular fibrillation, and is a benign arrhythmia in this sense.

Ventricular fibrillation, by far the main cause of sudden cardiac death, is understandably of supreme importance.

PREMATURE VENTRICULAR CONTRACTIONS

Mechanism

When an irritable focus in the ventricles discharges before the arrival of the next anticipated impulse from the SA node (or other supraventricular pacemaker) the resulting beat is called a *premature ventricular contraction* (PVC). The ectopic focus stimulates the ventricles directly (without traversing the normal conduction pathway) and produces a wide, distorted QRS complex—one of the main characteristics of a PVC. The SA node is not usually affected by the PVC and continues to discharge independently, on schedule; however, the P waves are seldom visible, being hidden in the abnormal QRS complex. Following the PVC there is a *complete compensatory pause* before the next sinus impulse comes along to initiate a normal ventricular beat. (A complete or fully compensatory pause means that the interval between the beat preceding the PVC and the beat following it is exactly equal to two cardiac cycles. When the interval is less than two cardiac cycles, as with premature atrial or junctional contractions, the compensatory pause is described as incomplete.)

PVCs are the most common of all arrhythmias associated with acute myocardial infarction and are thought to represent a sign of ventricular irritability.

Danger in Acute Myocardial Infarction

1. PVCs reflect myocardial irritability and are of particular importance because they may initiate repetitive ventricular firing in the form of ventricular tachycardia or ventricular fibrillation. The sequence of PVCs → ventricular tachycardia → ventricular fibrillation is most apt to occur when PVCs occur in any of the five following forms:

    a. when PVCs occur frequently, especially six or more times per minute
    b. when every second beat is a PVC (bigeminy)
    c. when the PVC strikes on the T wave of the preceding complex (the "R on T" pattern)
    d. when PVCs originate from more than one irritable focus in the ventricle (multiple PVCs)
    e. when there are two consecutive PVCs (couplets or pairs).

2. Since PVCs develop in 90% of all patients with acute myocardial infarction, their mere presence has little significance in their own right. PVCs are of concern if they increase in frequency or occur as one of the five dangerous forms described above.

3. Overdosages of digitalis frequently cause PVCs. This relationship is suggested especially when PVCs occur as bigeminy.

4. Hypokalemia also predisposes to PVCs. Patients receiving powerful diuretic agents and those on long-term therapy often lose sufficient potassium to induce PVCs.

5. *RISK:* If PVCs appear infrequently, the threat of provoking serious ventricular arrhythmias is not great. However, if these ectopic beats occur with increasing frequency or are of a dangerous type, they should be considered as a serious warning of impending ventricular tachycardia or ventricular fibrillation.

Clinical Features

1. Many patients are aware of PVCs and describe the sensation as "palpitations" or "skipping of the heart." The greater the frequency of these ectopic beats, the more likely the patient is to notice them.

2. When listening to the heart or taking the pulse, a relatively long pause is noted immediately after the premature beat. This delay (called a complete compensatory pause) is characteristic and is practically diagnostic of the arrhythmia.

PREMATURE VENTRICULAR CONTRACTIONS
IDENTIFYING ECG FEATURES

1. **Rate:**   Often normal, but PVCs can occur at any rate.
2. **Rhythm:**   The premature beat and the compensatory pause that follows it create an irregularity in the rhythm. Characteristically, the interval between the beat preceding and the beat following a PVC is equal to two normal beats (a complete compensatory pause, as shown in Figure 12.1 below).
3. **P waves:**   Although the SA node discharges independently of the PVC, the P wave is usually hidden in the QRS complex.
4. **P-R interval:** A PVC does not have a P-R interval because the ventricle is stimulated directly and there is no conduction from the atrium to the ventricles.
5. **QRS:**   The QRS complex is always widened and distorted in shape. The particular configuration of the QRS complex depends on the site of the ventricular focus. The T wave is usually oppositely directed from the QRS complex.

Isolated Premature Ventricular Contraction (Figure 12.1)

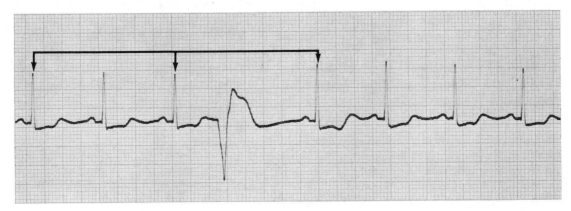

Rate:	About 80/minute.
Rhythm:	Irregular because of PVC.
P waves:	Not seen in PVC; normal in the other cardiac cycles.
P-R interval:	Absent in the PVC because the impulse originates in the ventricle. (Conduction of the remaining beats is normal.)
QRS:	The ectopic complex is widened and bizarre in configuration, and the T wave is *oppositely* directed from the QRS complex.
Comment:	The interval between the beat preceding the PVC and the beat following the PVC is equal to the time of two normal beats (arrows) and represents a full compensatory pause.

Treatment

1. Lidocaine is the primary agent used to control PVCs. Suppression of the irritable ventricular focus can be achieved promptly in most instances by administering 50-100 mg lidocaine as a rapid intravenous injection ("push dose"). This should be followed by a continuous infusion of lidocaine given at a rate of 2-3 mg/minute (20-30 microdrops/minute of a solution containing 3000 mg lidocaine in 500 cc glucose solution) in order to control further myocardial irritability. If the PVCs are not controlled with this regimen, a second or third IV bolus of lidocaine (50-100 mg) can be administered at 15 minute intervals. The total dosage, however, should not exceed 500 mg/hour.
2. If adequate doses of lidocaine fail to suppress PVCs, procainamide (Pronestyl) can be given intravenously as a second line treatment. Although sometimes successful in this situation, the drug has the disadvantage of producing hypotension and has a higher incidence of side-effects than lidocaine. (The methods of administration and side-effects of procainamide are described in Chapter 16, Antiarrhythmic Drugs.)
3. Occasionally neither lidocaine or procainamide in customary doses is effective in inhibiting PVCs. In this circumstance it is unwise to increase the dosages beyond their recommended levels since overdosages of both drugs can produce serious toxic effects. Resistance to drug therapy often indicates a depletion of myocardial potassium and for this reason it is useful to administer an intravenous infusion of potassium (40 mEq KCl in 500 cc dextrose solution), particularly if there is evidence of hypokalemia.
4. Oral antiarrhythmic agents are often effective in controlling ventricular ectopic activity. However their action is too slow for acute situations and therefore they are reserved for maintenance therapy. The most commonly used drugs for this purpose are procainamide (500 mg every 4 hours), quinidine (400 mg every 6 hours), and dispyramide (150 mg every 6 hours). Long-acting procainamide is also available.
5. If PVCs develop during treatment with digitalis or diuretics the possibility of drug-induced ectopic beats must always be considered. In this circumstance the drugs may have to be discontinued and potassium administered.

Nursing Role

1. Identify PVCs and distinguish these ventricular ectopic beats from less serious atrial or junctional premature contractions.
2. Carefully assess the relative frequency of PVCs during successive time intervals to ascertain any change in number. Also identify the type of PVC noted (i.e., multifocal, couplet).
3. If PVCs occur in any of the most threatening forms, the physician should be notified and lidocaine should be administered immediately.
4. When an infusion of lidocaine is used to control PVCs, adjust the rate of flow to suppress ectopic activity with the minimal dosage.
5. If lidocaine is given repeatedly or in large doses, seek signs of overdosage as manifested by petit mal or grand mal seizures or drowsiness. If procainamide is being administered, the blood pressure should be monitored frequently to detect hypotension.
6. In the event PVCs develop during digitalis therapy, advise the physician before administering the next dose of digitalis.

CASE HISTORY

A 51-year-old woman with an acute myocardial infarction showed evidence of PVCs from the time of her admission to the unit. These ectopic beats occurred at a rate of 1-2/minute. During the next several hours the nurse noted that the PVCs gradually increased in frequency and that bigeminy had developed. The physician was advised of this change and a push dose of lidocaine (75 mg) was given. The PVCs disappeared within a minute of the injection. An intravenous infusion of lidocaine was then started. Two hours later the PVCs reappeared and the nurse increased the rate of infusion from 1 mg to 2 mg/minute, after which the PVCs disappeared.

FIVE DANGEROUS FORMS OF PREMATURE VENTRICULAR CONTRACTIONS

1. Frequent PVCs Occurring More Than 6/Minute (Figure 12.2)

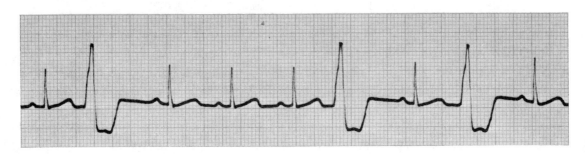

Rate:	About 90/minute.
Rhythm:	Irregular, as the result of PVCs.
P waves:	Not identified in ectopic beats.
P-R interval:	Absent in PVCs. The remaining beats are conducted normally from the SA node.
QRS:	The PVCs are very wide (0.16 second) and distorted in shape, indicating their ventricular origin.
Comment:	There are 3 PVCs in this 6-second strip. At this frequency, about 30 PVCs would occur per minute—a serious sign of ventricular irritability.

2. Bigeminy (Alternate PVCs or Coupled Rhythm) (Figure 12.3)

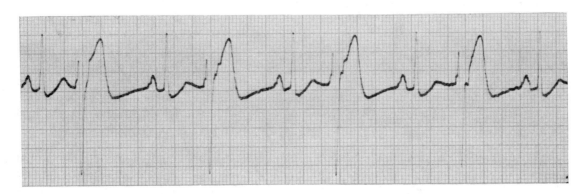

Rate:	About 90/minute.
Rhythm:	Irregular due to bigeminy (coupled beats).
P waves:	Not seen in the PVCs.
P-R interval:	There is no P-R interval in the ectopic beats. The ventricles are stimulated directly by an ectopic focus.
QRS:	Grossly distorted in PVCs and obviously different from the beats originating in the SA node.
Comment:	Bigeminy may warn of more dangerous ventricular arrhythmias. It is often a forerunner of ventricular tachycardia.

3. The R on T Pattern (Figure 12.4)

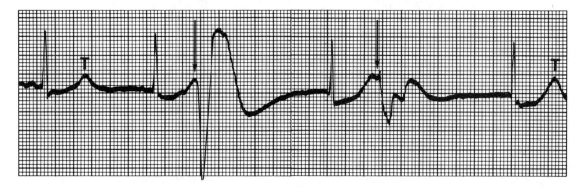

Rate:	About 60/minute.
Rhythm:	The ectopic beats create an irregularity in the basic sinus rhythm.
P waves:	Not seen in the PVCs.
P-R interval:	Absent. The ectopic beats arise in the ventricle. There is no conduction from the atrium and hence no P-R interval.
QRS:	The two ectopic beats are distorted and have different configurations. The difference in their shape indicates that more than one irritable focus is present in the ventricle (*multifocal PVCs*).
Comment:	Both PVCs strike directly on the T waves of the preceding complexes (arrows). When a PVC occurs at the time of the T wave (the R on T pattern) there is a high risk of precipitating ventricular fibrillation. This sequence is shown in the example below. Note the onset of ventricular fibrillation when an isolated PVC (arrow) strikes the T wave of the preceding beat.

Onset of Ventricular Fibrillation (Figure 12.5)

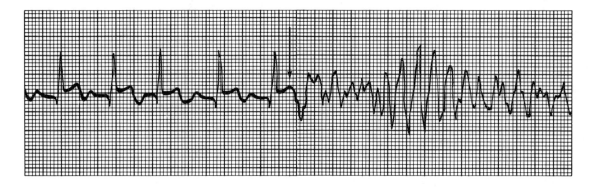

4. Multifocal PVCs (Figure 12.6)

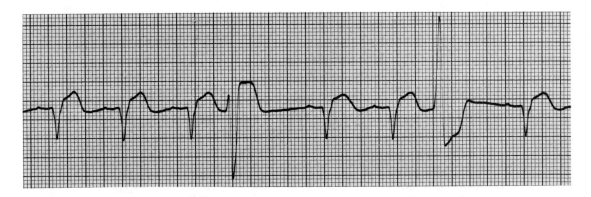

Rate:	About 80/minute.
Rhythm:	Irregular.
P waves:	No P waves are visible with the two PVCs.
P-R interval:	Not determinable with PVCs.
QRS:	The two PVCs show characteristically widened and distorted QRS complexes. However, their configuration (and direction) is distinctly different, indicating that they originated from different foci in the ventricle (multifocal PVCs).
Comment:	Multifocal PVCs usually reflect advanced ventricular ectopic activity and are considered more serious than PVCs that originate from a single focus (unifocal PVCs).

5. Consecutive PVCs (Figure 12.7)

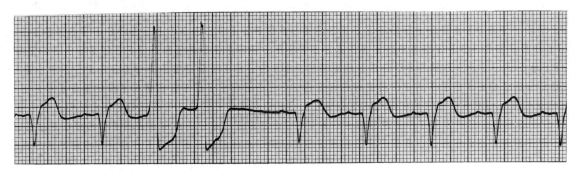

Rate:	About 90/minute.
Rhythm:	Irregular.
P waves:	Not visible in pair of PVCs.
P-R interval:	Not determinable in PVCs; otherwise P-R intervals are normal (0.18 second).
QRS:	Typically widened and distorted. PVCs occur consecutively for two beats.
Comment:	Two consecutive PVCs (usually called couplets or pairs) often lead to repetitive ventricular firing in the form of ventricular tachycardia or ventricular fibrillation.

VENTRICULAR TACHYCARDIA

Mechanism

Ventricular tachycardia can be considered as a series of three or more *consecutive* premature ventricular contractions occurring at a rapid rate (usually 140-250 beats/minute). The arrhythmia is due to a repetitive discharge of an ectopic focus in the ventricles, and usually reflects marked myocardial irritability.

The QRS complexes are wide and bizarre, typical of PVCs. Although the ventricular focus serves as the dominant pacemaker, the atria continue to discharge independently. As a result, the P waves (which are usually obscured) bear no relationship to the QRS complexes.

Occasionally ventricular tachycardia may develop without any warning signs, but most often the arrhythmia is preceded by frequent or dangerous types of PVCs. Ventricular tachycardia may terminate spontaneously, after just a few beats (a short run), or it may persist as a sustained rhythm. The latter condition is ominous since it produces serious hemodynamic effects and can degenerate into *ventricular fibrillation.*

Danger in Acute Myocardial Infarction

1. The seriousness of ventricular tachycardia depends primarily on the duration of the tachycardia. Short runs of ventricular tachycardia, lasting for only a few seconds, are seldom dangerous in their own right. However they represent a warning of sustained ventricular tachycardia and the possible development of ventricular fibrillation.

2. In contrast, when ventricular tachycardia persists and becomes an established rhythm, serious hemodynamic consequences can be expected. These are manifested by a marked reduction in cardiac output which leads to left ventricular failure, cardiogenic shock, and myocardial and cerebral ischemia. The hemodynamic deficit may be so great that sudden death can occur during ventricular tachycardia.

3. At any time during the course of ventricular tachycardia, the arrhythmia may suddenly change into ventricular fibrillation. For this reason ventricular tachycardia must be considered in the same life-threatening category as ventricular fibrillation.

4. *RISK:* Ventricular tachycardia, when sustained, is an extremely dangerous arrhythmia—a true emergency.

Clinical Features

1. Most patients are immediately aware of the sudden onset of rapid heart action and describe dyspnea, palpitations and lightheadedness. When angina accompanies these symptoms, as it usually does, the patient senses that a catastrophe has occurred, and marked apprehension is evident.

2. The blood pressure falls soon after the onset of ventricular tachycardia (often to hypotensive levels) and signs of left ventricular failure may develop with surprising rapidity if the tachycardia continues. These adverse hemodynamic effects are due to a reduction in cardiac output resulting from decreased ventricular filling time.

3. On many occasions ventricular tachycardia occurs as short runs lasting for only a few seconds before terminating spontaneously. These brief episodes may not produce any signs or symptoms.

VENTRICULAR TACHYCARDIA—IDENTIFYING ECG FEATURES

1. **Rate:**   Usually 140-220 beats/minute, but may be faster.
2. **Rhythm:**   The ventricular rhythm is essentially regular, but there may be a slight irregularity.
3. **P waves:**   The SA node continues to discharge *independently* during ventricular tachycardia, but the P waves bear no relationship to the QRS complexes. (The P waves can seldom be identified specifically, being buried in the QRS complexes.)
4. **P-R interval:** There is no conduction from the atria to the ventricles and, therefore, no P-R interval.
5. **QRS:**   Wide, slurred complexes, typical of repetitive PVCs.

Sustained Ventricular Tachycardia (Figure 12.8)

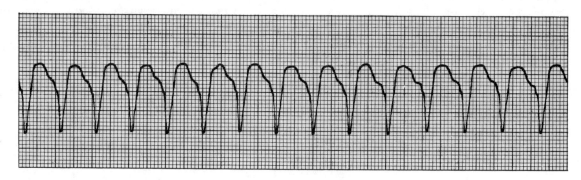

Rate:	About 150/minute.
Rhythm:	Regular.
P waves:	Not identified.
P-R interval:	Absent.
QRS:	Successive PVCs with widened, bizarre configuration.
Comment:	Sustained ventricular tachycardia is likely to degenerate into ventricular fibrillation. The arrhythmia must be terminated without delay.

Ventricular Tachycardia Stopping Spontaneously (Figure 12.9)

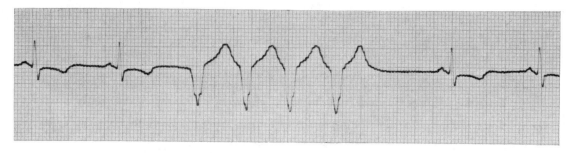

Rate:	About 130/minute (during brief burst of ventricular tachycardia).
Rhythm:	Slightly irregular during ventricular tachycardia.
P waves:	Not identified during ventricular tachycardia.
P-R interval:	Normal before and after salvo of ventricular tachycardia.
QRS:	The four consecutive PVCs (comprising the short run of ventricular tachycardia) are wide and distorted. They contrast sharply with the beats of sinus origin.
Comment:	This brief episode of ventricular tachycardia stopped spontaneously without treatment and was followed by normal sinus rhythm. Short bursts of this type are the most common form of ventricular tachycardia.

Treatment

1. Ventricular tachycardia must be terminated promptly and never allowed to persist. The first step is to administer 100 mg lidocaine intravenously as a bolus injection. If successful, additional lidocaine should be given in the form of a continuous intravenous infusion, at a rate of 2-4 mg/minute, to prevent recurrent episodes of ventricular tachycardia.

2. Failure to convert ventricular tachycardia to normal sinus rhythm with a bolus injection of lidocaine should be considered an indication for immediate *precordial shock,* particularly if the patient experiences angina or shows evidence of hypotension or heart failure. Further attempts with injections of lidocaine (or other drugs) are ill-advised in this situation. As a general rule, if ventricular tachycardia persists after the bolus injection is completed, the next step should be cardioversion.

3. At least 50% of all episodes of ventricular tachycardia are of short duration and stop spontaneously without treatment. The transiency of these attacks, although reassuring at the moment, should not afford great comfort since there is a high risk of additional episodes of ventricular tachycardia or the sudden onset of ventricular fibrillation. Consequently, even when ventricular tachycardia occurs as a short run, vigorous antiarrhythmic treatment is nevertheless indicated. An infusion containing 3000 mg lidocaine in 500 cc glucose solution should be started promptly. The flow should be set initially at 2 mg/minute and adjusted subsequently (2-4 mg/minute) to suppress ventricular ectopic activity.

4. In some instances ventricular tachycardia is refractory to lidocaine (and other conventional drugs) or recurs soon after cardioversion. In this circumstance bretylium tosylate may be administered intravenously to terminate or prevent recurrent attacks.

Nursing Role

1. When the high-rate alarm sounds and ventricular tachycardia is identified, an emergency situation exists. A planned treatment program must be initiated at once.

2. Go to the bedside and examine the patient. If he is *unconscious,* proceed immediately with precordial shock (see Chapter 14).

3. If the patient is conscious, assess his clinical state, especially for the presence of dyspnea, angina, and hypotension.

4. Call the physician immediately.

5. Prepare a syringe containing 100 mg lidocaine and administer the drug intravenously as a bolus injection.

6. If the injection of lidocaine is successful in terminating the arrhythmia, an infusion of lidocaine should be started with a flow of 2-4 mg/minute.

7. If unsuccessful, and the patient is *not* in distress, a second bolus injection (100 mg) may be administered.

8. Bring the defibrillator to the bedside. *Remember that ventricular fibrillation may develop at any time.*

9. If ventricular tachycardia occurs as a short run and terminates spontaneously start an intravenous infusion of lidocaine (2-4 mg/minute) to prevent recurrent episodes.

CASE HISTORY

A 47-year-old man with an acute myocardial infarction was admitted to the CCU in no distress. Just after the monitor electrodes had been attached and an intravenous infusion of dextrose solution started, the high-rate alarm sounded. The nurse recognized immediately that ventricular tachycardia had developed. She examined the patient who complained of recurrent chest pain. In accordance with the standing orders of the unit, the nurse prepared a syringe containing 100 mg lidocaine, which she injected rapidly into the existing intravenous line. The ventricular tachycardia stopped within 30 seconds. The physician was notified of this event and instructions were given regarding a continuous lidocaine infusion.

Rapid Ventricular Tachycardia (Figure 12.10)

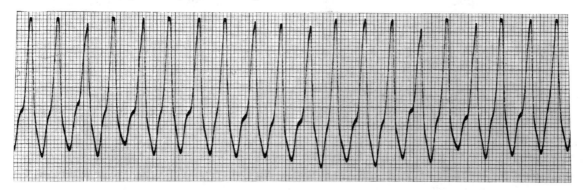

Rate:	About 200/minute.
Rhythm:	Slightly irregular.
P waves:	Not identified.
P-R interval:	Absent. The ventricles are stimulated directly by an ectopic focus at a rate of 200/minute. There is no atrioventricular conduction.
QRS:	The complexes are widened and distorted in shape.
Comment:	This very rapid ventricular rate is extremely detrimental to the pumping efficiency of the heart; it must be terminated immediately.

Extreme Ventricular Tachycardia (Ventricular Flutter) (Figure 12.11)

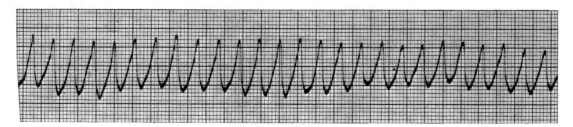

Rate:	About 270/minute.
Rhythm:	Slightly irregular.
P waves:	Not visible.
P-R interval:	Absent.
QRS:	The very rapidly occurring complexes resemble a helix (similar to a stretched, coiled spring).
Comment:	This extreme form of ventricular tachycardia is sometimes designated ventricular flutter. In many instances it is an immediate forerunner of ventricular fibrillation and must be treated with the same urgency as ventricular fibrillation—by means of precordial shock (defibrillation).

ACCELERATED IDIOVENTRICULAR RHYTHM

Mechanism

Like ventricular tachycardia, accelerated idioventricular rhythm is characterized by a series of consecutive ventricular ectopic beats. However, the ventricular rate is only 50-100/minute, in contrast to the rapid rate (140-250/minute) of ventricular tachycardia. Also, accelerated idioventricular rhythm begins and ends gradually unlike ventricular tachycardia. Because of these latter characteristics the arrhythmia has been called slow ventricular tachycardia or nonparoxysmal ventricular tachycardia. Neither of these terms is appropriate and the arrhythmia is best described as *accelerated idioventricular rhythm.*

Accelerated idioventricular rhythm denotes that the ventricles initiate impulses on their own (idioventricular), without stimulation from a higher center; but instead of discharging at the inherent rate of ventricular tissue (25-40 beats/minute), the pacemaker fires at an accelerated rate of 50-100/minute. The ventricular pacemaker takes command only if its rate exceeds the sinus rate. This occurs most often as the result of momentary slowing of the SA node. As soon as the sinus rate increases the ventricular focus is subdued. Probably the most common cause of accelerated idioventricular rhythm is ischemia of the SA node after myocardial infarction. The arrhythmia may also be a manifestation of digitalis toxicity.

Danger in Acute Myocardial Infarction

1. Accelerated idioventricular rhythm develops in about 20% of patients with acute myocardial infarction. It is a transient arrhythmia, lasting for only a few seconds to a minute (usually 3-30 beats), and produces no hemodynamic effects.
2. In the great majority of cases, accelerated idioventricular rhythm is uncomplicated and does not lead to more serious ventricular arrhythmias.
3. Only rarely is accelerated idioventricular rhythm associated with ventricular tachycardia. In these instances the ventricular rate increases suddenly after a few idioventricular beats.
4. *RISK:* Accelerated idioventricular rhythm is a benign arrhythmia. It has no serious consequences and does not affect prognosis except in rare instances when it occurs together with ventricular tachycardia.

Clinical Features

1. Because the rate is usually normal and there is no hemodynamic deficit, accelerated idioventricular rhythm produces no symptoms.
2. Although accelerated idioventricular rhythm and ventricular tachycardia both consist of a repetitive series of ventricular ectopic beats, the two arrhythmias are readily distinguishable on the basis of their ventricular rates.

Treatment

1. Accelerated idioventricular rhythm seldom requires treatment; it is usually a self-limiting arrhythmia.
2. If episodes of accelerated idioventricular rhythm occur frequently or are associated with independent premature ventricular beats, atropine (1 mg) may be administered intravenously to accelerate the SA node, and allow it to regain control.
3. In the event accelerated idioventricular rhythm leads to ventricular tachycardia, 100 mg lidocaine should be injected intravenously at once (as described in previous pages).
4. Digitalis therapy should be discontinued if there is any suspicion that the arrhythmia is digitalis-induced.

Nursing Role

1. The detection of accelerated idioventricular rhythm requires careful cardiac monitoring. Without close observation the arrhythmia may go unnoticed since it usually lasts for only a few seconds and does not trigger the low- or high-rate alarms.
2. Document the arrhythmia, determine the ventricular rate, and distinguish it from ventricular tachycardia.
3. Observe the monitor closely for additional episodes of accelerated idioventricular rhythm and for the possible development of ventricular tachycardia.
4. If the patient is being treated with digitalis, consult the physician before administering the next dose.

ACCELERATED IDIOVENTRICULAR RHYTHM
IDENTIFYING ECG FEATURES

1. **Rate:** 50-100/minute.
2. **Rhythm:** Regular (or nearly regular).
3. **P waves:** The atria are stimulated independently by the SA node or by retrograde conduction from the ventricles. However P waves are seldom visible, being buried in the QRS complexes.
4. **P-R interval:** Not measurable during accelerated idioventricular rhythm.
5. **QRS:** Wide and distorted, typical of ventricular ectopic beats.

Accelerated Idioventricular Rhythm (Figure 12.12)

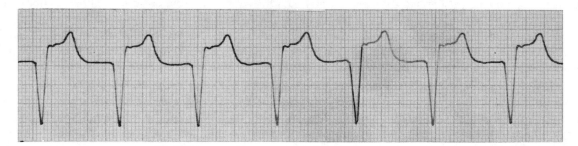

Rate:	About 70/minute.
Rhythm:	Regular.
P waves:	Not identified specifically.
P-R interval:	Not measurable.
QRS:	Wide (0.16 second), distorted.
Comment:	Accelerated idioventricular rhythm resembles ventricular tachycardia but is readily distinguishable by the slower rate (less than 100/minute).

Accelerated Idioventricular Rhythm (Figure 12.13)

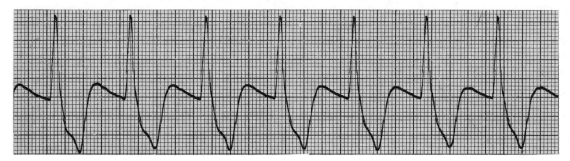

Rate:	About 70/minute.
Rhythm:	Regular.
P waves:	None visible.
P-R interval:	Not measurable.
QRS:	Very wide, distorted and bizarre in shape.
Comment:	Accelerated idioventricular rhythm begins when the SA node slows or fails to discharge and ends when normal sinus rhythm returns. The arrhythmia usually lasts for only a few beats.

CASE HISTORY

Sixteen hours after admission to the CCU, a 52-year-old man with an acute inferior myocardial infarction developed a series of 8 consecutive ventricular ectopic beats. At first glance the nurse thought these ectopic beats represented ventricular tachycardia, but a rhythm strip showed that their rate was 76/minute. Recognizing that the arrhythmia was accelerated idioventricular rhythm, the nurse did not administer lidocaine as she would have done if the arrhythmia was ventricular tachycardia.

VENTRICULAR FIBRILLATION:
A DEATH-PRODUCING ARRHYTHMIA

Ventricular fibrillation is the most common cause of *sudden* death in patients with coronary heart disease. As noted, this lethal arrhythmia is triggered in most instances by PVCs or ventricular tachycardia. However, ventricular fibrillation can arise *spontaneously* without preceding signs of ventricular irritability, and therefore there is always a threat of sudden death in patients with acute myocardial infarction. Once ventricular fibrillation develops, the only hope for survival is the instant application of resuscitative techniques.

Within the CCU the program to resuscitate the "dead" patient is distinctly different from that utilized elsewhere in the hospital.* *In the CCU the first step in resuscitation is to terminate ventricular fibrillation by precordial shock (defibrillation).* This means that external cardiac compression, mouth-to-mouth ventilation, the administration of oxygen, and other cardiopulmonary resuscitative measures are deliberately bypassed in favor of immediate defibrillation. It is sometimes difficult for nurses and physicians to realize that there is no reason to initiate external cardiac compression and mouth-to-mouth ventilation when ventricular fibrillation occurs in the CCU. These techniques are only interim measures used in other settings to sustain the circulation until ventricular fibrillation can be terminated electrically. In the CCU, where everything is in readiness to halt the arrhythmia immediately, supportive measures have little importance and in fact do no more than waste precious time. *When a patient develops ventricular fibrillation in the CCU, precordial shock must be given without delay by the first person reaching the bedside, and should precede any and all other steps!*

This reversal of the customary management of cardiac arrest (as practiced in the CCU) in no way minimizes the value of cardiopulmonary resuscitation as a lifesaving measure. The ability to sustain an adequate circulation by means of external cardiac compression and mouth-to-mouth ventilation has been of inestimable help in combating sudden death outside the prepared setting of a specialized unit. The greatest usefulness of these methods is in sustaining vital organ perfusion until resuscitative equipment can be brought to the patient. All medical and paramedical personnel should be thoroughly competent in performing cardiopulmonary resuscitation.

Mechanism

The individual muscle fibers which jointly comprise the ventricular wall are normally stimulated simultaneously and contract in unison. The fibers then recover together and rest until the next impulse causes another contraction. In ventricular fibrillation an extraordinary electrical force arising within the ventricle repeatedly stimulates these muscles at a rate so extremely rapid that the recovery period disappears and the individual muscle fibers merely twitch continuously, but do not contract. Since the muscular twitching (ventricular fibrillation) is completely ineffective in propelling blood from the ventricles, the circulation stops abruptly and *death follows within minutes.* Immediately after the onset of ventricular fibrillation, the patient becomes unconscious (and convulsions frequently occur) because of inadequate cerebral oxygenation.

The exact mechanism that triggers ventricular fibrillation is not known. Although this lethal arrhythmia may develop spontaneously, there is usually evidence of myocardial irritability in the form of PVCs before the onset of this catastrophic event. It is generally believed that following myocardial infarction the injured myocardium is sensitized so that a minimal electrical stimulus can initiate ventricular fibrillation. The electrical stimulus responsible for this chain reaction is often a PVC which strikes during the vulnerable phase of the cardiac cycle (at the time of the T wave).

Ventricular fibrillation can develop in patients with acute myocardial infarction who have no obvious complications at the time. This form of ventricular fibrillation is defined as *primary ventricular fibrillation.* In contrast, if this lethal arrhythmia occurs as a terminal rhythm in a patient dying of advanced left ventricular failure, it is classified as *secondary ventricular fibrillation.* This distinction is very important because death can be predictably prevented by prompt defibrillation in nearly all instances of *primary* ventricular fibrillation, while the secondary form is seldom responsive to resuscitation because of the underlying heart failure. Primary ventricular fibrillation reaches its peak incidence within the first few hours of myocardial infarction and decreases thereafter, but the threat always remains.

---

*The previously accepted definition of death, namely the cessation of the heartbeat, peripheral pulses, and respiration has become obsolete since many patients have been restored to useful life despite these signs of circulatory arrest. A more meaningful definition must include irreversible damage to the brain as the ultimate criterion of death. The need to define death more precisely has assumed great importance since the advent of organ and heart transplantation where death of the donor must be clearly delineated for legal and moral purposes.

VENTRICULAR FIBRILLATION—IDENTIFYING ECG FEATURES

The ECG pattern is characterized by a rapid, repetitive series of *chaotic* waves originating in the ventricles; the waves have no uniformity and are bizarre in configuration. PQRST waves cannot specifically be identified. The complexes differ from each other and occur in completely irregular fashion. A typical example of ventricular fibrillation is seen in Figure 12.14.

These grossly irregular bizarre waves can hardly be mistaken for any other arrhythmia. The only other possibility to account for such gross distortion is a malfunction of the monitor (or the electrocardiograph machine) or a loose electrode.

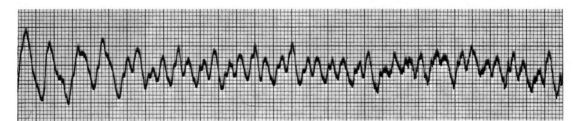

Figure 12.14

The Onset of Ventricular Fibrillation (R on T Pattern) (Figure 12.15)

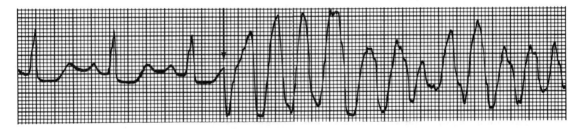

Comment: A premature ventricular contraction striking the T wave of the preceding complex (arrow) precipitates ventricular fibrillation.

Danger in Acute Myocardial Infarction

1. Death occurs within a few minutes after the onset of ventricular fibrillation unless the arrhythmia is terminated. The exact duration of life with primary ventricular fibrillation depends on several factors, probably the most important of which is the patient's age. For example, an 80-year-old man may die less than a minute after the onset of ventricular fibrillation, whereas a much younger patient may survive 3 minutes or more before death becomes irreversible. For this reason the precise time available for successful resuscitation cannot be defined. *The average time is probably 2 minutes.*
2. Although ventricular fibrillation can still be terminated after this crucial 2-minute period, irreversible brain damage may have developed.
3. *RISK: SUPREME DANGER! Death is inevitable unless resuscitation is accomplished immediately.*

Clinical Features

1. The patient loses consciousness almost instantly after the onset of ventricular fibrillation. *It is safe to assume that a conscious patient does not have ventricular fibrillation.*
2. Peripheral pulses cannot be detected, no heart sounds are audible, and the blood pressure is unobtainable—all signs of circulatory collapse.
3. The pupils dilate rapidly and convulsions may occur as a result of cerebral anoxia.
4. Cyanosis develops quickly and total *cessation of circulation* is evident.

Treatment

The treatment program for primary ventricular fibrillation consists of four phases.

1. *Recognition.* The first step in treating ventricular fibrillation is to identify the arrhythmia immediately. Ventricular fibrillation activates the alarm system of the monitor instantly, alerting the staff. The electrocardiographic pattern of ventricular fibrillation is unmistakable: a series of chaotic waves which lack any uniformity and have a bizarre configuration (Figure 12.16). If the arrhythmia cannot be definitely identified immediately (for example, because of the possibility of artifact from a loose electrode), no time should be wasted in observing the monitor additionally. Instead, the nurse should proceed at once to the bedside and determine if the patient is unconscious as the result of ventricular fibrillation. If the patient is found to be unconscious and peripheral pulses are not detectable, the planned treatment program to terminate ventricular fibrillation should be initiated instantly.

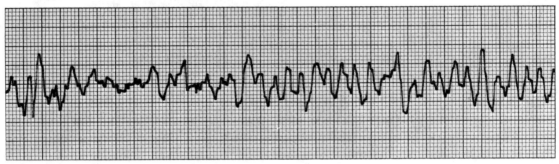

Figure 12.16

2. *Termination of ventricular fibrillation.* Defibrillation (precordial shock) is the first and only means for terminating ventricular fibrillation and restoring an effective heartbeat. The shock should be delivered by the first person to reach the bedside, whether a nurse or a physician. The sooner the shock is administered, the greater the chance for recovery. In any case, defibrillation must be accomplished within two minutes; otherwise the procedure may be ineffective, particularly in elderly patients. Also, any delay in reestablishing an effective heartbeat may result in permanent brain damage secondary to prolonged cerebral ischemia. For these reasons, precordial shock should precede all other life-saving measures in the CCU, including cardiopulmonary resuscitation. Remember that the primary objective is to terminate ventricular fibrillation in the shortest time possible.

    The technique of precordial shock is essentially standardized (as described in Chapter 14), however there is some controversy about the actual energy level required for defibrillation. For many years defibrillators were designed to store up to 400 watt-seconds energy and to deliver a maximum energy of about 300 watt-seconds. Although this level of delivered energy seemed clinically effective in most instances, experimental studies showed that large animals required more energy for defibrillation than smaller ones. On this basis it was assumed that the power setting for defibrillation should be based on the patient's body weight and therefore that the energy requirement for heavy patients might exceed the 300 watt-seconds delivered by conventional defibrillators. As a result, several defibrillators were marketed which were capable of delivering 500 watt-seconds or more energy. Although this issue is still unsettled, the trend toward high energy defibrillators is abating. Current opinion indicates that an energy setting of 400 watt-seconds with a maximum deliverable energy of 360 watt-seconds (the present capabilities of conventional defibrillators) is safe and effective. Defibrillation with higher energies is probably no more efficacious and may, in fact, be dangerous, causing cardiac damage.

3. *Correction of acidosis.* Ventricular fibrillation invariably produces metabolic acidosis, regardless of the brevity of cardiac arrest. The acidosis results from failure to perfuse tissues during the period of circulatory collapse allowing lactic acid to accumulate. (Acidosis also develops during CPR, but in this circumstance it is usually due to hypoventilation rather than perfusion failure.) In any event untreated metabolic acidosis is hazardous, especially since it reduces the threshold for recurrent ventricular fibrillation. Consequently, sodium bicarbonate should be administered immediately after ventricular fibrillation has been terminated. However, recent studies indicate that large doses of sodium bicarbonate (as used in the past) are not necessary and may in fact provoke alkalosis. The currently recommended dose of sodium bicarbonate is 1 mEq/kg initially, followed by half this dose every ten minutes, if necessary. Serial blood gas determinations should be performed until acid-base balance is assured.

4. *Prevention of recurrence of ventricular fibrillation.* The myocardial irritability which leads to ventricular fibrillation in the first place may produce subsequent episodes of this lethal arrhythmia. In other terms, the cause of the original electrical instability of the myocardium is still present and must be treated vigorously if further episodes of ventricular fibrillation are to be prevented. The main approach to prevention involves a continuous infusion of lidocaine (3000 mg in 500 cc glucose solution), administered at a rate designed to inhibit or at least minimize PVCs.

Bretylium tosylate may be used for recurrent resistant episodes of ventricular fibrillation. This drug raises the threshold for ventricular fibrillation and at the same time makes defibrillation easier to accomplish. However, bretylium is usually reserved for patients in whom lidocaine is ineffective.

Nursing Role

1. Ventricular fibrillation will trigger the alarm system of the monitor. (Either the high- or low-rate alarm may sound.)

2. Identify the bizarre irregular pattern of ventricular fibrillation. Even if in doubt do not waste time with further monitor observation. Allow the electrocardiographic record to run continuously to document the event.

3. Go to the bedside and examine the patient. If he is conscious and responds to your call, ventricular fibrillation is *not* the problem. If the patient is unconscious, ascertain the absence of peripheral pulse and heart sounds.

4. If assistance is available, ask that the emergency system call be sounded and that an automatic time be activated.

5. Turn on the power switch of the defibrillator and, depending on the type of equipment, set the energy dial at 400 watt-seconds of stored energy or 300-360 watt-seconds of delivered energy. Make certain that the synchronizer switch (used for elective cardioversion) is in the *off* position (see Chapter 14).

6. *Perform defibrillation immediately. Do not wait for the arrival of a physician or other personnel before proceeding.* Remember that survival after ventricular fibrillation is directly dependent on the rapidity with which the shock is delivered.

    The steps in defibrillation are as follows:
    a. Make certain the machine is *on;* that the delivered energy level is 300-360 watt-seconds; and that the synchronizer is *off.*
    b. Apply a generous amount of electrode paste to the defibrillator paddles and spread the jelly evenly by approximating the surfaces of the paddles.
    c. Hold the paddles tightly against the chest wall. The exact position of the paddles is not important as long as the current will traverse the axis of the heart.
    d. Trigger the discharge mechanism of the defibrillator.

7. Immediately after the shock is delivered, observe the monitor to see if the fibrillation has terminated. (If an oscilloscope is not visible from the bedside, the prompt return of peripheral pulses or the return of consciousness indicates successful defibrillation.)

8. If ventricular fibrillation persists after the initial attempt, a second or third shock should be given promptly.

9. If precordial shock has not been successful after three attempts (an unlikely situation with the use of proper technique), additional shocks are probably unwarranted at this time. Instead, external cardiac compression and mouth-to-mouth ventilation should be started without further delay. During the period of cardiopulmonary resuscitation, sodium bicarbonate should be injected rapidly and then defibrillation attempted again. Bretylium tosylate may also be utilized at this situation (see Chapter 16).

10. Unsuccessful defibrillation after all of these measures usually implies that ventricular fibrillation is secondary to advanced left ventricular failure. Survival in this circumstance is unlikely. (Failure to terminate primary ventricular fibrillation indicates that the resuscitation attempt was started too late—a situation that should never occur in a CCU.)

CASE HISTORY

Note: The following case history describes the first instance of lifesaving defibrillation performed by a nurse in the absence of a physician. This event took place in 1963 and became the precedent for the now established practice of defibrillation by nurses.

A 72-year-old male was admitted to the CCU of the Presbyterian-University of Pennyslvania Medical Center with a history of chest pain that had subsided by the time of his arrival. He had no complaints; in fact, he wanted to go home. An ECG showed an acute myocardial infarction. Physical examination was normal, and there was no evidence of complications. He remained in normal sinus rhythm with a rate ranging from 60 to 74 beats/minute. Occasional premature ventricular beats were noted.

Some 60 hours after admission, in the middle of the night, the monitor alarm sounded. The nurse instantly recognized ventricular fibrillation on the oscilloscope and ran to the bedside where the patient was found to be unconscious. She immediately called the physician and set a timing device for 2 minutes. She turned on the defibrillator, set the energy level at 400 watt-seconds, and applied electrode paste to the defibrillator paddles. The 2-minute-interval timer sounded, the physician had not arrived. (The practice at that time was for the nurse to proceed with defibrillation herself only if a physician had not arrived within 2 minutes.) The nurse then defibrillated the patient without further delay. Normal sinus rhythm was established almost immediately (Figure 12.17). The patient survived and was still alive 10 years later.

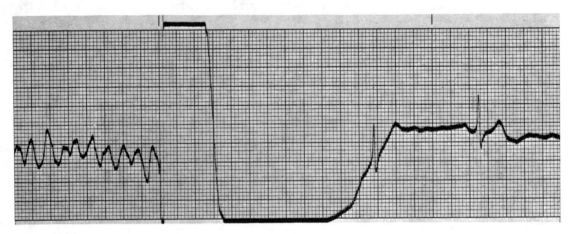

Figure 12.17

OTHER EXAMPLES OF
ARRHYTHMIAS ORIGINATING IN THE VENTRICLES

Ventricular Trigeminy (Figure 12.18)

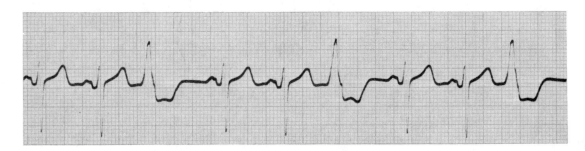

Rate:	About 90/minute.
Rhythm:	Irregular.
P waves:	Not identified with PVCs.
P-R interval:	Not measurable with PVCs.
QRS:	Every third beat is a PVC with widened, distorted QRS complexes.
Comment:	The occurrence of a PVC every third beat is described as ventricular trigeminy. (When PVCs occur every other beat, the arrhythmia is called ventricular bigeminy.)

Consecutive PVCs: Multifocal Couplet (Figure 12.19)

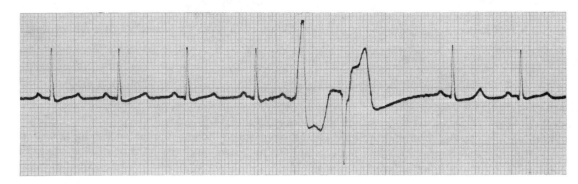

Rate:	About 80/minute.
Rhythm:	Irregular.
P waves:	Not identified with PVCs; otherwise normal.
P-R interval:	Not measurable with PVCs.
QRS:	Two PVCs with grossly different configurations (multifocal) occur consecutively to produce a couplet.
Comment:	Multifocal couplets of this type represent high-grade ventricular ectopic activity and warn of ventricular tachycardia or ventricular fibrillation.

Ventricular Tachycardia Beginning with R-on-T PVC (Figure 12.20)

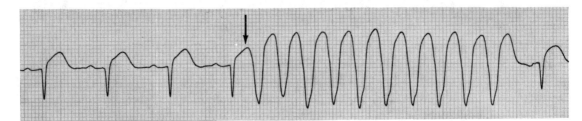

Rate:	About 200/minute during ventricular tachycardia.
Rhythm:	Regular during episode of ventricular tachycardia.
P waves:	Not visible during burst of ventricular tachycardia.
P-R interval:	Indeterminate.
QRS:	After 4 normal sinus beats, a PVC suddenly strikes the apex of the preceding T wave (R-on-T pattern) and precipitates an episode of ventricular tachycardia.
Comment:	This episode of ventricular tachycardia lasted for 10 beats before ending spontaneously.

PVCs Occurring as Couplets (Figure 12.21)

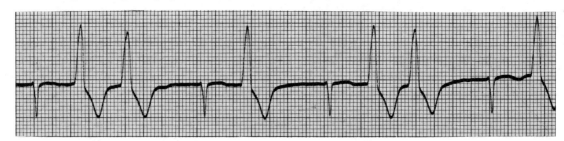

Rate:	About 100/minute.
Rhythm:	Irregular.
P waves:	Not identified in PVCs (or other beats, perhaps because of lead placement).
P-R interval:	Not measurable.
QRS:	There are six wide, bizarre complexes, typical of PVCs.
Comment:	The high frequency of PVCs and the presence of 2 sets of couplets (pairs) in this brief 6-second strip should be considered a distinct warning of the possible development of a life-threatening ventricular arrhythmia.

Ventricular Tachycardia: 3-beat (Figure 12.22)

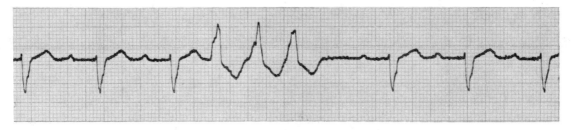

Rate:	About 90/minute.
Rhythm:	Irregular.
P waves:	Not visible in PVCs; normal otherwise.
P-R interval:	Prolonged (0.28 second) in sinus beats. Not measurable in PVCs.
QRS:	About 0.12 second in sinus beats. Wide and distorted in PVCs.
Comment:	Three consecutive PVCs at a fast rate fulfill the criterion for the diagnosis of ventricular tachycardia. When the episode consists of only 3 PVCs it is often called 3-beat ventricular tachycardia to distinguish it from longer (more serious) runs. The first-degree heart block (P-R interval 0.28 second) and widened QRS complexes (0.12 second) observed in this tracing are not related to the episode of ventricular tachycardia.

Ventricular Tachycardia: Sustained (Figure 12.23)

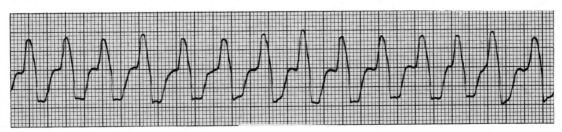

Rate:	About 140/minute.
Rhythm:	Regular.
P waves:	None identifiable.
P-R interval:	Not measurable.
QRS:	Consecutive PVCs, wide (0.20 second) and distorted.
Comment:	Sustained ventricular tachycardia must be terminated as soon as possible because of its adverse hemodynamic effects and the threat of ventricular fibrillation.

Accelerated Idioventricular Rhythm (Figure 12.24)

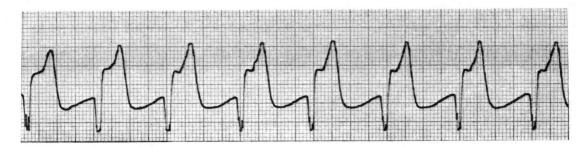

Rate:	About 80/minute.
Rhythm:	Regular.
P waves:	None visible.
P-R interval:	Not determinable.
QRS:	Wide and distorted.
Comment:	The series of 8 consecutive ventricular ectopic beats seen in this example should not be classified as ventricular tachycardia because they occur at a rate of only 80/minute. The preferred terminology is *accelerated idioventricular rhythm*, meaning that the beats originate in the ventricle but at a normal (non-tachycardic) rate.

Ventricular Fibrillation: Onset (Figure 12.25)

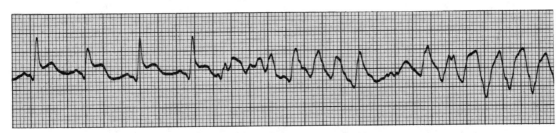

Rate:	Before the onset of ventricular fibrillation the heart rate is 110/minute.
Rhythm:	Chaotic beating with no rhythm once ventricular fibrillation begins.
P waves:	Normal prior to ventricular fibrillation.
P-R interval:	Normal until onset of ventricular fibrillation.
QRS:	When ventricular fibrillation begins, the QRS complexes are replaced by a series of chaotic waves that have no uniformity and are bizarre in configuration.
Comment:	Ventricular fibrillation may begin without any previous warnings, but antecedent PVCs are usually the case.

Artifact Mimicking Ventricular Fibrillation (Figure 12.26)

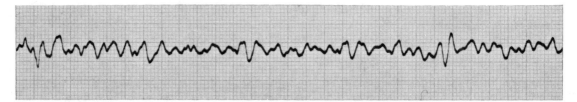

Comment: This strip seems to demonstrate typical ECG findings of ventricular fibrillation. However, the bizarre pattern was in fact due to a loose electrode! Remember: Go to the bedside immediately and examine the patient when ventricular fibrillation appears on the monitor.

13

Disorders of Conduction and Ventricular Standstill

FIRST-DEGREE AV HEART BLOCK
SECOND-DEGREE AV HEART BLOCK
Type 1 (Wenckebach) Block
Type 2 (Mobitz) Block
THIRD-DEGREE (COMPLETE) AV BLOCK
INTRAVENTRICULAR BLOCKS
Bundle Branch Blocks
PRIMARY VENTRICULAR STANDSTILL
SECONDARY VENTRICULAR STANDSTILL

As described previously, impulses normally arise in the SA node; travel by way of the internodal tracts to the atrioventricular (AV) node; pass through the AV node to the bundle of His, the left and right bundle branches, and their divisions (fascicles), to the Purkinje network; and terminate in the myocardial cells. Any interference or abnormal delay in the passage of impulses from the SA node through the Purkinje-myocardial junction is described as a *heart block*. Heart blocks can occur at any level of the conduction system, and it is customary to categorize these disorders into three groups according to the main anatomic sites of involvement (Figure 13.1):

1. Blocks in the SA node or atria
2. Blocks in the AV node or the surrounding junctional area (atrioventricular or junctional blocks)
3. Blocks in the His-Purkinje system (intraventricular or subjunctional blocks).

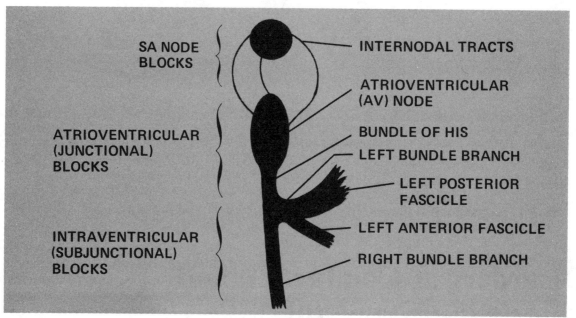

Figure 13.1.

BLOCKS IN THE SA NODE OR ATRIA

When an impulse is blocked within the SA node or in the internodal tracts the electrical stimulus does not reach the atria or the ventricles. As a result, the entire PQRST complex is absent. Blocks in the SA node or internodal tracts cannot be specifically distinguished electrocardiographically or clinically from sinoatrial (SA) arrest, a disorder of impulse formation discussed previously (see Chapter 9). Therefore blocks involving the SA node are not considered separately in this section.

ATRIOVENTRICULAR (JUNCTIONAL) BLOCKS*

Blocks interfering with conduction of impulses between the atria and ventricles usually develop because of ischemic injury to the AV node or AV junctional tissue. Less commonly, increased parasympathetic (vagal) activity or drugs (especially digitalis) produce these disturbances.

Atrioventricular blocks are categorized into first-degree, second-degree, and third-degree (complete) AV block, a classification based on the extent of the conduction defect between the atria and the ventricles. In first-degree block, the AV node merely delays impulses before they enter the intraventricular conduction system, but each impulse is conducted to the ventricles. In second-degree AV block, where nodal involvement is greater, some atrial impulses are actually blocked in the AV node or AV junction and are not conducted beyond this point. In third-degree (complete) AV block, the more seriously affected AV node prevents transmission of all impulses from the atria to the ventricles. (In this circumstance the inherent automaticity of the ventricles produces ventricular contractions in the absence of stimulation from supraventricular centers.) These three forms of atrioventricular block are discussed individually in this chapter.

INTRAVENTRICULAR (SUBJUNCTIONAL) BLOCKS

Disturbances in conduction occurring *below* the level of bifurcation of the bundle of His are categorized as intraventricular or subjunctional blocks.

When these blocks develop during the acute phase of acute myocardial infarction they generally reflect ischemic damage to the conduction pathways (particularly in the interventricular septal area). However, intraventricular blocks may exist before acute myocardial infarction. In this circumstance the block is a consequence of chronic degeneration or fibrotic scarring of the bundle branches and intraventricular network.

Until recently it was believed that the bundle of His consisted of two branches, the left bundle branch and the right bundle branch. Histological studies have shown, however, that the left bundle branch is comprised of two

---

*As shown in Figure 13.1, the AV junctional area extends from the level at which the internodal tracts enter the AV node to the point where the His bundle divides into its left and right bundle branches. In this discussion the term AV block includes blocks in the AV junctional area as well as in the AV node itself.

parts, an anterior and a posterior fascicle. For this reason the bundle of His is considered to have three branches (or fascicles), any of which can be blocked individually or in combination. Several types of intraventricular block may develop in this trifascicular system, as shown schematically in Figure 13.2.

1. Block of the right bundle branch (RBBB)
2. Block of the *main* left bundle branch (LBBB)
3. Block of the *anterior* fascicle of the left bundle branch (called left anterior hemiblock or LAH)
4. Block of the *posterior* fascicle of the left bundle branch (called left posterior hemiblock or LPH)
5. Block involving the right bundle branch and one of the fascicles of the left bundle branch (called bifascicular block since two of the three branches are involved)
6. Blocks involving all three branches of the bundle of His (called trifascicular blocks).

The diagnosis and differentiation of all of these various forms of intraventricular block require a 12-lead ECG (and sometimes even more sophisticated studies of electrical conduction called His-Bundle electrograms). Consequently it is not possible to ascertain the precise type of intraventricular block from a single monitor lead used in the CCU. Because interpretation of 12-lead ECGs is outside the customary nursing role, no attempt will be made here to discuss the diagnostic features of each type of intraventricular block. However, intraventricular blocks are characterized by wide QRS complexes (greater than 0.12 second); this one electrocardiographic finding, readily detectable on a cardiac monitor, should indicate to the nurse that a bundle branch block is present.

Intraventricular blocks developing as the result of acute myocardial infarction are more dangerous than atrioventricular blocks, particularly when more than one fascicle is involved. Bifascicular or trifascicular blocks often lead to complete heart block and ventricular standstill. Moreover, acute intraventricular blocks generally reflect extensive myocardial infarction involving the interventricular septum.

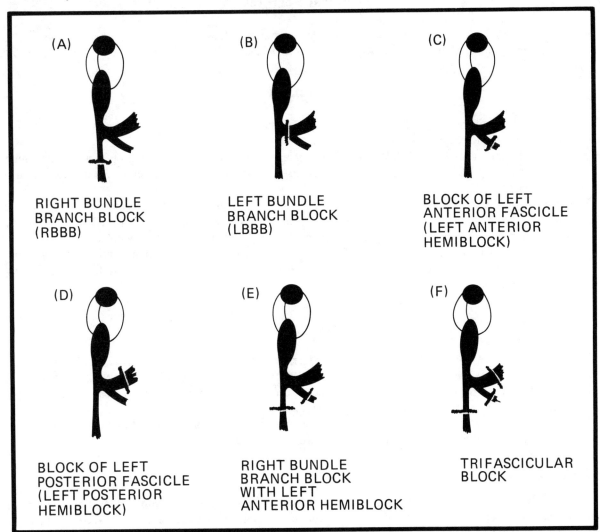

Figure 13.2. Types of Intraventricular Blocks.

FIRST-DEGREE AV HEART BLOCK

Mechanism

First-degree AV block denotes that conduction from the SA node to the ventricles is abnormally delayed within the AV node or junctional area. However, each sinus impulse reaches the ventricles and causes a ventricular response (i.e., each P wave is followed by a QRS complex). The delay in conduction usually results from ischemia of the AV node, but digitalis, antiarrhythmic agents and increased vagal activity can also produce this type of AV block.

Danger in Acute Myocardial Infarction

1. First-degree AV block is not a serious arrhythmia in its own right. It does not reduce hemodynamic efficiency nor does it affect the rate or rhythm of the heart.
2. The arrhythmia is important because it usually indicates injury to the AV nodal area and may warn of impending second- or third-degree heart blocks. The latter blocks, which reflect *advanced* stages of AV nodal involvement, are far more dangerous and may lead to ventricular standstill.
3. *RISK:* First-degree AV block is often an early warning of more advanced heart block but is not a dangerous arrhythmia in itself.

Clinical Features

1. Prolonged AV conduction produces no symptoms or physical findings.
2. The diagnosis of first-degree AV block can be made only by ECG.

Treatment

1. If there is only a slight delay in AV conduction (P-R interval of 0.21 to 0.28 second) and the block does not increase, no treatment is necessary.
2. If the P-R interval is beyond 0.28 second or, more significantly, if it shows progressive lengthening, atropine (0.5 mg-1.0 mg intravenously) may be used in an attempt to accelerate conduction through the AV node.
3. If drug therapy is unsuccessful in controlling a *progressive* first-degree block or if the block is extreme (more than 0.5 second), insertion of a temporary transvenous pacing catheter may be indicated. This prophylactic approach reduces the risk of sudden development of complete heart block or asystole.
4. If first-degree heart block develops during the course of treatment with digitalis or any antiarrhythmic agent, the further use of these drugs should be carefully considered in view of their known ability to depress AV nodal conduction.

Nursing Role

1. When first-degree heart block is identified, record a rhythm strip and carefully measure the P-R interval. If the P-R interval is greater than 0.26 second or if it shows progressive lengthening, advise the physician.
2. Carefully observe the monitor for the appearance of second- or third-degree block. If these advanced forms of heart block develop, notify the physician immediately.
3. In patients with evidence of first-degree block who are receiving digitalis or other antiarrhythmic agents, discuss the further administration of these drugs with the physician.

CASE HISTORY

The day after his admission to the CCU, a 64-year-old man with an inferior myocardial infarction developed a first-degree heart block. The P-R interval was 0.24 second at first and then increased to 0.30 second. The nurse notified the physician about the progressive P-R prolongation and atropine (0.5 mg intravenously) was ordered. The P-R interval decreased to 0.26 second and remained stable thereafter.

FIRST-DEGREE AV HEART BLOCK
IDENTIFYING ECG FEATURES

1. **Rate:** Usually normal.
2. **Rhythm:** Regular.
3. **P waves:** Normal, originating in the SA node.
4. **P-R interval:** *Prolonged* beyond 0.20 second. This prolongation is due to a delay in the passage of the impulse through the AV node.
5. **QRS:** Normal. Intraventricular conduction is not disturbed.

First-Degree AV Heart Block (Figure 13.3)

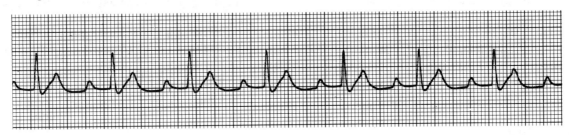

Rate:	About 70/minute.
Rhythm:	Regular.
P waves:	Normal.
P-R interval:	Prolonged (0.26 second).
QRS:	Normal (0.08 second).
Comment:	The prolongation of the P-R interval indicates a delay in conduction between the SA node and ventricle, usually in the AV node.

First-Degree AV Block (Figure 13.4)

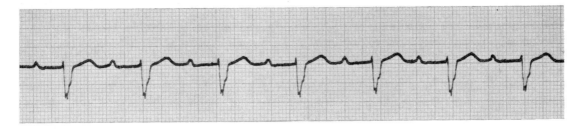

Rate:	About 70/minute.
Rhythm:	Regular.
P waves:	Normal.
P-R interval:	Prolonged to 0.32 second.
QRS:	Slightly widened, but normal (just less than 0.12 second).
Comment:	Conduction through the AV node can often be accelerated by intravenous atropine, as evidenced by shortening of the P-R interval.

SECOND-DEGREE AV HEART BLOCK
Type 1 (Wenckebach) Block

Mechanism

In second-degree AV block, some impulses from the SA node do not reach the ventricles because they are blocked within (or sometimes below) the AV node. When this happens a P wave is *not* followed by a QRS complex and a ventricular beat is absent (dropped).

Type 1 (Wenckebach) second-degree block is characterized by progressive lengthening of the P-R intervals preceding the blocked beat. Conduction through the AV node becomes more difficult with each successive impulse until finally an atrial impulse is completely blocked in the AV node and a QRS complex fails to appear. The pause resulting from the dropped beat allows the conduction system to recover momentarily and then the entire sequence of progressive P-R prolongation is repeated.

The most common cause of Wenckebach-type second-degree block is ischemic damage to the AV node. In most instances this process is temporary. Digitalis and increased vagal tone can also produce Type 1 second-degree block.

Danger in Acute Myocardial Infarction

1. Type 1 (Wenckebach) block is usually caused by ischemic injury to the AV node and therefore may progress to third-degree (complete) AV block. However, it rarely leads to ventricular standstill or sudden death because a pacemaker in the junctional area assumes command and stimulates the ventricles.
2. Wenckebach block is most often a *temporary* disorder of conduction associated with inferior myocardial infarction; it generally subsides spontaneously within 72-96 hours.
3. Unless the ventricular rate is very slow, circulatory efficiency is seldom affected and Wenckebach block is generally well tolerated.
4. *RISK:* Type 1 (Wenckebach) second-degree AV block is usually a *temporary* disorder of conduction that may lead to third-degree (complete) heart block but rarely to ventricular standstill and sudden death.

Clinical Features

1. Symptoms depend primarily on the frequency of blocked beats and the resulting ventricular rate. Unless the rate is markedly slow (below 50/minute) the patient is usually unaware of the presence of this conduction disorder.
2. Although Type 1 block produces an irregular rhythm (when ventricular beats are dropped), the diagnosis can be established only by ECG findings, not by physical examination.

Treatment

1. Since Type 1 (Wenckebach) blocks seldom progress to ventricular standstill many physicians believe that no therapy is required. Others, however, adopt a more cautious attitude and prefer to insert a temporary transvenous pacemaker when the conduction disorder is identified, particularly if it is associated with a slow ventricular rate.
2. If the ventricular rate is less than 50/minute, isoproterenol (Isuprel) can be used in an attempt to increase conduction through the AV node. An intravenous infusion of this drug (1 mg in 250 cc 5% glucose solution) may be administered. Atropine (1 mg intravenously) sometimes decreases the degree of AV block but is less dependable than isoproterenol.
3. If Wenckebach block persists for more than 3 or 4 days, temporary pacemaker insertion may be indicated.
4. If there is any suspicion that digitalis or quinidine is implicated, these drugs should be stopped promptly.

SECOND-DEGREE AV BLOCK (TYPE 1 WENCKEBACH) IDENTIFYING ECG FEATURES

1. **Rate:** The ventricular rate is usually slow but may be normal.
2. **Rhythm:** Irregular because of dropped beats.
3. **P waves:** Because some sinus impulses are blocked in the AV node, the number of P waves always exceeds the number of QRS complexes.
4. **P-R interval:** There is *progressive* prolongation of the P-R interval until a sinus impulse is blocked and a QRS complex fails to appear (a dropped beat). Following the dropped beat, the P-R interval shortens and then the entire sequence is repeated. (The sequence is called a Wenckebach period.)
5. **QRS:** Normal.

Wenckebach-Type Second-Degree AV Block (Figure 13.5)

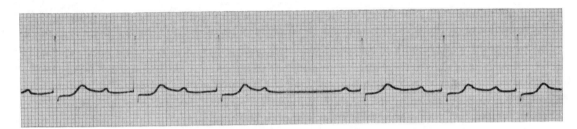

Rate:	Ventricular rate is about 60/minute.
Rhythm:	Irregular because of blocked beat.
P waves:	Normal in configuration and occur at regular intervals. The number of P waves exceeds the number of QRS complexes.
P-R interval:	The P-R interval increases during the first 3 beats. Then, a P wave is blocked and a QRS complex does not occur. The first P-R interval after the blocked beat is much shorter, and then lengthening begins again.
QRS:	Normal.
Comment:	The sequence of progressive lengthening of the P-R interval until a ventricular beat is dropped is the key diagnostic feature of Wenckebach-type block.

Nursing Role

1. When second-degree heart block is identified, determine whether it is a Type 1 (Wenckebach) or Type 2 block. The two types can be distinguished by analyzing the P-R intervals preceding the dropped beats: the P-R intervals lengthen progressively with Type 1 block and are of constant duration with Type 2 block (as described in the following pages).
2. Determine the heart rate and the frequency of dropped beats. Symptoms (angina, dyspnea, lightheadedness) may occur with slow ventricular rates.
3. Notify the physician of your findings.
4. If the physician decides to observe the patient without any treatment, monitor the heart rate carefully and watch for signs of third-degree (complete) AV heart block.
5. If the ventricular rate is 50 or less per minute, atropine or isoproterenol may be ordered. Document the response to therapy.
6. Prepare for temporary pacemaker insertion if there is no response to drug treatment or if the patient is symptomatic.
7. Withhold digitalis, quinidine, or procainamide until the physician has been consulted.

Wenckebach-Type Second-Degree AV Block (Figure 13.6)

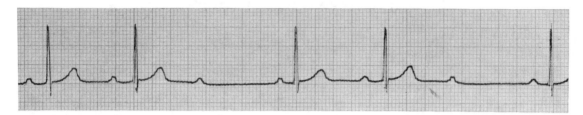

Rate:	Ventricular rate is about 50/minute while the atrial rate is about 70/minute.
Rhythm:	Irregular.
P waves:	Normal configuration. The third and sixth P waves are blocked in the AV node.
P-R interval:	On two occasions, progressive lengthening of the P-R intervals occurs for two beats before a P wave is blocked.
QRS:	Normal (0.06 second).
Comment:	There are two Wenckebach cycles in this 6-second strip. As a result of the non-conducted beats the ventricular rate is reduced to about 50/minute.

CASE HISTORY

Eighteen hours after admission to the CCU, a 48-year-old man with an inferior myocardial infarction developed a Type 1 (Wenckebach) second-degree heart block. There were no signs of left ventricular failure and the patient had no complaints. The nurse advised the attending physician of this development, and he requested a cardiology consultation to determine the need for a temporary transvenous pacemaker. The consultant felt that a temporary pacemaker was not required since the ventricular rate was 72/minute and there were no other complications. He advised that atropine be administered if the rate dropped below 60/minute. The clinical course was uneventful and the heart block disappeared after 48 hours.

SECOND-DEGREE AV HEART BLOCK
Type 2 (Mobitz) Block

Mechanism

Like Type 1 (Wenckebach) block, Type 2 (Mobitz) block is characterized by failure of some sinus impulses to conduct to the ventricles. However, in contrast to Type 1 (Wenckebach) block the P-R intervals do not lengthen progressively before the dropped beats. In other words, in Type 2 (Mobitz) block the P-R intervals of the preceding beats are of *constant* duration and suddenly a sinus P wave is blocked.

Impulses may be blocked occasionally or at regular intervals. When the dropped beats occur regularly, for example, after every second, third, or fourth P wave, the conduction defect is called a 2:1, 3:1 or 4:1 second-degree AV block.

Type 2 (Mobitz) block is much less common than Type 1 (Wenckebach) block, but is far more serious. It results from injury to the conduction system *below* the AV junction, involving the bundle branches and Purkinje system.

Danger in Acute Myocardial Infarction

1. Type 2 (Mobitz) block may progress abruptly to complete heart block or ventricular standstill. Since the block is *below* the AV junction (subjunctional block), a junctional pacemaker cannot take over in the event of a long series of blocked sinus beats. Only the inherent automaticity of the ventricles (at a rate of 30-40/minute) is left to sustain the heart beat.

2. When impulses are blocked regularly during Type 2 (Mobitz) block (e.g., 2:1 AV block), the heart rate may be too slow to maintain effective circulation and angina or congestive failure can develop.

3. Type 2 (Mobitz) block is usually (but not always) associated with anterior or anteroseptal infarction and because of extensive ventricular damage left ventricular failure may complicate the clinical course.

4. *RISK:* Type 2 (Mobitz) block is a very serious disorder of conduction that often presages complete heart block or ventricular asystole.

Clinical Features

1. Symptoms are related to the ventricular rate. With rates under 50/minute, patients may experience angina, dyspnea or cerebral insufficiency.

2. Type 2 (Mobitz) block can only be identified (and distinguished from Type 1 block) by ECG.

Treatment

1. Because of the unpredictable course of Type 2 block and the ever present threat of sudden complete heart block or ventricular standstill, a temporary transvenous pacemaker should be inserted when this conduction disorder is identified.

2. Isoproterenol may be administered before pacemaker insertion can be accomplished, particularly if the ventricular rate is slow.

3. Atropine is seldom useful in this condition and can be detrimental. Although it usually increases the atrial rate, it does not decrease the degree of block. As a result, more P waves may be blocked, causing a further reduction in the ventricular rate.

4. Digitalis and antiarrhythmic drugs should be discontinued in the presence of Type 2 block.

Nursing Role

1. Distinguish Type 2 (Mobitz) from Type 1 (Wenckebach) second-degree AV block by measuring the P-R intervals preceding the dropped beats.

2. Notify the physician promptly.

3. Prepare for the insertion of a temporary pacemaker.

4. Observe the monitor carefully for the sudden appearance of complete heart block or ventricular asystole.

5. Withhold digitalis and antiarrhythmic agents.

CASE HISTORY

A 64-year-old man was admitted to the CCU because of an acute anterior wall myocardial infarction. The original rhythm strip revealed normal sinus rhythm, but the P-R interval was 0.24 second (first-degree AV block). About 1 hour later the slow-rate alarm sounded, and the nurse noted that the heart rate had suddenly decreased from 90 to 45/minute. On examining the rhythm strip, it was apparent that there were two P waves for each QRS complex and that a 2:1-type second-degree heart block had developed. It was also noted that the QRS complex was widened (0.12 second). The nurse advised the physician of these findings, and it was decided that a temporary transvenous pacemaker should be inserted, particularly in light of the widened QRS complexes and the potential threat of progression to complete heart block (or ventricular standstill).

SECOND-DEGREE AV BLOCK (TYPE 2 MOBITZ)
IDENTIFYING ECG FEATURES

1.	**Rate:**	The ventricular rate is usually slow, but depends on the frequency of blocked beats.
2.	**Rhythm:**	When the block occurs at regular intervals (e.g., 2:1 AV block) the rhythm is regular. If blocked beats occur occasionally, the rhythm at the time is irregular.
3.	**P waves:**	More numerous than QRS complexes, but normal in configuration.
4.	**P-R interval:**	The P-R interval of the beats preceding a blocked beat are of *constant* duration.
5.	**QRS:**	Usually widened, indicating the block is *below* the AV junction.

Mobitz II Second-Degree AV Block (Figure 13.7)

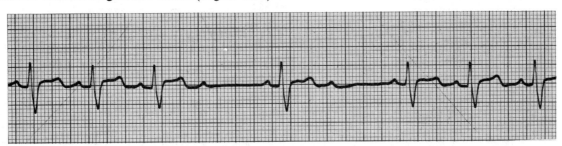

Rate:	Ventricular rate is about 70/minute. Atrial rate is about 90/minute.
Rhythm:	Irregular because of 2 blocked beats.
P waves:	Normal in shape and occur regularly. The fourth and sixth P waves are blocked and not conducted to the ventricles.
P-R interval:	The P-R intervals are of constant duration and do *not* lengthen before the blocked beats.
QRS:	Widened (0.14 second), indicating that an intraventricular conduction defect is present (a common finding in Mobitz II blocks).
Comment:	The distinguishing characteristic of a Mobitz II block is a constant P-R interval before and after the blocked beats, unlike the changing P-R intervals of Wenckebach-type second-degree AV block.

Second-Degree AV Block (2:1 Type) (Figure 13.8)

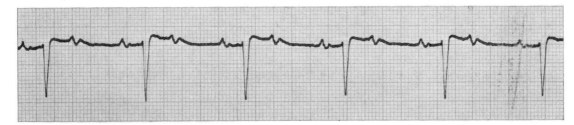

Rate:	Ventricular rate is 56/minute. Atrial rate is 112/minute.
Rhythm:	Regular.
P waves:	There are *two* P waves in each R-R interval. The first of these P waves (which occurs just before the T waves) is blocked.
P-R interval:	Mildly prolonged (0.22 second). The P-R intervals are constant.
QRS:	Normal (0.08 second). No QRS complex follows blocked P wave.
Comment:	The ventricular rate is one-half the atrial rate because every other P wave is blocked (2:1 block).

THIRD-DEGREE (COMPLETE) AV BLOCK

Mechanism

In third-degree AV block, all impulses from the atria are blocked and *none* reach the ventricles. The block may occur above or below the bifurcation of the Bundle of His. Regardless of the site of the block, the atria and ventricles beat *independently,* each controlled by a separate pacemaker. The SA node serves as the pacemaker for the atria, while the ventricles are governed by a ventricular focus at an inherent rate of 30-40/minute. (If the block is *above* the bifurcation of the His Bundle the ventricles may be stimulated by a junctional escape pacemaker at a rate of 40-60/minute.) In either case there is no relationship between P waves and QRS complexes—a condition called *atrio-ventricular dissociation.* In patients with acute myocardial infarction, complete heart block is almost invariably due to ischemic injury to either the AV junctional area or the conduction system below it. Only rarely is digitalis toxicity responsible for the block.

Danger in Acute Myocardial Infarction

1. An *independent* ventricular pacemaker is not dependable and may fail abruptly, causing ventricular standstill. Also, the slow ventricular rate predisposes to ventricular tachycardia or ventricular fibrillation by allowing more rapid foci in the ventricles to gain control.
2. Complete heart block almost always causes a marked reduction in cardiac output because the ventricular rate is constant at 30-40 beats/minute and cannot increase to meet circulatory demands. Consequently, left ventricular failure and myocardial ischemia are common hemodynamic complications of complete block.
3. A gross reduction in blood flow to the brain, resulting from the very slow heart and low cardiac output, may cause episodes of syncope with or without convulsion (Stokes-Adams attacks). Lesser degrees of cerebral ischemia are manifested by confusion and lightheadedness.
4. As a general rule, complete heart block occurring within or about the AV node is less dangerous than subjunctional blocks. With blocks at the AV nodal level, a junctional escape pacemaker may maintain the ventricular rate at 40-60/minute.
5. *RISK:* Complete heart block, especially at the subjunctional level, is an *extremely dangerous* arrhythmia. It represents a clear warning of impending ventricular standstill or ventricular fibrillation.

Clinical Features

1. Complete heart block can be suspected from clinical examination. The key finding is a very slow, regular heart rate (usually less than 40/minute) that remains *constant* and does not fluctuate with activity (a fixed heart rate).
2. Signs of cerebral ischemia, ranging from confusion and lightheadedness to syncope and convulsions, are common during complete heart block.
3. Symptoms and signs of left ventricular failure are usually present, as is hypotension.

Treatment

1. The only dependable method of treating complete heart block is transvenous cardiac pacing. This procedure should be undertaken as soon as third-degree block is identified.
2. While preparing for the insertion of the pacemaker, an intravenous infusion of isoproterenol (Isuprel), 1 mg in 250 cc glucose solution, should be given slowly. Occasionally, isoproterenol may reduce the degree of AV block and increase the heart rate. Despite the apparent effectiveness of drug therapy, sudden recurrence of complete block often occurs, and therefore it is wise to insert a transvenous pacemaker in all patients who develop complete heart block.
3. Cardiac pacing should be continued until normal sinus rhythm returns, and the pacing catheter should remain in place for at least 5 days thereafter.
4. Rarely, complete heart block persists because of *irreversible* damage to the conduction system. In this circumstance a permanent pacemaker is required.
5. Because complete heart block is often preceded by lesser degrees of AV block, the treatment of this arrhythmia should begin ideally when *progressive* heart block is first identified (as explained in the description of second-degree block).

THIRD-DEGREE (COMPLETE) AV BLOCK
IDENTIFYING ECG FEATURES

1. Rate: The ventricular rate is usually 30-40/minute (but can be 40-60/minute with a junctional escape pacemaker). The atrial rate, which is independent of the ventricular rate, is always faster.

2. Rhythm: Both atrial and ventricular rhythms are regular, but independent of each other.

3. P waves: There are more P waves than QRS complexes. Because atrial stimulation is unaffected, the size and shape of the P waves are normal.

4. P-R interval: Because the atria and ventricles have separate pacemakers, there is no relationship between P waves and QRS complexes (atrio-ventricular dissociation). Therefore, the P-R interval is inconstant.

5. QRS: Configuration of the complex depends on the site of the block and the location of the ectopic ventricular pacemaker. If the block and the ectopic pacemaker are near the AV node the QRS complex may be normal. In contrast, when the block and the pacemaker are subjunctional the QRS complexes are widened and distorted.

Complete Heart Block with Wide QRS Complexes (Figure 13.9)

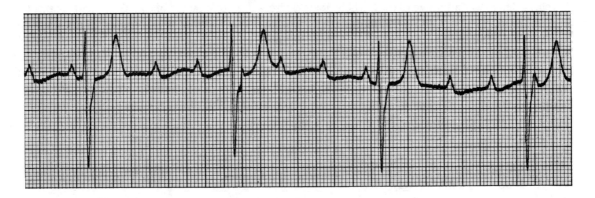

Rate: Ventricular rate is about 40/minute. Atrial rate is about 130/minute.

Rhythm: Regular.

P waves: Occur at regular intervals, independent of QRS complexes, at a rate of 130/minute.

P-R interval: There is no relationship between P waves and QRS complexes; therefore the P-R intervals are inconstant.

QRS: Wide and distorted, indicating their ventricular origin.

Comment: No impulses from the SA node or AV junction reach the ventricles (complete heart block), and the only remaining pacemaker is ventricular (at a rate of about 40/minute).

Nursing Role

1. Identify this slow-rate arrhythmia and distinguish it from marked sinus bradycardia, junctional rhythm, and second-degree AV block. Document the disorder with a rhythm strip.
2. Notify the physician immediately after this arrhythmia is recognized.
3. Prepare an infusion containing 1 mg isoproterenol in 250 cc dextrose solution.
4. Because of the threat of ventricular fibrillation developing in the presence of the slow ventricular rate, a defibrillator should be brought to the bedside and made ready for use.
5. Keep a syringe containing 100 mg lidocaine at the bedside.
6. Prepare for the insertion of a transvenous pacemaker (see Chapter 14).
7. Assess the patient's clinical condition repeatedly, with particular emphasis on signs or symptoms that indicate left ventricular failure.
8. Diligently observe the monitor for premature ventricular contractions; these ectopic beats may forewarn of ventricular tachycardia or fibrillation.
9. If a transvenous pacemaker has been inserted previously for prophylactic reasons (because of second-degree AV block or block in the His-Purkinje system), verify that the pacemaker is functioning properly.
10. If ventricular standstill develops, initiate cardiopulmonary resuscitation (CPR) immediately. Sound an emergency alarm.

CASE HISTORY

A 56-year-old man was admitted to the CCU in acute distress. He complained of substernal pain, shortness of breath, and a feeling of faintness. On examining the patient the nurse found that the blood pressure was 96/68, and that the pulse rate was only 36/minute. A rhythm strip confirmed the nurse's clinical suspicion of complete heart block. The physician was notified promptly of these findings, and it was decided that a temporary transvenous pacemaker should be inserted without delay to increase the heart rate. The physician requested that an intravenous infusion of isoproterenol be given while preparations were being made to insert a pacing catheter. When the heart was paced at a rate of 75/minute, there was marked clinical improvement, reflecting increased cardiac output. A rhythm strip recorded during the course of cardiac pacing is shown in Figure 13.10.

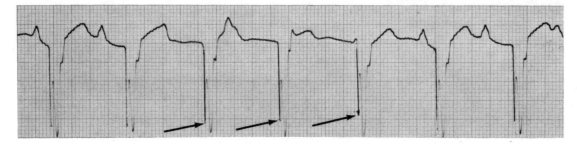

Figure 13.10

Although the complete heart block still exists (as evidenced by the random position of the P waves) the ventricular rate is now controlled by the pacemaker. The pacing stimuli occur 75 times/minute, creating a ventricular response at this rate.

Complete Heart Block with Normal QRS Complexes (Figure 13.11)

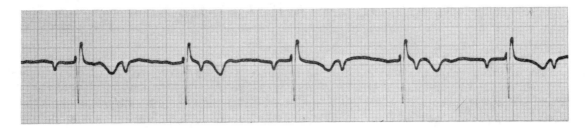

Rate:	The ventricular rate is about 50/minute. The atrial rate is about 80/minute.
Rhythm:	Regular.
P waves:	Occur at regular intervals, but none are conducted to the ventricles. The P waves are inverted in this particular lead.
P-R interval:	Inconstant, reflecting independent atrial and ventricular rhythms.
QRS:	Normal (0.10 second).
Comment:	The heart rate (about 50/minute) and the normal QRS complexes (0.10 second) indicate that a pacemaker just below the AV junction has assumed control. Compare this example with the one above in which a ventricular pacemaker is in command.

Complete Heart Block Leading to Ventricular Tachycardia and Fibrillation (rhythm strip was continuous but has been divided and reduced in scale for purposes of full reproduction.)

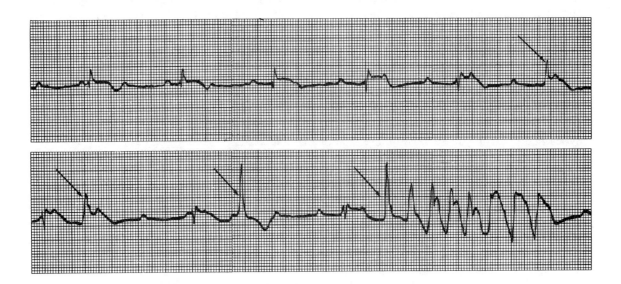

Comments:	The electrocardiographic sequence seen above demonstrates one of the greatest dangers of complete heart block: the development of *ventricular fibrillation*. In the presence of the very slow ventricular rate associated with complete heart block, PVCs developed (arrows). These ectopic beats caused repetitive ventricular firing and ventricular fibrillation (lower strip).

INTRAVENTRICULAR BLOCKS
BUNDLE BRANCH BLOCKS

Mechanism

All blocks occurring below the bifurcation of the Bundle of His are categorized as intraventricular (or subjunctional) blocks. A bundle branch block refers to an obstruction or delay in conduction through one of the main branches of the His bundle.

Normally, sinus impulses, after traversing the AV node and Bundle of His, are conducted down the left and right bundle branches and stimulate the respective ventricles simultaneously. The total time for depolarization of both ventricles, as represented by the width of the QRS complex, is less than 0.12 second.

When one of the bundle branches is blocked impulses travel through the intact branch and stimulate the ventricle it supplies on schedule. The ventricle affected by the bundle branch block is activated indirectly by impulses crossing through the interventricular septum from the unaffected side. The delay caused by this circuitous route for complete ventricular activation (i.e., both ventricles) is manifested electrocardiographically by widening of the QRS complex beyond 0.12 second—the characteristic feature of a bundle branch block.

The most common cause of bundle branch block is chronic degeneration or fibrotic scarring of the intraventricular conduction system. Consequently, bundle branch blocks are often present before acute myocardial infarction, particularly in elderly patients, and have no relation to the attack itself. Bundle branch blocks that develop as a complication of acute infarction usually reflect extensive myocardial damage involving the interventricular septum and the bundle branches.

Danger in Acute Myocardial Infarction

1. Intraventricular blocks that develop *acutely* as a result of myocardial infarction are associated with a high mortality because of the extensive nature of the infarction. Death may be due to electrical failure (ventricular standstill) or circulatory (power) failure.
2. There is a high risk of sudden electrical failure when more than one of the three intraventricular pathways are blocked. For example, a right bundle branch block in conjunction with a block of the anterior fascicle of the left bundle branch (collectively called a bilateral bundle branch block) may progress abruptly to complete heart block or ventricular standstill. (In this circumstance the only remaining conduction pathway to the ventricle is the posterior fascicle of the left bundle branch.)
3. *RISK:* Bundle branch block is a very serious disorder when the block develops as a consequence of acute myocardial infarction and involves more than one bundle branch.

Clinical Features

1. Bundle branch block causes no symptoms because the heart rate and rhythm are not affected.
2. The presence of a bundle branch block can be recognized by very wide QRS complexes on a single cardiac monitoring lead. However, the location of the block (i.e., a right, left bundle branch, or a fascicular block) can only be determined by means of a 12-lead ECG.
3. A left bundle branch block obscures the characteristic electrocardiographic signs of acute myocardial infarction; therefore the diagnosis of acute infarction in this situation depends primarily on enzyme studies. A right bundle branch block does not affect the ECG signs of infarction.

Treatment

1. A temporary transvenous pacemaker should be inserted prophylactically when a bundle branch block develops acutely after myocardial infarction in an attempt to combat sudden complete heart block or ventricular standstill.
2. Chronic bundle branch blocks that are present before acute myocardial infarction generally require no treatment. However, some clinicians believe that a temporary pacemaker should be inserted for chronic blocks that involve more than one bundle branch (bilateral bundle branch block).
3. There is no drug treatment for intraventricular blocks.
4. Infrequently, overdosages of antiarrhythmic drugs, particularly quinidine, may produce intraventricular blocks. In this circumstance the block may disappear after the drug is discontinued.

BUNDLE BRANCH BLOCK—IDENTIFYING ECG FEATURES

1. Rate:		Usually normal, but sometimes bundle branch block is rate-related, appearing and disappearing with changes in the heart rate.
2. Rhythm:		Regular.
3. P waves:		Normal.
4. P-R interval:		Normal, because impulses reach the *uninvolved* ventricle without delay.
5. QRS:		*Always* widened to at least 0.12 second and the configuration of the complex is distorted. After the uninvolved ventricle is stimulated the impulses must then be transmitted through the interventricular septum to activate the blocked side. This delay in activation causes the QRS complexes to be wide and notched.

Bundle Branch Block (Figure 13.12)

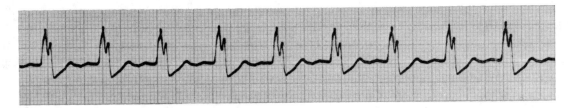

Rate:	About 90/minute.
Rhythm:	Regular.
P waves:	Normal.
P-R interval:	Normal (0.18 second). The impulse from the SA node passes through the uninvolved bundle without delay and activates one ventricle normally.
QRS:	The complex is abnormally widened (more than 0.12 second), indicating that the time for *total* ventricular activation is prolonged. (The impulse must pass through the interventricular septum to stimulate the blocked ventricle.)
Comment:	With a single monitor lead it is usually not possible to distinguish which of the bundle branches is blocked. This localization, which has prognostic importance, is made with a 12-lead ECG, from which the respective patterns can be readily identified. The monitor lead indicates only that an intraventricular conduction defect is present.

Nursing Role

1. If an intraventricular block (manifested on the monitor by a widened QRS complex) develops acutely, document the conduction disturbance with an ECG strip and notify the physician of this change.
2. Obtain a 12-lead ECG at this time so that the physician can localize the site of the block and the number of fascicles involved. (As noted, these facts *cannot* be ascertained from the monitor strip alone.)
3. Because it is likely that a temporary transvenous pacemaker will be inserted, prepare for this procedure.
4. Carefully observe the patient's clinical condition. This observation is particularly important since intraventricular blocks are usually associated with extensive infarctions and the risk of multiple complications is great.
5. If the patient develops an intraventricular block during the course of drug therapy, discuss the problem with the physician before the next dose is administered.

Bundle Branch Blocks (Figure 13.13)

(A)   (B)   (C)

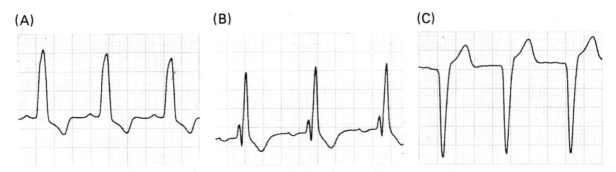

Comment: The three different ventricular complexes shown above are more than 0.12 second in duration, indicating an intraventricular conduction defect in each example. The configuration of the QRS complexes varies with the type of block and the lead locations.

CASE HISTORY

A 70-year-old woman was admitted to the CCU with a history of severe substernal pain of 2 hours' duration. The nurse noted a widened QRS complex on the initial rhythm strip. A 12-lead ECG demonstrated a left bundle branch block. The admitting physician stated that this pattern had been present for at least 3 years. Because of the LBBB, the diagnosis of acute myocardial infarction could not be made definitely at the time. Despite this uncertainty, the patient was treated as if an acute infarction had occurred. The question was resolved within a few days when enzyme studies confirmed the diagnosis of acute myocardial infarction.

VENTRICULAR STANDSTILL
A DEATH-PRODUCING ARRHYTHMIA

Ventricular contraction depends on an effective electrical stimulus. If for some reason electrical stimuli to the ventricles are of inadequate intensity or if they cease entirely, the ventricles stop contracting. This state is designated *ventricular standstill* or ventricular asystole. There is some confusion regarding the proper terminology of this catastrophe. The terms ventricular standstill, ventricular asystole, cardiac standstill, and cardiac arrest are used interchangeably to designate cessation of heart action. At the bedside, without an ECG, one cannot distinguish ventricular standstill from ventricular fibrillation since both arrhythmias are characterized by the absence of audible heart sounds. It is common practice, therefore, to classify cessation of the circulation as *cardiac arrest* even though ventricular fibrillation may actually be at fault. In the CCU, where the lethal arrhythmia can be specifically identified, it is poor practice to use the general term cardiac arrest when the arrhythmia is in fact either ventricular standstill or ventricular fibrillation. The net effect of ventricular standstill is the same as with ventricular fibrillation: sudden death.

Like ventricular fibrillation, ventricular standstill may develop as a primary electrical disorder, called *primary ventricular standstill,* or as a terminal arrhythmia during advanced heart failure *(secondary ventricular standstill).* The latter mechanism is far more common.

In primary ventricular standstill, sinus (or atrial) impulses are discharged normally and produce P waves. Suddenly, however, all of these impulses are blocked and none reach the ventricles. Despite the seeming suddenness of ventricular standstill, the catastrophe is preceded in practically all instances by some form of *subjunctional* heart block, usually a bifascicular block. Because an inherent ventricular pacemaker does not come to the rescue, ventricular activation stops and all QRS complexes disappear on the ECG (while P waves continue). When ventricular stimulation ceases, unconsciousness develops immediately and death occurs within a very brief period unless effective ventricular action can be restored by CPR. On some occasions, ventricular standstill is a transient phenomenon with conduction and ventricular stimulation returning spontaneously after a few seconds. These intermittent episodes are characterized by syncope and are called *Stokes-Adams attacks.*

In contrast to primary ventricular standstill, secondary ventricular standstill is always associated with circulatory failure and is a terminal event in patients dying of cardiogenic shock or advanced left ventricular failure. In these conditions inadequate tissue perfusion results in hypoxia, acidosis, and electrolyte imbalance, all of which depress electrical conductivity. At a critical point, the heart's electrical activity becomes insufficient to stimulate the myocardium and ventricular standstill develops. This secondary type of standstill seldom yields to resuscitative techniques (including cardiac pacing) because the oxygen-deprived myocardium is unable to respond to any stimulation. In other words, the basic circulatory deficit that affected electrical conductivity in the first place is still present. Death from secondary ventricular standstill usually occurs gradually; electrical activity may continue, but muscle contractions are weak and ineffective in propelling blood from the ventricles. This state is described as mechanical or power failure—in contrast to failure of electrical stimulation and conduction.

Mechanism

As noted, when all impulses from the SA node or atria fail to reach the ventricles and an inherent ventricular focus does not take over as an escape pacemaker, ventricular stimulation stops and circulation ceases. This condition is called *ventricular standstill.* Primary ventricular standstill is the result of a conduction disorder, usually involving two or three fascicles of the bundle branches. The underlying cause of secondary ventricular standstill is hypoxia, which depresses impulse formation, conduction and myocardial responsiveness to stimulation.

Danger in Acute Myocardial Infarction

1. Primary ventricular standstill results in sudden death unless an effective heartbeat can be restored immediately by resuscitative measures. This death-producing arrhythmia however, is relatively rare compared to primary ventricular fibrillation.
2. Secondary ventricular standstill is almost inevitably fatal with current means of treatment. It seldom responds to resuscitation (including cardiac pacing) because the severely ischemic myocardium is unable to respond to any stimulation.
3. *RISK: Ventricular standstill is the most dreaded and the most dangerous of all arrhythmias.* Even with primary ventricular standstill the results from resuscitation are distressingly poor (in sharp contrast to the effectiveness of resuscitation from primary ventricular fibrillation). Consequently, *prevention* of ventricular standstill is of supreme importance.

Clinical Features

1. When primary ventricular standstill develops there is a sudden, complete cessation of circulation. No heartbeat can be heard, no pulses can be felt, the blood pressure cannot be obtained, and the patient loses consciousness immediately. *Death occurs within minutes.* The clinical picture is therefore identical to ventricular fibrillation; however the two lethal arrhythmias can be readily distinguished electrocardiographically.
2. Death from secondary ventricular standstill usually occurs gradually during the course of cardiogenic shock or left ventricular failure. Electrical activity often continues (in the form of wide QRS complexes) but the ventricles do not respond. Thus the circulation stops even though QRS complexes are still evident on the ECG. This condition is called *electro-mechanical dissociation.*

Treatment

The treatment and resuscitation program has four phases:

1. *Recognition.* When primary ventricular standstill occurs, the low-rate alarm of the monitoring system is activated. The electrocardiographic pattern is characterized by the absence of ventricular (QRS) complexes, while atrial activity (P waves) persists (Figure 13.14). If the ECG pattern cannot be identified instantly, no further time should be spent observing the monitor. The nurse should proceed immediately to the bedside to see if the patient is unconscious.

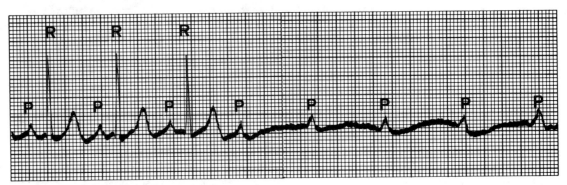

Ventricular Standstill (Figure 13.14)

2. *Termination of ventricular standstill.* If the patient is unconscious and there is no evidence of circulation, the nurse or physician who reaches the bedside first should strike the patient's chest with a forceful blow directly over the sternum. Occasionally this simple step, if performed within seconds of the onset of ventricular standstill, will cause resumption of the heartbeat.

    If the blow to the chest is ineffective, external cardiac compression and mouth-to-mouth ventilation should be initiated instantly and continued while the following measures are carried out.

    a. An emergency alarm should be sounded to summon the personnel to assist in the resuscitative attempt.

    b. After an airway has been established to administer oxygen and while effective external cardiac compression is being performed in an effort to maintain cerebral circulation, cardiac pacing should be attempted. The technique of cardiac pacing is described in the following chapter.

   c. Epinephrine (5 cc of a 1:10,000 solution) may be injected directly into the heart in an effort to stimulate electrical activity.

3. *Correction of lactic acidosis.* Lactic acidosis must be anticipated in every patient who develops ventricular standstill. Sodium bicarbonate should be administered intravenously as soon as possible and repeated as necessary (depending on blood gas values) while cardiopulmonary resuscitation is in progress. Unless the acidosis is corrected, the heart will not respond to pacing or other measures.

4. *Prevention of recurrence.* If resuscitation is successful, cardiac pacing should be continued until signs of heart block or bradycardia have disappeared. A transvenous pacemaker should be left in place for at least 1 week after sinus rhythm has been reestablished.

Nursing Role

When a Transvenous Pacemaker Has NOT Been Inserted Prophylactically

1. When the low-rate alarm sounds, attempt to identify the ECG pattern on the monitor. Is the arrhythmia ventricular fibrillation or ventricular standstill?
2. Go to the bedside at once and examine the patient. If the patient is awake and conscious it is quite certain that a false alarm has occurred.
3. If the patient is unconscious and has no peripheral pulses or heartbeat, sound the emergency alarm system.
4. Deliver a sharp blow to the chest wall directly over the sternum. This simple procedure may sometimes reestablish the heartbeat and is always worth trying.
5. If the heartbeat does not return immediately after the blow to the chest, begin the planned program of cardiopulmonary rescitation (CPR).
6. Continue external cardiac compression and mouth-to-mouth ventilation until other personnel provide assistance.
7. While CPR is in progress, one member of the team should prepare a syringe containing 40 mEq sodium bicarbonate for immediate intravenous injection.
8. Bring all necessary equipment for cardiac pacing to the bedside for immediate use by the physician.
9. In the event of failure with other measures, the physician may inject 5 cc of 1:10,000 epinephrine directly into the heart. Prepare a syringe with an intracardiac needle for this purpose. (Epinephrine may also be administered intravenously in this circumstance.)

When a Transvenous Pacemaker Has Been Inserted Prophylactically

1. As noted previously, ventricular standstill is usually preceded by some form of heart block. Thus the development of ventricular standstill cannot actually be considered as unexpected; only the onset is sudden. By recognizing the warning conduction disorder and inserting a transvenous pacemaker prophylactically, it should be possible, at least in some instances, to prevent the occurrence of primary ventricular standstill. As soon as a QRS complex fails to appear, a demand pacemaker automatically begins to discharge impulses and stimulates the ventricles to contract.
2. The nursing role in cardiac pacing is described in the next chapter.

CASE HISTORY

A 78-year-old man was admitted to the CCU with signs of advanced left ventricular failure. The ECG revealed an anteroseptal myocardial infarction, and a rhythm strip showed sinus tachycardia with a rate of 124/minute. He was treated with furosemide (Lasix), rotating tourniquets, oxygen, and intravenous digoxin. The response to therapy was poor, and the patient continued to exhibit marked dyspnea. During the course of treatment the heart rate slowed abruptly to 58/minute, and a junctional rhythm was recognized on a monitor strip. A transvenous pacemaker was inserted, but pacing was ineffective and the ventricles did not respond to stimulation (because of severe hypoxia). About 5 minutes later the patient lost consciousness. The nurse was unable to record a blood pressure, and no peripheral pulses were palpable. The monitor now showed isolated, broad, distorted QRS complexes occurring about 10 times/minute. Resuscitation attempts were unsuccessful. The cause of death was advanced left ventricular failure. The terminal rhythm was secondary ventricular standstill.

PRIMARY VENTRICULAR STANDSTILL—IDENTIFYING ECG FEATURES

1. **Rate:**   At the onset of ventricular standstill the ventricles cease to contract and there is no heartbeat.
2. **Rhythm:**   No ventricular beats.
3. **P waves:**   Usually normal; they continue independently despite the cessation of ventricular activity.
4. **P-R interval:**   Atrial activity may persist, but the impulses are not conducted to the ventricle and there is no P-R interval.
5. **QRS:**   None.

Primary Ventricular Standstill (Figure 13.15)

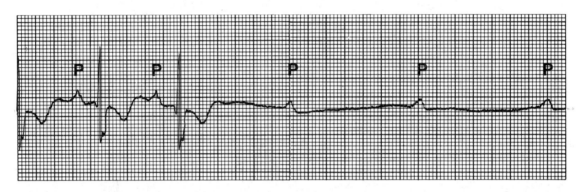

Rate:	After the third QRS complex, ventricular activation ceases and there is no heartbeat.
Rhythm:	There is no cardiac rhythm because of total cessation of ventricular contractions.
P waves:	Atrial activity continues after ventricular standstill.
P-R interval:	Although the atria are stimulated, no impulses reach the ventricles.
QRS:	Absent when the ventricular stimulation ceases.
Comment:	In this case, ventricular standstill developed in the presence of an intraventricular conduction defect. A 12-lead ECG showed a right bundle branch block as well as a block of the anterior subdivision of the left bundle branch (bundle branch block). A first-degree heart block is also apparent in the single-lead tracing shown above.

SECONDARY VENTRICULAR STANDSTILL—IDENTIFYING ECG FEATURES

1. **Rate:**   Electrical activity in the ventricles may continue, producing infrequent QRS complexes (rate 10-30/minute).
2. **Rhythm:**   The isolated electrical activity in the ventricle is insufficient to stimulate ventricular contraction, and so there is no heartbeat or peripheral pulses.
3. **P waves:**   Absent, since atrial death has occurred (downward displacement of pacemaker).
4. **P-R interval:**   No P-R interval. The QRS complexes arise from the ventricles.
5. **QRS:**   Wide, slurred complexes occur at a very slow rate.

Secondary Ventricular Standstill (Figure 13.16)

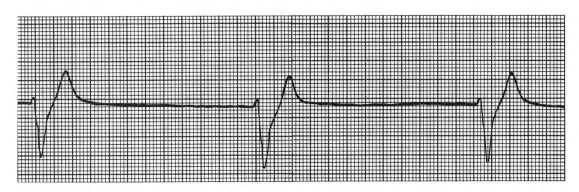

Rate:	Isolated ventricular electrical activity at a rate of less than 30/minute.
Rhythm:	The occasional ventricular complexes do not actually constitute a cardiac rhythm. They represent isolated electrical activity, but are not associated with effective ventricular contractions.
P waves:	Absent.
P-R interval:	Absent. There is no conduction through the heart.
QRS:	Very wide and distorted.
Comment:	Cardiac pacing is seldom effective in secondary ventricular standstill. The myocardium is unable to respond to the electrical stimulus because of hypoxia.

Dying Heart (Figure 13.17)

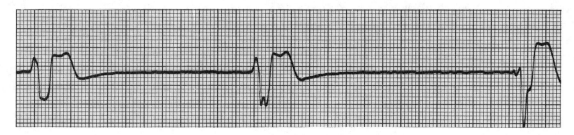

Comment: Although there is occasional electrical activity in the ventricles, true stimulation of the myocardium does not occur. The bizarre, distorted ventricular complexes may continue for several minutes even though the patient is clinically dead. This ECG pattern is common among patients dying of advanced left ventricular failure and is described as a dying heart pattern.

OTHER EXAMPLES OF DISORDERS OF CONDUCTION

Prolonged P-R Interval (First-Degree AV Heart Block) with Intraventricular Conduction Defect (Figure 13.18)

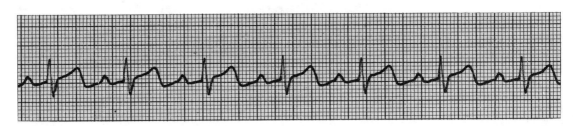

Rate:	About 70/minute.
Rhythm:	Regular.
P waves:	Normal.
P-R interval:	Prolonged (0.24 second).
QRS:	Widened (0.14 second).
Comment:	This example demonstrates a first-degree AV heart block (P-R interval of 0.24 second) as well as an intraventricular conduction defect (QRS greater than 0.12 second). The presence of more than one conduction disorder usually indicates diffuse disease of the conduction system.

Short P-R Interval: Lown-Ganong-Levine Syndrome (Figure 13.19)

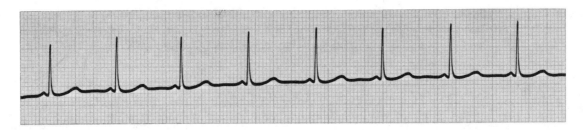

Rate:	About 80/minute.
Rhythm:	Regular.
P waves:	Occur regularly and precede each QRS complex.
P-R interval:	Less than 0.10 second (0.08 second).
QRS:	Normal.
Comment:	The very short P-R interval (0.08 second) seen in this example is a manifestation of *accelerated conduction* from the SA node to the ventricle, usually through an anomalous (shorter-than-normal) pathway. Early stimulation of the ventricles that results from accelerated conduction is often described as the *preexcitation syndrome*.

Short P-R Interval: Wolff-Parkinson-White Syndrome (Figure 13.20)

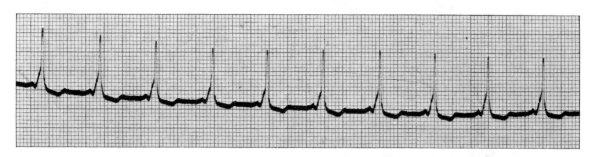

Rate:	About 100/minute.
Rhythm:	Regular.
P waves:	Normal and precede each QRS complex.
P-R interval:	Shortened (0.06 second).
QRS:	Widened (0.14 second) with slurring and notching of the upstroke of the R wave (called a delta wave).
Comment:	The combination of a short P-R interval in conjunction with a widened QRS complex and initial slurring of the R wave (delta wave) is called the *Wolff-Parkinson-White syndrome.* It is one form of the preexcitation syndrome (see above) and is associated with a high incidence of paroxysmal tachycardias.

Type 1 (Wenckebach) Second-Degree AV Block (Figure 13.21)

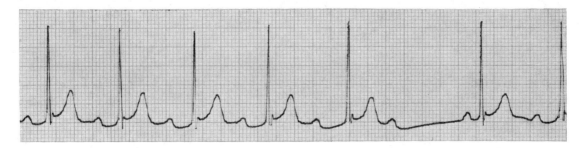

Rate:	About 70/minute.
Rhythm:	Irregular as the result of a blocked beat.
P waves:	Normal, and precede each QRS complex.
P-R interval:	The P-R intervals lengthen progressively for the 5 beats until a P wave is blocked. After the blocked beat the cycle starts again.
QRS:	Normal (0.08 second).
Comment:	Progressive lengthening of the P-R intervals until finally a beat is dropped is usually the result of transient injury to the AV node. This type of second-degree block (Wenckebach) is far less serious than Mobitz II second-degree block, which usually occurs below the AV node and may lead to ventricular standstill.

Type 1 (Wenckebach) Second-Degree AV Block (Figure 13.22)

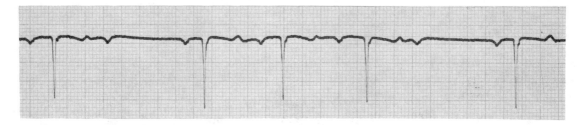

Rate:	About 50/minute.
Rhythm:	Irregular.
P waves:	Normal (inverted in this lead) and occur at regular intervals.
P-R interval:	Vary from 0.20 second to 0.32 second, depending on various stages of Wenckebach cycle.
QRS:	Normal (0.06 second). Two QRS complexes are absent because the corresponding impulses were blocked in the AV node.
Comment:	The key to the interpretation of this conduction disorder is the gradual prolongation of the P-R intervals in the 3 beats in the center of the strip. Without this important observation, the disturbance might be classified incorrectly as a Mobitz II block. (The inverted waves in this example are due to lead placement.)

Second-Degree AV Heart Block: 2:1 Type (Figure 13.23)

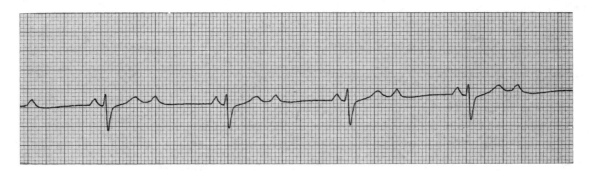

Rate:	Ventricular rate is 44/minute. Atrial rate is 88/minute.
Rhythm:	Regular.
P waves:	The P waves are normal and occur at regular intervals. However, every other P wave is blocked.
P-R interval:	Constant at 0.16 second.
QRS:	Normal (0.10 second).
Comment:	That every other P wave is blocked indicates that this is a 2:1 second-degree AV block. (The atrial rate is twice the ventricular rate.) The P-R intervals are constant. The normal width of the QRS complexes suggests that the block is junctional rather than subjunctional in location.

Third-Degree (Complete) AV Heart Block (Figure 13.24)

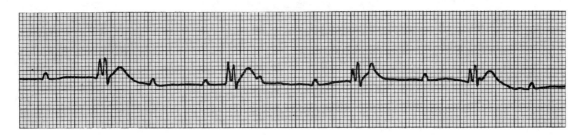

Rate:	The ventricular rate is 44/minute. The atrial rate is 100/minute.
Rhythm:	Regular.
P waves:	Normal, and occur regularly.
P-R interval:	Variable because of dissociation between atria and ventricles.
QRS:	Widened (0.14 second), indicating that they originate in the ventricles.
Comment:	The sinus node continues to discharge normally (at a rate of 100/minute), but all of the impulses are blocked. The ventricles discharge independently at a rate of 44/minute. The two rhythms are dissociated (atrioventricular dissociation) and bear no relation to each other.

Intraventricular Conduction Defect (Figure 13.25)

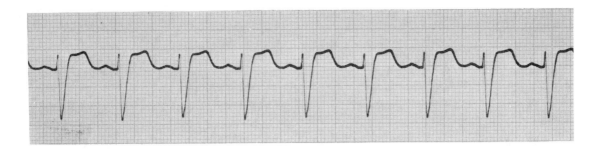

Rate:	About 90/minute.
Rhythm:	Regular.
P waves:	Normal and precede each QRS complex.
P-R interval:	Normal (0.20 second).
QRS:	Widened (0.16 second).
Comment:	The broad QRS complexes preceded by normal P waves indicate an intraventricular conduction defect. However, it cannot be determined from this single lead if the disorder is a right or left bundle branch block; a 12-lead ECG is necessary.

Ventricular Standstill (Figure 13.26)

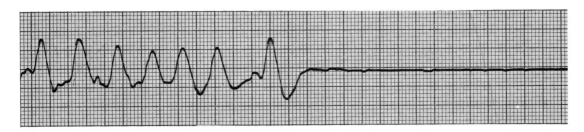

Comment:	This example shows the sudden cessation of all ventricular activity (ventricular standstill) during an episode of ventricular tachycardia. Just before this terminal arrhythmia occurred there was evidence of a complete heart block, which allowed the ventricular tachycardia to develop. The underlying cause of ventricular standstill, however, was complete heart block.

14

The Electrical Treatment of Arrhythmias: Cardiac Pacing and Precordial Shock

CARDIAC PACING

If for some reason the inherent electrical system of the heart does not generate impulses or fails to conduct impulses to the ventricles, it is possible to stimulate the myocardium and induce ventricular contraction by means of electrical impulses from an external source. This stimulation is achieved by using a battery-powered device called a pacemaker, which discharges repetitive electrical impulses so that an effective heart rate can be maintained and life preserved. The impulses are delivered to the heart by way of a catheter electrode, which is passed through the venous system into the right ventricular cavity. This technique is known as transvenous pacing.*

---

*Before the introduction of transvenous pacing in the early 1960's, pacing was accomplished by means of a large electrode placed on the chest wall. This method of stimulation (called external pacing) is no longer used because it was not predictably effective. Furthermore the magnitude of electrical current required to effect ventricular contractions through the closed chest wall is so great that the stimulus causes local pain, intense spasms of the skeletal muscles, and (with prolonged use) skin burns. Another technique that is now seldom used is transthoracic pacing. In this form of pacing the myocardium is stimulated by a thin wire electrode inserted directly into the ventricular wall by way of a needle introduced through the rib cage. The advantage of this method is the rapidity with which pacing can be initiated in catastrophic situations. However with the ability to prevent primary ventricular standstill by prophylactic pacemaker insertion (in patients with advanced heart block), transthoracic pacing is rarely required, except perhaps as a desperate measure during cardiopulmonary resuscitation.

Conduction disturbances resulting from acute myocardial infarction are most often transient in nature and usually disappear during the healing phase of the attack; therefore, cardiac pacing is used only as a temporary measure in this circumstance. By contrast, in patients with chronic, irreversible heart block (unrelated to myocardial infarction) permanent cardiac pacing is required. Permanent pacing, which involves surgical implantation of a pacemaker under the skin, has no application in the treatment of the acute phase of myocardial infarction and therefore is not discussed further here. The following description focuses on temporary transvenous pacing.

Transvenous Pacing

The heart can be safely and effectively stimulated by electrical impulses delivered through a small electrode positioned in the right ventricular cavity. The transvenous pacing electrode is introduced into a peripheral vein and then advanced through the venous system to the vena cava and the right atrium, and finally lodged against the endocardial surface of the right ventricle. The electrical stimuli are furnished by a small battery-powered generator (pacemaker). This technique is called transvenous pacing.

The prime purpose of transvenous pacing is to *prevent* primary ventricular standstill. This lethal arrhythmia seldom develops spontaneously (see Chapter 13); in most instances it is preceded by second- or third-degree heart block, or by bundle branch block involving more than one fascicle. By inserting a transvenous pacemaker when these advanced forms of heart block are detected, ventricular standstill can often be avoided.

In addition to this fundamental indication, transvenous pacing is also employed in the treatment of persistent bradyarrhythmias. It is a common practice to accelerate the heart rate deliberately by transvenous pacing when marked sinus bradycardia or a slow junctional rhythm resists customary drug therapy and compromises the cardiac output.

Temporary pacing is also used to control resistant ectopic rhythm (for example, frequent premature ventricular contractions or recurrent ventricular tachycardia) which are rate-related. By pacing the heart at a rate *faster* than its existing rate, premature beats can often be suppressed. This principle of arrhythmia control is called *overdriving* the heart.

Equipment for Transvenous Pacing

A transvenous pacing system consists of two basic components:

1. *A pulse generator* (battery-operated) serves as the source of electrical impulses. Both the rate and the intensity of these impulses can be regulated by control mechanisms.
2. An insulated wire *catheter* that carries the current from the pulse generator (pacemaker) to one or two small electrodes situated in the distal end of the catheter. The electrodes are in contact with the endocardial surface of the myocardium and permit the ventricle to be stimulated directly.

The Pulse Generator. There are two types of pacemakers: set-rate and demand. The differences between these pacing systems and their respective functions are discussed in the following paragraphs.

The Set-Rate Pulse Generator. This device, the first available for cardiac pacing, is seldom used in most CCUs at the present time. Nevertheless it is important to consider the design and operation of set-rate pacemakers to understand the newer pacemakers now in use. Very simply, these pulse generators initiate impulses at a fixed or set rate. For example, if the rate dial of the pacemaker is positioned at 60/minute, an impulse is fired every second (60 impulses/minute). Each pacing impulse (manifested on the ECG as a "pacing spike") stimulates the myocardium to produce a QRS complex as shown in Figure 14.1. The resulting QRS complexes are widened and have the configuration of a left bundle branch block pattern. (This pattern is understandable since the electrode delivering the stimulus to the myocardium is in the right ventricle and the impulse must be transmitted from this site to the left ventricle, creating a delay in complete ventricular activation.)

Although set-rate pacing is a dependable method for myocardial stimulation, it has one serious drawback that limits its usefulness in elective cardiac pacing: the instrument disregards the existing electrical activity of the heart and continues to discharge impulses at a fixed rate. Thus a natural beat from the heart and an artificial pacing stimulus may occur at the same time, as demonstrated in Figure 14.2. This

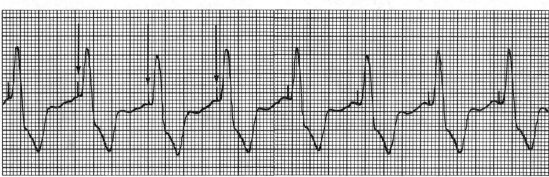

Figure 14.1.

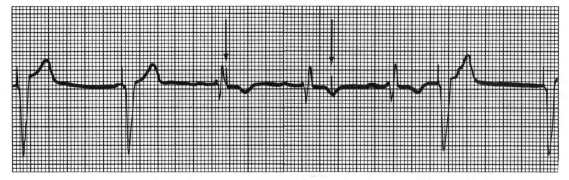

Figure 14.2.

phenomenon is called *competition.* Note that after two paced beats, three natural beats arise from the SA node. The set-rate pacemaker nevertheless continues to discharge impulses during this period (arrows).

When the natural and paced rhythms compete in this way there is a potential threat of inducing serious ventricular arrhythmias. This is particularly true when the pacing stimulus happens to hit on the T wave of the preceding natural beat. The arrival of the pacing stimulus during the period of the T wave, the *vulnerable period,* may create repetitive firing in the form of ventricular tachycardia or, worse, ventricular fibrillation. In other words, set-rate pacing has the same theoretical danger of inducing ventricular fibrillation as does a premature contraction striking a T wave. An example of ventricular fibrillation developing as the result of a set-rate pacing stimulus striking the T wave of a preceding natural beat is depicted in Figure 14.3.

Although competition certainly does not result in ventricular arrhythmias in all or even most instances (as evident in Figure 14.4, where the pacing stimulus hits the T wave of a premature ventricular contraction without provoking repetitive firing), this potential danger nevertheless exists. The risk of inducing ventricular fibrillation is distinctly increased in the presence of myocardial ischemia, and it is for this reason that set-rate pacing is undesirable in the treatment of acute myocardial infarction.

The Demand Pulse Generator. To avoid the potential risk of competition, associated with fixed-rate pacing, a more sophisticated pulse generator was developed. Instead of discharging impulses at a fixed rate, irrespective of the heart's inherent electrical activity, these pacemakers are designed to be noncompetitive and to discharge only on *demand.*

The principle of demand pacemaking is as follows: the pacemaker fires an impulse only if a QRS complex does *not* occur within a preset time interval. If a heartbeat does occur within this designated period the pacemaker recognizes this electrical activity and deliberately withholds the pacing impulse. On this basis a pacing impulse cannot strike the T wave of a premature ventricular contraction since the pacemaker will sense the ectopic beat (which occurs within the preset time interval) and accordingly will not discharge an impulse. On the other hand, if the pacemaker does *not* sense a natural or ectopic beat, it discharges impulses at a preset rate. An example of how a demand pacemaker functions is shown in Figure 14.5. Note that the pacemaker stops discharging impulses when a series of natural beats occur (all of which fall within the preset time interval). However, when the interval is again exceeded because a natural beat did not occur on schedule the pacemaker begins to discharge again.

For a pacemaker to function on demand it must receive an electrocardiographic signal indicating that a natural or ectopic beat has occurred; it is this signal that inhibits the pacemaker from discharging unwanted impulses. This information is obtained by having the catheter tip (which is in contact with the endocardial surface of the right ventricle) serve as an exploring electrode to detect each QRS complex. The electrical activity of the heart is transmitted back through the

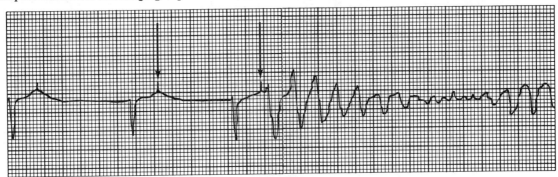

Figure 14.3.

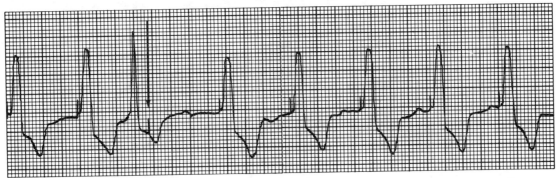

Figure 14.4.

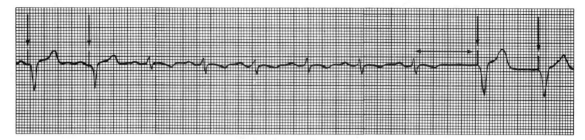

Figure 14.5.

catheter to a sensing device within the pacemaker. The pacing catheter thus serves to relay electrocardiographic signals to the pacemaker as well as to send pacing impulses from the instrument to the myocardium (Figure 14.6).

Catheter Electrodes. There are two basic types of catheter electrodes: those with a single electrode incorporated in the tip of the catheter (unipolar electrode) and those with two electrodes positioned about 1 cm apart at the distal end of the catheter (bipolar electrode), as shown in Figure 14.7. As with any electrical circuit the electrical impulse must flow between two poles (or electrodes) in order to stimulate the heart. With a unipolar catheter only one electrode (the negative pole) is within the heart, and a second electrode (the positive pole) is required to complete the circuit. This latter electrode usually consists of a wire suture placed in the skin of the chest wall.

The bipolar catheter electrode, which is used far more commonly than the unipolar system, obviates the need for a secondary skin electrode since both electrodes are incorporated into the catheter itself.

Because of this dual electrode system bipolar catheters are of greater diameter (larger gauge) than unipolar catheters and therefore may be more difficult to insert. Nonetheless bipolar catheters are preferable to unipolar types because the presence of two adjacent electrodes within the heart enhances the likelihood of direct contact with the endocardial surface of the right ventricle, a requirement for successful pacing. With the unipolar catheter the electrode may easily become displaced from the ventricular wall and thus interrupt effective pacing.

Technique of Transvenous Pacing

Catheter Insertion. The pacing electrode can be introduced into the venous system through an antecubital, femoral, jugular, or subclavian vein. Selecting the vein to be used for this purpose is essentially a matter of individual preference; there are advocates for each approach. Although an arm vein is usually the easiest to enter percutaneously, the route to the

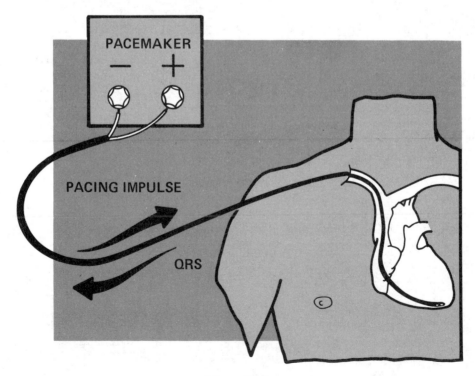

Figure 14.6.

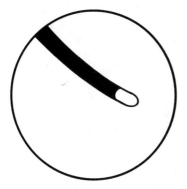 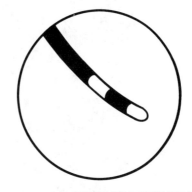

UNIPOLAR TYPE ELECTRODE   **BIPOLAR TYPE ELECTRODE**

Figure 14.7.

heart is long and torturous, often making it difficult to advance the catheter into the ventricle. Furthermore, any movement of the arm may result in displacement of the catheter after it has been properly positioned. The jugular and subclavian veins, being closer to the superior vena cava, are shorter, more direct routes to the right ventricle. For this reason, and because displacement of the catheter is less likely, these latter sites are generally preferred.

Introduction of the Catheter Electrode. Once a particular vein has been selected, the surrounding skin area must be scrupulously prepared as for any surgical procedure. The area is draped to prevent contamination.

Several specially designed needles are available for catheter insertion. Most of these placement units consist of a large-bore needle (with a stylus) and a thin plastic sheath which fits over this cannula (Figure 14.8). After the skin is infiltrated with a local anesthetic, the unit is inserted into the vein; the needle (and stylus) is then removed, leaving the plastic sheath positioned in the vein.

The catheter electrode is introduced through this plastic sheath into the vein and advanced to the right ventricle. After the electrode is in proper position within the ventricle, the plastic conduit is removed so that the catheter extends directly through the skin opening. In instances where needle penetration of the skin or vein is difficult, a small surgical "cut-down" incision can be made to facilitate entry to the vein.

Passage of the Catheter Electrode. Regardless of the site of introduction, the catheter is advanced slowly to the superior vena cava, into the right atrium, through the tricuspid valve, and to the right ventricle, where it is positioned against the endocardial surface. The pathway of the catheter (as shown on a chest x-ray) is noted in Figure 14.9. Two methods are

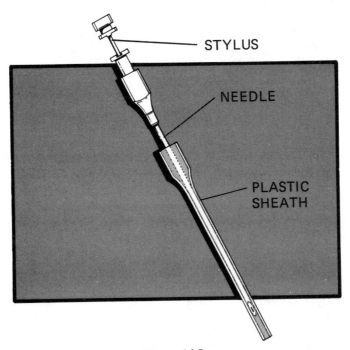

STYLUS

NEEDLE

PLASTIC SHEATH

Figure 14.8.

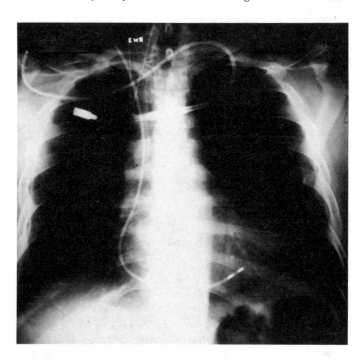

Figure 14.9. Transvenous pacing catheter in right ventricle. Note that this is a bipolar catheter.

available to guide the catheter to its ultimate position in the ventricle. The first involves fluoroscopy, where the radiopaque catheter is directly visualized during its passage. Although this technique is very desirable, most CCUs are not equipped with the expensive apparatus needed for this purpose (i.e., a portable fluoroscope with an image intensifier). Therefore when a catheter is to be positioned with this technique, patients have to be moved to either an x-ray department or a cardiac catheterization laboratory. This separation of the patient from the prepared setting of the CCU poses obvious risks, but this method is popular because it facilitates electrode positioning.

The catheter can also be guided to the right ventricle by electrocardiographic means. This method can be performed in the CCU and avoids the danger of moving the patient. The principle of this "blind" technique of insertion is as follows: as the electrode is being advanced to the heart an electrocardiogram can be recorded *through* the catheter by attaching its free end to the chest lead (V lead) terminal of the ECG machine. In other words, the catheter tip serves as an exploring electrode from within the heart. The resulting tracing is called an *intracavitary* electrocardiogram. Because the ECG patterns from the vena cava, the atrium, and the right ventricle have different configurations, it is possible to identify the position of the electrode in this way. Typical ECG patterns from these various locations are shown in Figure 14.10 (A-F). Note the large distinctive complexes recorded when the catheter enters the ventricle (14.10D). When this method of electrocardiographic guidance is used it is necessary to connect all of the limb leads

to the patient just as if a customary electrocardiogram were to be recorded. The only difference is that the chest (V) lead, rather than being used as a skin electrode, is joined to the free end of the catheter with an alligator clamp.

Attachment of the Catheter Electrode to the Pacemaking Device. As shown in Figure 14.11, the pacemaker has two terminals for connection of the electrodes; these are clearly marked as positive (+) and negative (−). When a unipolar electrode is used, the free end of the catheter is attached to the negative (−) terminal of the pacemaker, and the wire from the skin electrode (suture) to the positive (+) terminal. With a bipolar catheter electrode the two wires extending from the catheter can be connected to the terminals without concern about positive or negative poles.

Rate of Pacing. The pacing rate is governed by several principles. First, the number of pacing stimuli per minute must exceed the existing heart rate. In complete heart block, for example, where the inherent cardiac rate may be 30-40/minute, the pacing rate would be set at 60-70/minute. Second, it is undesirable to pace the heart at an overly fast rate since the oxygen demand of the myocardium is increased with rapid pacing and patients may experience angina. Furthermore, when the heart is paced rapidly the time for ventricular filling is decreased and cardiac output may be adversely affected. Therefore the pacing rate must be adjusted for each patient so that pumping efficiency is not reduced while the underlying arrhythmia is being controlled.

ECG PATTERNS DURING PACEMAKER INSERTION

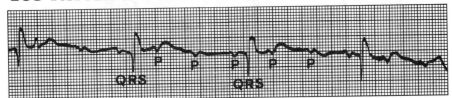

Figure 14.10(A). The ECG reveals complete heart block. The catheter tip is in the vena cava. The P waves are small and inverted.

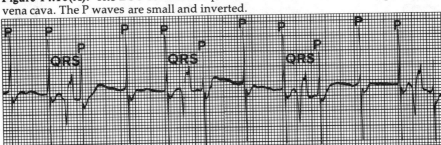

Figure 14.10(B). The catheter tip is now in the right atrium. Note the very tall, biphasic P waves recorded from this intra-atrial position.

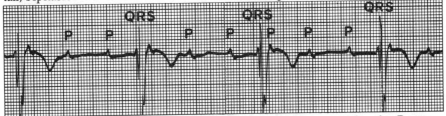

Figure 14.10(C). As the catheter advances toward the ventricle, the P waves diminish in size while the QRS complexes become larger.

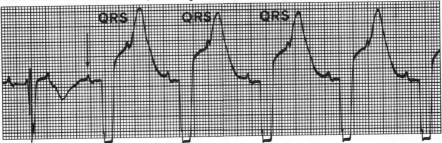

Figure 14.10(D). The catheter tip passes from the right atrium to the right ventricle (arrow), as indicated by the sudden appearance of very large QRS complexes.

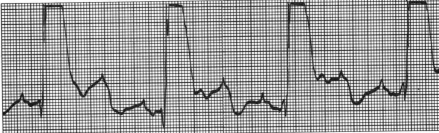

Figure 14.10(E). The tip of the catheter is now wedged against the endocardial wall of the right ventricle. In this position the ST segment is markedly elevated.

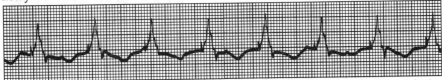

Figure 14.10(F). After the catheter has been properly positioned and the pacemaker turned on, a standard ECG reveals effective pacing.

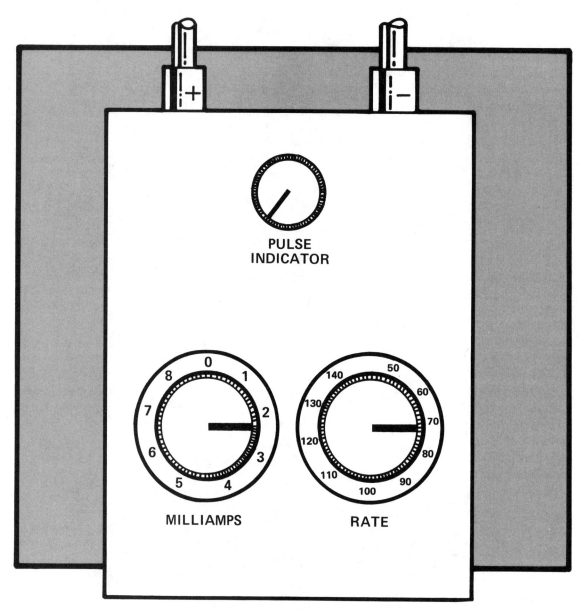

Figure 14.11.

Energy of Pacing. In determining the energy or intensity of the stimulus required for cardiac pacing it is necessary to consider a fundamental characteristic of myocardial contractility: when the heart is stimulated by an electrical impulse it responds (contracts) either completely or not at all (the "all-or-none" law). The lowest electrical energy that will cause myocardial contraction is called the *threshold level.* If the intensity of a pacing stimulus is less than the threshold level contraction will *not* occur. Conversely, a pacing stimulus greater than the threshold level will not produce a stronger contraction since the muscle already contracts to its fullest extent at the threshold point. In other words, there is a critical level of electrical energy below which contraction will not occur and above which it is not augmented.

Therefore, in setting the intensity of the pacing impulse it is necessary to first determine the threshold level. This is accomplished as follows: after the catheter has been positioned correctly and attached to the pacemaker, the energy control dial is increased gradually from the lowest milliampere setting to a point where a QRS complex is noted with each stimulus. This setting is the threshold level.

When a catheter electrode is properly positioned and the electrode is in good contact with the endocardium, the threshold level in most patients is usually less than 2 milliamperes. If the threshold is much higher, for example 6 or 8 milliamperes, it is likely that the catheter is poorly situated in the ventricle and that repositioning of the tip is required. Because the threshold is not constant at all times, and varies with the contact of the electrode tip and the endocardium (as well as other factors), it is customary to set the initial energy level for pacing at twice the threshold value to overcome this variation. For example, if the threshold is found to be 1 milliampere, the final setting for the pacing stimulus should be 2 milliamperes.

Duration of Pacing. As already noted, transvenous pacing is employed fundamentally as a prophylactic measure when advanced forms of heart block or bradyarrhythmias (refractory to drugs) exist. Because these particular arrhythmic disturbances are almost always of a transient nature in acute myocardial infarction, cardiac pacing is required only on a temporary basis until a normal rate and rhythm have returned. While the exact duration of these rhythm disturbances varies with the site of infarction and the rate of healing (among other factors), most of these disorders last less than 10 days and pacing is seldom necessary beyond this period. After normal sinus rhythm has returned, it is customary to leave the pacing catheter in place for another week in case the arrhythmia returns. Following this additional period, the pacing catheter is removed.

Problems With Temporary Transvenous Pacing

Several difficulties may be encountered during the course of temporary pacing. The most common of these are as follows:

Displacement of the Catheter Tip. For pacing to be effective the catheter electrode must remain proximate to the inner wall of the right ventricle. Displacement of the tip of the catheter is frequent during temporary pacing and is the most common cause of pacing failure. Displacement occurs with greater frequency when the catheter has been introduced via an arm vein (motion of the arm tends to move the entire catheter), but dislodgment of the tip may result from a change of body position regardless of the insertion site.

Displacement of the pacing electrode may be suspected when each pacing stimulus fails to produce a QRS complex. This means that the pacing impulse is ineffective and is not capturing the heartbeat. An example of *loss of capture* is shown in the ECG in Figure 14.12. It is apparent that none of the pacing spikes (arrows) stimulate the ventricle to produce QRS complexes. Once displacement has occurred the catheter usually has to be repositioned in the ventricle to achieve effective pacing, although occasionally changing the position of the patient in bed will restore the catheter to its proper position.

Sensing Errors. As discussed previously, competition of rhythms can be expected when fixed-rate pacemakers are used. The problem is particularly common when the heart is being paced because of temporary heart block or other slow-rate arrhythmias, and normal sinus rhythm returns suddenly. In this circumstance the natural and paced rhythms (which may now be of similar rates) compete with each other. Although theoretically competition should not develop during demand pacing, the problem can in fact occur. This competition usually results when the sensing mechanism of the pacemaker fails to recognize spontaneous heartbeats. Unless the R wave transmitted back to the sensing mechanism is of sufficient amplitude (voltage), the pacemaker will not sense the beat and will discharge an impulse; this results in competition. When competition is caused by improper sensing the catheter tip must be moved to a different location in the right ventricle to obtain a better R wave signal for the sensing mechanism.

Loss of Pacing Artifact. If the pacing stimulus does not produce an artifact (spike) on the ECG it can be presumed that one of the components of the pacing system has failed. The source of the problem is usually not difficult to identify. If the pulse indicator (on the face of the pacemaker) shows no movement it implies that either the batteries are exhausted or the pulse generator is broken. If, on the other hand, the pulse indicator dial shows that the pacemaker is functioning, it can be reasoned that impulses, while originating normally, are not reaching the heart. This condition may develop because of a broken wire within the catheter or, more simply, because the catheter terminal has become disconnected from the pulse generator.

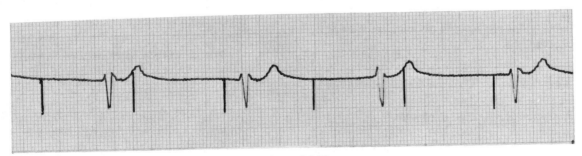

Figure 14.12.

Perforation of the Ventricular Wall by the Catheter Tip. Since the catheter electrode is deliberately placed against the inner surface of the ventricular wall it is understandable that the catheter tip may embed itself in the myocardium, particularly when the catheter remains in the heart for many days. In some patients the catheter actually burrows through the full thickness of the myocardium and finally perforates the right ventricular wall. However, this untoward event produces surprisingly few effects. Because the blood pressure within the right ventricle is normally quite low (unlike the high pressure within the left ventricle), perforation of the right ventricular chamber seldom produces any hemodynamic consequences. Moreover, if there is bleeding into the pericardium the amount of blood is generally trivial and does not produce cardiac tamponade.

That perforation of the ventricular wall has occurred can be suspected by noting a sudden loss of capture after a period of successful pacing. On some occasions the catheter perforation is recognized by the appearance of contractions of the diaphragm or the chest wall. This muscle twitching (which is usually obvious to the patient) signifies that the catheter electrode has perforated the right ventricle and has traveled to the diaphragm or the intercostal muscles. The diagnosis can often be confirmed by means of a chest x-ray, which shows the catheter tip outside the right ventricle. In the event of perforation it is necessary to withdraw the catheter gently and reposition it in the right ventricle.

Thrombophlebitis and Skin Infection. Since pacing catheters must often remain in the venous system for prolonged periods, there is always the possibility that thrombophlebitis may develop from mechanical irritation of the vein wall. The likelihood of this inflammatory reaction is perhaps greater when smaller veins are used as insertion sites (e.g., arm veins); however other factors undoubtedly contribute to this complication. If thrombophlebitis is marked, the catheter must be removed and another one inserted in a different vein.

Because the skin puncture site is in effect an open wound, local infection may occur. The risk can be minimized (almost excluded) by adherence to strict surgical asepsis at the time of catheter placement and by the routine use of antibiotic (neomycin) ointment subsequently.

The Nursing Role in Cardiac Pacing

Preparation for Catheter Insertion

1. When a decision has been made to pace the heart temporarily it is important to explain to the patient why the procedure is necessary and how it will be performed. The explanation should emphasize the preventive benefit of being able to control the heart rate as desired with pacing. Allow the patient time to ask questions or to express his concerns.
2. If cardiac pacing is to be performed on an elective basis (e.g., in a patient with second-degree heart block) it is customary to have an operative permit signed by the patient. In emergency situations this measure can be disregarded.
3. When the catheter is to be positioned by electrocardiographic (rather than fluoroscopic) means, the limb lead electrodes should be attached to all of the extremities and a separate ECG machine brought to the bedside. After the catheter has been inserted into the venous system, the chest (V) lead terminal is connected to the free end of the pacing catheter by means of an alligator clamp. This exploring electrode records an intracavitary tracing from which the position of the catheter electrode can be determined. It is essential that *all of the equipment used be grounded properly* to prevent the threat of electrocution by extraneous electrical current passing through the catheter to the heart. Some institutions use battery-powered electrocardiographic machines to reduce this danger.
4. A syringe containing 100 mg lidocaine should be prepared and placed at the bedside. In addition, the nurse should verify the patency of the preexisting "keep-open" intravenous line. This preparedness is essential to combat any ventricular irritability that may develop suddenly while the catheter is being positioned within the heart.
5. A defibrillator should be available for immediate use in the event (even though unlikely) that the catheter may induce ventricular fibrillation.

Catheter Insertion

1. The skin surrounding the intended site of catheter insertion is prepared with soap, alcohol, and a skin antiseptic, as with any surgical procedure. An "eye sheet" is used to drape the area, leaving only the operative site exposed. In addition, the patient's face is covered with a loose drape to prevent breath contamination. (Pathogens from the mouth and nose are a far greater source of wound infection than bacteria found on the skin.)
2. The needle placement set and the appropriate catheter should be sterile and ready for use. Sterilization can be accomplished by the use of bactericidal solutions or preferably a gas technique; autoclaving should not be used because

of the plastic materials contained in the catheter and needle sheath.

3. A local anesthetic (procaine or lidocaine) is used to infiltrate the skin before the large-bore needle is inserted into the vein.

4. As the catheter is advanced into the heart the ECG must be monitored with great care to detect premature ventricular beats that may develop. Consequently the ECG must be observed *continuously* during the insertion procedure. This is accomplished with usual cardiac monitoring equipment (when the catheter is placed by fluoroscopy) or with an ECG machine (when placement is guided by an intracavitary electrode).

5. After the physician has placed the catheter in a proper position, and effective capture of the heartbeat has been achieved, the catheter must be secured to the skin. This may be accomplished by placing a suture around the catheter and through the skin or, more simply, by adhesive tape. An antibiotic ointment (neomycin or bacitracin) is then applied to the skin entry site and a dry dressing firmly affixed.

Subsequent Care

During the course of cardiac pacing the major responsibility of the nurse is to verify that the pacemaker system is functioning properly and effectively. As noted, several problems may arise during temporary pacing, and careful observation of the patient and the monitor is essential to detect these disturbances as soon as they occur.

Loss of Capture. If there is loss of capture the nurse should notify the physician immediately because the pacing stimulus is wholly ineffective in this situation. Depending on the underlying arrhythmia for which pacing is being used, loss of capture can be associated with serious consequences. For example, if pacing fails during complete heart block, ventricular standstill may result (Figure 14.13).

Absence of Pacing Artifacts. A second situation demanding emergency action is the sudden disappearance of pacing artifacts on the ECG (Figure 14.14). In many instances the cause of this crisis can be promptly identified and corrected by the nurse. The first step in solving the problem is to make certain the catheter terminals have not become disconnected from the pacemaker device. If these connections are found to be secure, the next thing to do is to ascertain that an adequate stimulus is being generated by the battery. If there is no movement of the pulse indicator, the pacemaker batteries may be exhausted and a different pacemaker should be attached. (To prevent the catastrophe of battery failure a careful record should be kept of the number of hours each pacemaker is actually used. While the effective battery life of most pulse generators is presumably 800 hours, it is good practice to change batteries routinely after 600 hours of use.) If pacemaker malfunction cannot be corrected instantly, cardiopulmonary resuscitation should be initiated without delay.

Competition. Of less importance than loss of capture or pacemaker failure is the development of competition between the paced and natural cardiac rhythms. If competition occurs during fixed-rate pacing it may indicate that normal sinus rhythm has returned. The presence of competition during demand pacing suggests difficulty with the sensing system of the pacemaker unit. In either instance the nurse should apprise the physician of this undesirable rhythm.

Perforation of Ventricle. That the catheter tip has perforated the right ventricle may be suspected when there is a sudden loss of capture. However, this finding is not diagnostic since loss of capture is most often the result of simple displacement of the catheter tip within the ventricular cavity. A more important finding is the appearance of contractions of the diaphragm or muscles of the chest wall which occur synchronously with pacing impulses. This complication should be reported to the physician immediately.

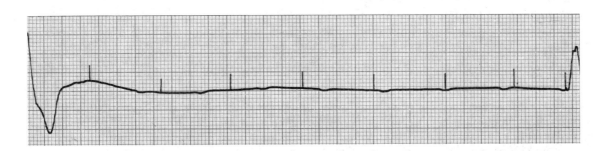

Figure 14.13.

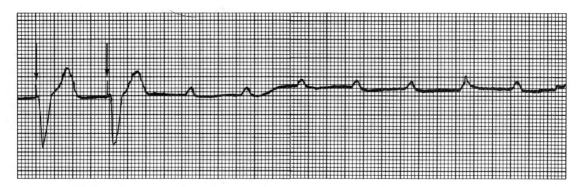

Figure 14.14.

Thrombophlebitis and Skin Infection. The nurse should carefully examine the catheter insertion site for signs of local infection. An antibiotic ointment should be applied daily. In changing the dressing care must be taken not to move the catheter. In addition to skin infections, signs of thrombophlebitis should be sought, particularly when the catheter has been introduced through an arm vein or has been in place several days.

PRECORDIAL SHOCK

Precordial shock is used either as a lifesaving emergency method for terminating ventricular fibrillation (defibrillation) or as an elective procedure to convert certain atrial and ventricular tachyarrhythmias to normal rhythm (cardioversion). The principle of precordial shock in treating ventricular fibrillation is straightforward: a high-voltage shock of very brief duration (only a few thousandths of a second) delivered through the chest wall is capable of abruptly stopping the chaotic electrical activity within the heart that produced the lethal arrhythmia. Once the bizarre fibrillatory rhythm is terminated in this way, the heart's natural pacemaker regains command and an effective beat is reestablished. This same principle is utilized in elective cardioversion where brief depolarization of the entire heart (at a particular time in the cardiac cycle) halts the ectopic pacemaker and allows the SA node to assume control again.

While enormous electrical energy (about 7000 volts) is required to defibrillate the heart through the chest wall, this electrical force is so very short in duration that the current does not injure the myocardium.

Equipment for Precordial Shock

Precordial shock to terminate ventricular fibrillation can be delivered by an alternating current (AC) or a direct current (DC) defibrillator. Although both types of defibrillators are effective for this particular purpose, the DC defibrillator can also be used for elective precordial shock. Because of this greater versatility, DC machines are now used routinely in CCUs, and AC defibrillators are obsolete.

A DC defibrillator builds and stores thousands of volts in a capacitor within seconds and discharges this energy on demand in less than 5 milliseconds. The stored energy is delivered to the heart through a circuit consisting of two electrodes (or paddles, as they are commonly called) which are held against the chest wall. The paddles are large in diameter (usually 3-4 inches), allowing the electrical discharge to pass through a wide area of skin, preventing electrical burns. To facilitate passage of current through the skin, a thick layer of conductive paste is applied to the skin and electrode surfaces before the energy is discharged. The handles of the paddles are insulated to protect the operator from leakage of current.

The electrical energy is discharged by pressing a button switch incorporated in the handles of the electrodes. The amount of current delivered by the defibrillator can be adjusted according to need by a dial setting on the machine. This electrical force is measured in watt-seconds (w/s) or joules; the scale ranges from 1-400 w/s with conventional equipment.

As noted in the discussion of ventricular fibrillation (Chapter 12) defibrillating equipment that can deliver much higher energies (400-1000 w/s) is also available. These high energy devices are based on the allegation that patients weighing more than 80 kg, for example, can not be predictably defibrillated by conventional defibrillators. However, prospective studies designed to answer this question show that shocks delivering 74-360 w/s were effective in 95% of instances. In all, little benefit was achieved with very high energy defibrillators and it is now believed that conventional defibrillators, which deliver about 300 w/s energy, are more suitable.

Synchronized and Nonsynchronized Precordial Shock

When precordial shock is used electively to convert atrial and ventricular tachyarrhythmias (cardioversion), it is important that the electrical discharge be *synchronized* with the cardiac cycle. This need can be appreciated on the following basis: when any electrical impulse, even a premature ventricular contraction, strikes during the vulnerable period of the cardiac cycle (i.e., during the time of the T wave, as shown in Figure 14.15) there is a potential danger of inducing *ventricular fibrillation*. The same threat may exist if a precordial shock (or a pacemaker impulse) arrives during the critical interval of the vulnerable period. To avoid this hazard, precordial shock is deliberately synchronized so that the electrical force is delivered at a point in the cardiac cycle when the heart is refractory to stimulation; this nonvulnerable (refractory) period corresponds to the time of the QRS complex. The equipment for precordial shock is so designed that the discharge energy can be synchronized with the safe (refractory) period of the cardiac cycle. When the synchronizer switch is *on* and the discharge button is triggered, the instrument waits until the next R wave before delivering its energy. On the other hand, if the synchronizer is *off*, discharge occurs the instant the machine is triggered, without reference to the cardiac cycle.

It is essential to understand clearly just when precordial shock should or should not be synchronized. *In terminating ventricular fibrillation with precordial shock (defibrillation), the synchronizer switch must be in the* off *position.* If the synchronizer switch is on in this circumstance, the machine will *not* fire because it waits for a QRS complex, which of course is nonexistent during ventricular fibrillation.

Conversely, when precordial shock is employed *electively* to convert other arrhythmias (e.g., atrial fibrillation) the synchronizer must be *on* to avoid the possibility of the discharge striking during the vulnerable period and inducing ventricular fibrillation.

Energy of Discharge

As indicated, the level of discharge energy is adjustable and must be set for the particular arrhythmias being treated. For ventricular fibrillation a delivered energy of 300-350 w/s is nearly always effective. For elective cardioversion the precise energy setting varies with several factors. First, it is known that certain arrhythmias are more responsive to precordial shock than others and require less energy for conversion. For example, atrial flutter can generally be terminated with minimal electrical force (e.g., 10-30 w/s) whereas atrial fibrillation is often more resistant and demands a higher energy setting. Second, cardioversion may provoke ventricular arrhythmias among patients receiving digitalis, and for this reason high energies are usually avoided in this circumstance. Third, factors such as the patient's body build, weight, and the presence of emphysema may increase the voltage demands. Many physicians prefer to attempt cardioversion using very low energies at first (e.g., 20 w/s or less) and, if the trial is unsuccessful, to increase the level on successive attempts until cardioversion is finally accomplished; others employ higher energies (e.g., 200 w/s or more) initially.

Technique of Elective Cardioversion and the Nursing Role

Preparation for Procedure

1. The procedure should be explained to the patient by a member of the nurse-physician team. Because the word shock has frightening connotations, it is wise to avoid this term when describing the treatment.

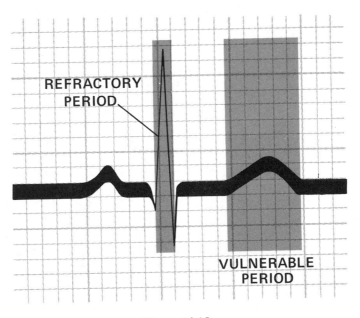

Figure 14.15.

2. In many institutions it is customary to have an operative permit signed by the patient when elective cardioversion is to be performed.

3. All necessary equipment and materials should be at the bedside. This includes the machine which delivers the synchronized shock, along with syringes, antiarrhythmic drugs, and anesthetic agents.

4. Although elective cardioversion is a remarkably safe procedure when properly performed, it is theoretically possible that the shock might induce ventricular fibrillation. For this reason emergency equipment for cardiopulmonary resuscitation should be in readiness. A syringe containing 100 mg lidocaine should always be at the bedside for immediate use to combat premature ventricular contractions that may develop after cardioversion.

5. Prior to the procedure an intravenous pathway must be established and its patency verified. This conduit is used to administer the anesthetic agent and any antiarrhythmic drugs that may be necessary.

6. In order for the electrical shock to be properly synchronized with the R wave of the cardiac cycle, it is necessary to use electrocardiographic electrodes for sensing R waves. These electrodes should be placed on all four extremities. (With some equipment the ECG electrodes are unnecessary because the customary monitoring electrodes serve this purpose.)

Setting the Machine for Cardioversion

1. The synchronizer switch is turned *on* so that the discharge of energy will coincide with the R wave of the cardiac cycle.

2. Because synchronization cannot be achieved unless the ventricular complexes are of sufficient amplitude to trigger the discharge, the "gain" dial may have to be adjusted to obtain R waves of adequate size (as evidenced by a flashing light or other signal). If complexes of sufficient height cannot be obtained by increasing the gain, a different lead must be used to obtain taller waves (e.g., changing from a lead II to a lead I position).

3. For safety it is wise to verify that proper synchronization will occur when the machine is fired. This is accomplished by a test mechanism within the machine which indicates where the discharge will fall in the cardiac cycle when the shock is actually delivered.

4. The energy (watt-seconds) to be used for the cardioversion attempt is set at the desired level by the physician.

Anesthesia

Although precordial shock itself creates little actual pain because of the extremely short duration of the stimulus, the sensation (and the associated generalized muscle contraction) is nevertheless frightening and unpleasant for most patients. Because an analgesic effect is required for only a few seconds, very short-acting agents—e.g., sodium methohexital (Brevital) or diazepam (Valium)—are given intravenously just before the shock is delivered.

Paddle Electrodes: Preparation and Placement

1. Prior to the procedure the paddles should be carefully cleaned with scouring powder to remove metallic oxides that form on the surface of the electrodes and interfere with the flow of current.

2. A thick layer of conducting jelly is placed on the face of the electrodes and distributed evenly. Additional electrode paste is applied to the chest wall where the paddles will be held. Unless there is an adequate amount of jelly at the electrode-skin interface, serious skin burns can occur.

3. One paddle is placed in the right sternal area and the other on the left lateral chest wall. The precise location of the paddles is not critical as long as the flow of current traverses the heart (Figure 14.16). An alternative method of paddle placement is to position one electrode (a special flat paddle) under the left scapula and to hold the other paddle directly over the upper sternum (Figure 14.17). In this way the flow of current passes directly through the heart in an anterior-posterior direction.

4. Before the energy is discharged it is important to ascertain that the conducting paste remains localized at the electrode sites and has not spread over the chest wall. Excess jelly should be wiped dry before proceeding, or the current will flow across the skin surface (rather than through the heart), creating a large spark and perhaps causing a burn.

5. The paddles must be pressed firmly and evenly against the chest wall; failure to preserve good contact results in dissipation of energy. Furthermore, tilting of the paddles may cause skin burns.

6. Since there is a theoretical threat that the electrical force being delivered to the patient could pass through the bed and reach the operator or others, it is wise to have all personnel stand clear of the bed at the moment of discharge.

7. The discharge switch is pressed, and the effect is immediately evident by a sudden generalized

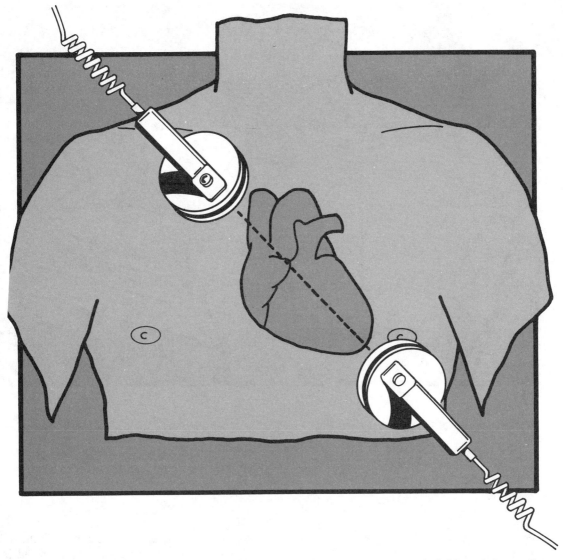

Figure 14.16. Placement of paddles. One is in the right sternal area and the other on the left lateral chest wall.

contraction of the patient's muscles. Observation of the oscilloscope will confirm whether normal rhythm has been restored.

8. In some instances premature ventricular contractions are noted following cardioversion, and lidocaine should be administered promptly to combat this cardiac irritability.
9. In the extremely unlikely event that the cardioversion attempt causes ventricular fibrillation, the synchronizer switch must be turned *off,* the energy increased to 400 watt-seconds, and a second shock delivered instantly to defibrillate the patient. Remember that defibrillation cannot be accomplished if the synchronizer is *on!*

Technique of Emergency Defibrillation

Although the method for defibrillation has been described in the discussion of ventricular fibrillation,

it is important to review this procedure with particular emphasis on the differences between defibrillation and elective cardioversion.

1. Defibrillation is a lifesaving technique and must be accomplished within a minute or so to be successful. This means that precordial shock must always be the *initial* step in treatment (within the setting of a CCU), and that no time should be wasted with other measures, such as the administration of oxygen or closed chest massage. The first person reaching the bedside, whether a physician or nurse, should proceed to defibrillate the patient at once.
2. The discharge energy should be set at its maximum delivered energy level: about 300-350 w/s; the use of less energy is pointless in this dire emergency.
3. It is absolutely essential that the synchronizer switch be in the *off* position for defibrillation so

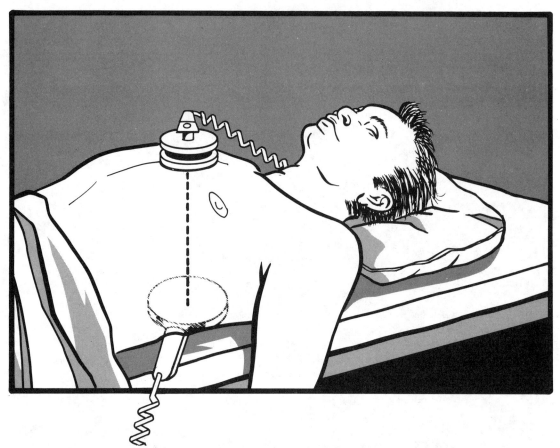

Figure 14.17. Alternative placement of paddles. A special flat paddle is placed under the left scapula, and another paddle is held directly over the upper sternum.

that the discharge will occur the instant the trigger is pressed.

4. Conductive jelly is applied to the electrode surfaces, and the paddles are held firmly against the chest wall in the same manner described for elective cardioversion.

5. If for some reason defibrillation is unsuccessful, precordial shock should be repeated immediately. With some equipment it is necessary to recharge the capacitor by pressing an appropriate button before a second discharge can be delivered.
6. Be sure that no one is touching the bed or patient at the time precordial shock is delivered.

15

Electrocardiographic Diagnosis Of Myocardial Infarction, Injury and Ischemia

In addition to its use in interpreting arrhythmias, electrocardiography serves an equally important role in establishing the diagnosis of acute myocardial infarction, myocardial injury and myocardial ischemia. The electrocardiogram (ECG), although by no means infallible, remains an indispensable method for verifying these particular manifestations of coronary heart disease (CHD) and deserves top rank among even the newest diagnostic techniques. The purpose of this chapter is to briefly explain the application of electrocardiography in the diagnosis of CHD, focusing primarily on the identification and location of acute myocardial infarction.*

---

*In previous editions of this book we deliberately excluded details of the ECG diagnosis of acute myocardial infarction. Several reasons influenced our decision, but above all we felt that the broad and complex subject of 12-lead electrocardiography was beyond the intent and scope of an introductory book on intensive coronary care. Moreover, this aspect of electrocardiography is of much less importance to the success of coronary care nursing than the interpretation of arrhythmias. Also, there are several excellent texts available on 12-lead electrocardiography which offer detailed information to interested readers. Although our attitude about this matter has not changed greatly, it has become apparent nevertheless that many CCU nurses—especially experienced nurses—find it worthwhile to at least be able to recognize the ECG signs of acute myocardial infarction and other manifestations of CHD. Accordingly, this chapter is meant to provide the nurse with a basic concept of ECG diagnosis, which can be expanded as necessary.

THE 12-LEAD ELECTROCARDIOGRAM

Unlike arrhythmias, which most often can be identified from a single (monitoring) lead, the detection and localization of acute myocardial infarction (and other myocardial abnormalities) require a complete, 12-lead ECG. Myocardial ischemia, injury and necrosis are reflected electrocardiographically by disturbances in depolarization and repolarization, which appear in the QRS, ST segment and T wave portions of the ECG. Since disorders of depolarization and repolarization may be confined to only one segment of the myocardium, multiple leads are necessary to provide a comprehensive view of these electrical events throughout the heart.

A complete (12-lead) ECG consists of three standard (limb) leads, three augmented leads and six chest (precordial) leads.

The standard leads, designated leads I, II, and III, are *bipolar* leads. This means that they measure the *difference* in electrical potential between two recording sites, as shown in Figure 15.1. Lead I, for example, measures the difference in potential between the right arm and left arm electrodes. However, it provides no information about the actual potential under either electrode. (The actual potential is a more revealing determination than the difference in potential in assessing and localizing abnormal electrical forces.)

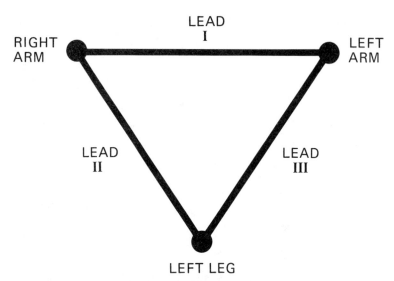

Figure 15.1. Bipolar limb leads.

The development of *unipolar* leads (in the early 1930s) permitted the routine measurement of actual electrical potentials at various electrode sites and, in doing so, expanded the scope and accuracy of electrocardiographic diagnosis in CHD. The concept of unipolar leads is as follows: the heart is considered to lie in the center of an equilateral triangle (Einthoven's triangle) formed by the three limb leads (Figure 15.2). Although the electrical forces generated by the heart differ in direction and magnitude in the three leads, these differences balance each other so that (if added together) their sum at any moment is zero. Thus, if the three limb leads are connected to a neutral electrode (or central terminal, as it is also called) the electrical potential of the neutral electrode will also be zero. Since this electrode has no electrical force at all it can be used as a standard of reference for comparing the *actual* electrical potential at other sites, using an exploring electrode. This arrangement, illustrated in Figure 15.3, in which there is a zero potential electrode at one end and an exploring electrode at the other is described as a unipolar lead.

The exploring electrode is attached to the limbs and to the chest wall to record actual electrical potentials from these particular sites. All of these unipolar leads are identified (prefaced) by the letter V, and are called *V leads*. Unipolar leads recorded from the extremities are of low voltage and therefore are electrically augmented. Hence, unipolar limb leads are called *augmented unipolar* leads and are designated by the symbol aV (a for augmented and V for unipolar). There are three augmented unipolar limb leads: aVR (right arm), aVL (left arm), and aVF (left leg). The six unipolar leads recorded from the chest (precordium) are designated V1 to V6, depending on the particular location of the electrode on the chest wall (Figure 15.4).

To summarize: a 12-lead electrocardiogram consists of 3 bipolar and 9 unipolar leads in the following categories:

Bipolar Leads	Unipolar Extremity Leads	Unipolar Chest Leads
Lead I	Lead aVR	Lead V1
II	aVL	V2
III	aVF	V3
		V4
		V5
		V6

A complete electrocardiogram depicting these 12 leads is shown in Figure 15.5.

DIAGNOSIS OF ACUTE MYOCARDIAL INFARCTION

An acute transmural myocardial infarction consists of three zones: 1) a central zone of necrosis or dead tissue, 2) a zone of injury surrounding the necrotic area and 3) a zone of ischemia peripheral to the zone of injury (Figure 15.6). Although not anatomically discrete entities, each of the three zones is characterized by a different ECG sign, and can be identified accordingly.

Electrocardiographic Signs of Myocardial Necrosis

Myocardial necrosis is reflected by the development of *deep, wide Q waves*. These pathological

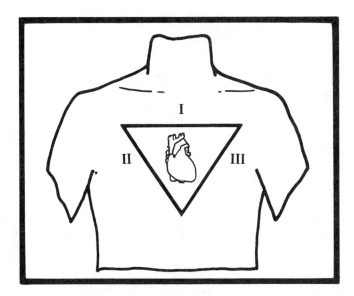

Figure 15.2. Einthoven's triangle formed by leads I, II and III with heart in the center.

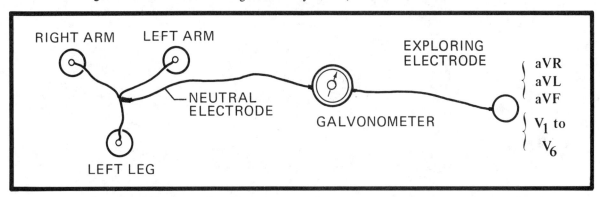

Figure 15.3. Arrangement for a unipolar lead. The exploring electrode is attached to the limbs (lead aVR, aVL and aVF) and to the chest wall (leads V1-V6).

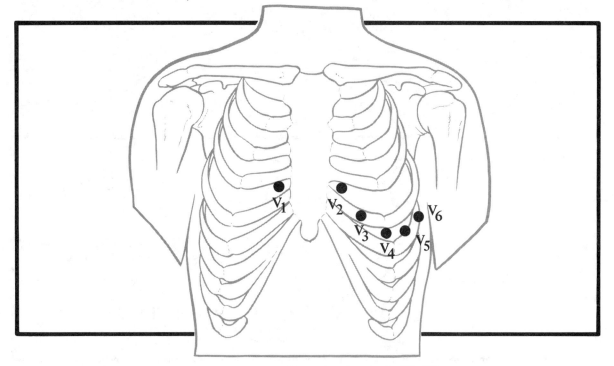

Figure 15.4. Location of unipolar chest leads (V1-V6).

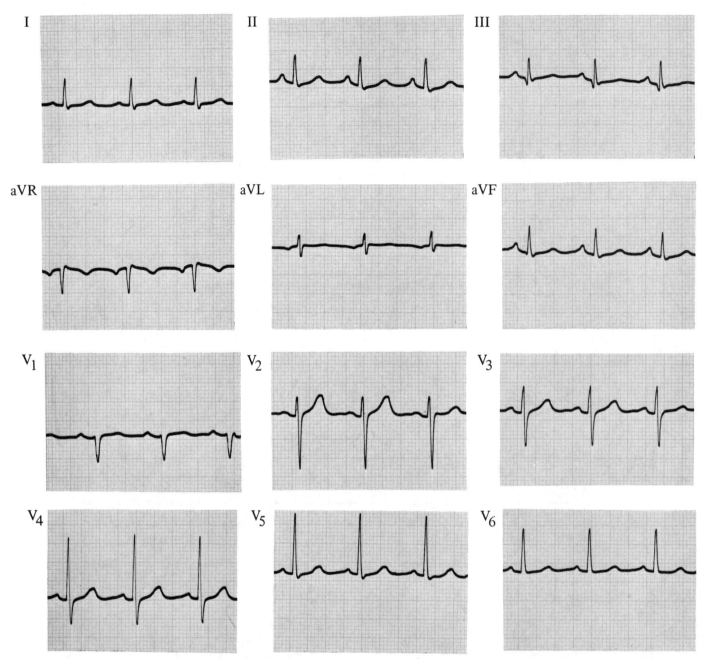

Figure 15.5. A complete (12-lead) electrocardiogram.

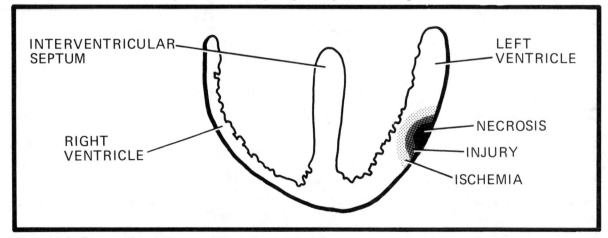

Figure 15.6. Cross-sectioned diagram of heart, showing the three zones (necrosis, injury, and ischemia) of acute myocardial infarction.

waves (which differ from normal, small Q waves) originate as follows: Necrotic tissue is electrically inert and generates no electrical forces. Electrically, the dead area can be considered a hole or a "window" in the myocardial wall. Thus an exploring electrode placed over the zone of dead tissue will in effect look through the hole and record electrical activity (depolarization) of the interventricular septum. The initial electrical forces of the septum (during depolarization) move *away* from the necrotic zone and therefore the electrode records a broad negative deflection, called the Q wave of myocardial infarction (Figure 15.7). Q waves are seen only in those leads that face the infarcted area.* The development of pathological Q waves may occur within an hour or so after an infarction or they may not appear until a few days later (which explains the need for repeated serial ECGs in determining the diagnosis of acute myocardial infarction). In any case, the presence of a deep, broad Q wave is considered the most definite evidence of an acute transmural myocardial infarction.

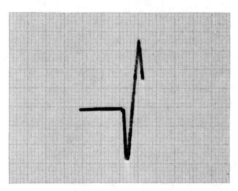

Figure 15.7. Diagram of pathological Q wave of acute myocardial infarction. This wide, deep Q wave differs from small, normal Q waves.

Electrocardiographic Signs of Myocardial Injury

Myocardial injury, often the earliest ECG manifestation of acute myocardial infarction, is reflected by changes in the ST segments. The ST segments may become elevated or depressed, depending on the site of the infarcted area and the lead in which it is recorded. Leads that face the injured area show *elevated* ST segments (Figure 15.8). These elevated ST segments usually develop a convex shape and are

described as coved ST segments (Figure 15.9). In contrast, electrodes that face away from the infarction record depression of the ST segments. The depressed segments (recorded from the opposite side of the injured area) represent a mirror image of the injured region and are categorized as *reciprocal* changes (Figure 15.10). In all, the distinctive ECG manifestation of myocardial injury is elevated, coved ST segments in leads facing the injured area. Reciprocal changes, which are not diagnostic in their own right, may or may not occur.

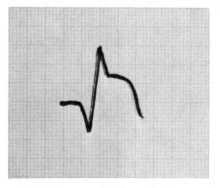

Figure 15.8. Diagram showing ST segment elevation resulting from myocardial injury.

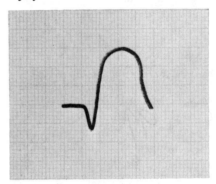

Figure 15.9. Diagram showing elevated ST segment with a coved configuration.

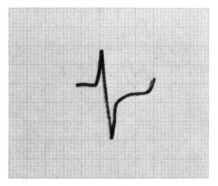

Figure 15.10. Diagram illustrating ST segment *depression* in a lead that faces away from injured area. Depressed ST segments represent a mirror image of the elevated ST segments and are called reciprocal changes.

---

*As explained in Chapter 8, electrical forces moving toward a positive electrode produce an upright deflection while forces moving away from the electrode result in a negative deflection. Since the septal forces move away from the electrode, the deflection is negative (i.e., a Q wave).

Electrocardiographic Signs of Myocardial Ischemia

The third (and least dependable) electrocardiographic indication of acute myocardial infarction is evidence of myocardial ischemia. The classic sign of myocardial ischemia is *inverted and sharply pointed T waves* that are symmetrical in shape, as shown in Figure 15.11. T wave inversion of this type indicates an abnormality in myocardial repolarization. However, a T wave is a nonspecific finding and may result from many causes unrelated to myocardial ischemia.

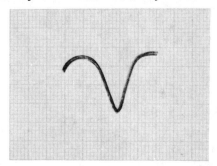

Figure 15.11. Diagram depicting typically inverted T wave of myocardial ischemia. Note that the inverted T wave is sharply pointed and resembles an arrowhead.

The Combined ECG Signs of Acute Myocardial Infarction

With a typical acute transmural myocardial infarction, signs of myocardial necrosis, injury, and ischemia may all be evident in certain leads. In other words, a deep, wide Q wave (myocardial necrosis), an elevated ST segment (myocardial injury) and an inverted, sharply pointed T wave (myocardial ischemia) may be noted on recordings from some leads. This combination of findings represents the classic pattern of acute myocardial infarction (Figure 15.12). It is

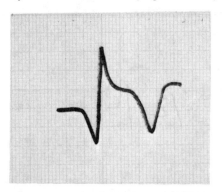

Figure 15.12. The combined ECG pattern of acute myocardial infarction consisting of deep, wide Q waves, elevated ST segments and sharply pointed inverted T waves.

important to recognize that not all of these ECG signs must be present to diagnose actue myocardial infarction. In fact, with small infarctions or transmural infarctions (mentioned later) Q waves or ST changes may never develop and the only ECG evidence of myocardial infarction is nonspecific T wave inversions. In these circumstances, enzyme studies may help confirm the clinical impression of acute infarction.

LOCALIZATION OF MYOCARDIAL INFARCTION

The location of a myocardial infarction influences the clinical course and outcome of the attack. For instance, the death rate is substantially higher among patients with anterior myocardial infarction than with inferior myocardial infarction, since anterior wall damage usually involves a larger muscle mass and therefore leads to pump failure more often. On the other hand, patients with inferior myocardial infarction are more likely to develop AV heart block because this type of infarction frequently involves the AV node itself. Thus it is important to know the site of an infarction when anticipating complications and planning a treatment program. Although the anatomic location of an infarction cannot be determined precisely by electrocardiography, the correlation is close enough so that the ECG can be regarded as a reliable means of localization for clinical purposes.

Myocardial infarction occurs mostly in the anterior and inferior walls of the left ventricle (Figure 15.13). Infarctions involving the posterior left ventricular wall, usually called true posterior infarctions, are rare by comparison and are simply mentioned here. Right

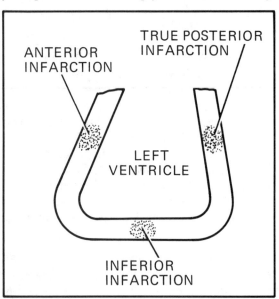

Figure 15.13. Main anatomical sites of acute myocardial infarction.

ventricular infarction, although more common than had been recognized in the past (as noted in Chapter 1), does not produce a typical ECG pattern which localizes the infarction specifically to the right ventricle. Accordingly, the ECG of right ventricular infarction is not considered in this discussion.

Anterior Myocardial Infarction

An anterior infarction is revealed by the presence of a characteristic infarction pattern (Q waves, elevated ST segments and inverted T waves) in the *precordial (V) leads* which face the infarction. Similar changes usually occur in leads aVL and lead I.

It is customary to classify anterior infarctions into three sub-groups, according to the particular ECG findings:

An *extensive anterior infarction* is manifested by an infarction pattern in *all* of the precordial leads, as well as in lead I and aVL (Figure 15.14). An *anteroseptal infarction*, involving the anterior wall at the septal area, is reflected by typical ECG signs in leads I, aVL and V1-V4 (in contrast to V1-V6 with an extensive anterior infarction). A diagram of an acute anteroseptal infarction is shown in Figure 15.15. An *anterolateral infarction* is revealed by an infarction pattern in V4-V6 (the outer precordial leads), and leads I and aVL (Figure 15.16).

Examples of 12-lead ECGs demonstrating acute anterior transmural myocardial infarctions are depicted in Figures 15.17 to 15.20.

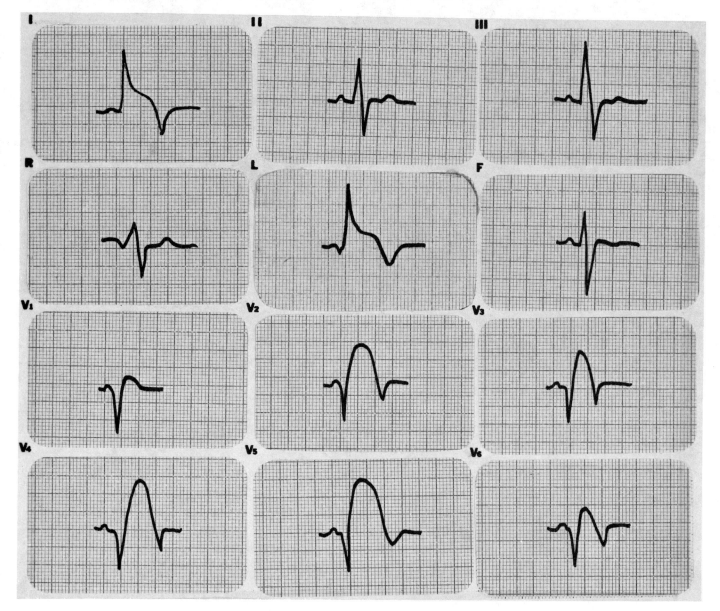

Figure 15.14. *Acute extensive anterior infarction.* Note that the electrocardiogram (diagrammatic) shows a typical infarction pattern in leads I, aVL, and *all* of the precordial leads (V1-V6).

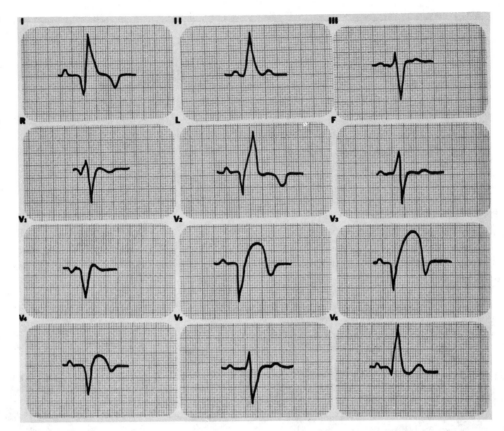

Figure 15.15. *Acute anteroseptal infarction.* The electrocardiographic features of an acute anteroseptal infarction, as shown in this diagram, are found in leads I, aVL, and leads V1 to V4.

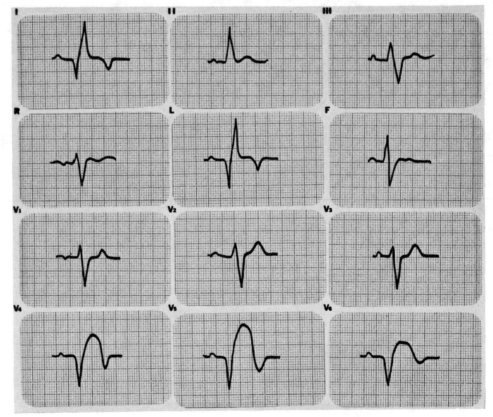

Figure 15.16. *Acute anterolateral infarction.* The electrocardiographic features of an acute anterolateral infarction, as shown in this diagram, are found in leads I, aVL, and V4 to V6.

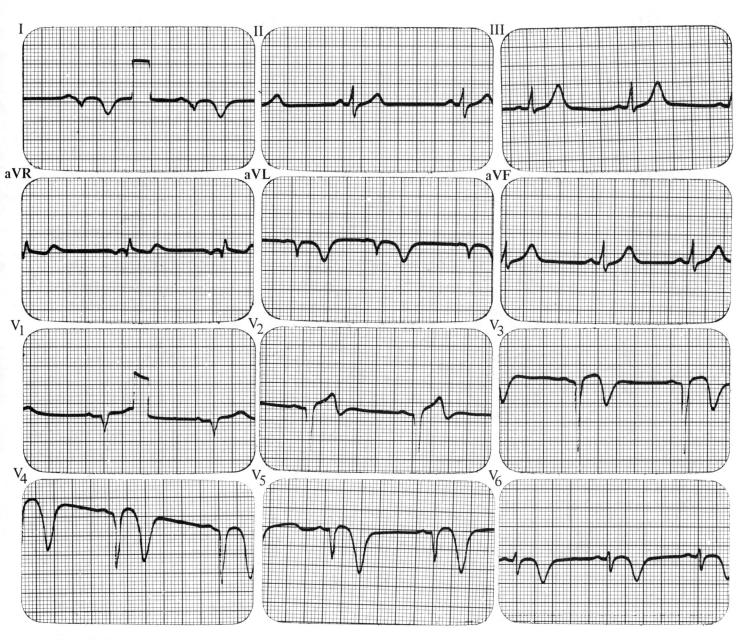

Figure 15.17. *Acute extensive anterior infarction.* Q waves are evident in leads I, aVL and V1-V5. Also, deep, symmetrical T wave inversions are seen in all of the precordial leads (V1-V6), and in leads I and aVL. (The rectangular wave in lead I represents an ECG standardization mark—10 mm in height.)

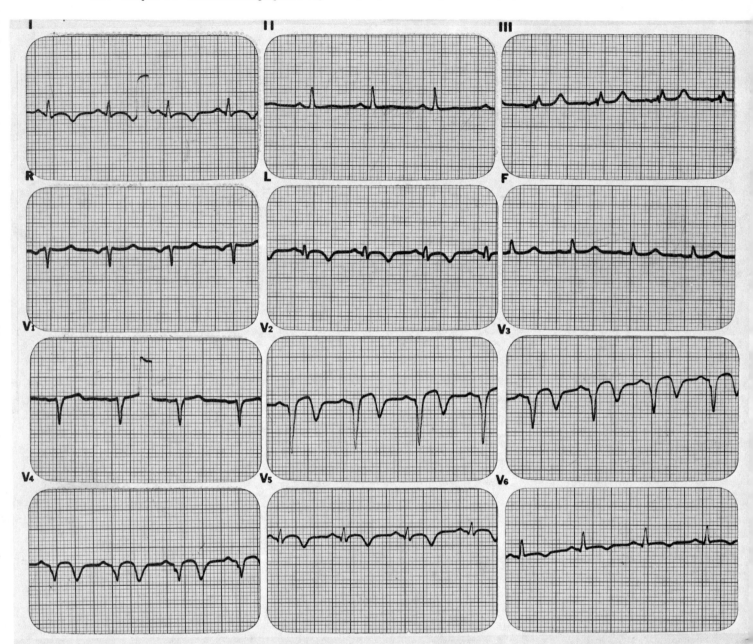

Figure 15.18. *Acute anterior myocardial infarction.* The precordial leads show deep Q waves in leads V1 through V4, and small Q waves in leads I, aVL and V5 and V6. Symmetrical T wave inversion is noted in all the anterior leads—leads I, aVL and V1-V6. These findings indicate extensive anterior wall damage.

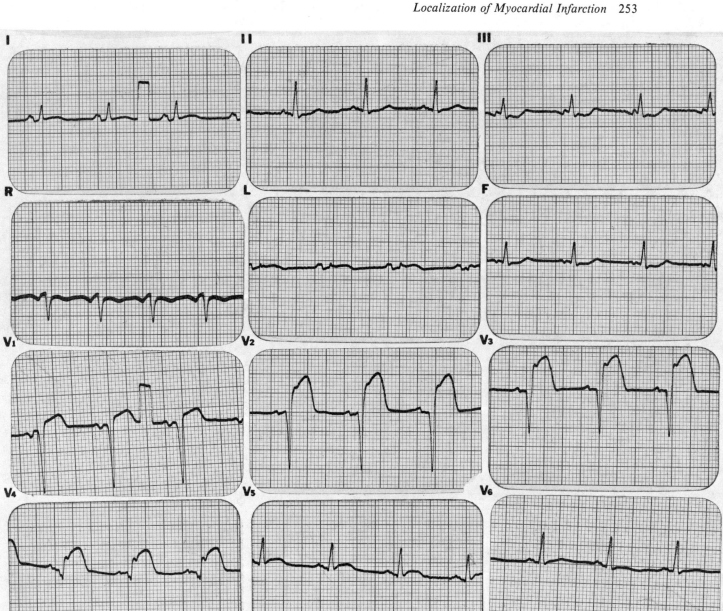

Figure 15.19. *Acute anteroseptal myocardial infarction.* There is marked ST segment elevation in leads V2, V3 and V4, which localizes the infarction to the anteroseptal area. Q waves have already developed in these leads, but T wave inversion has not occurred at this early stage of infarction.

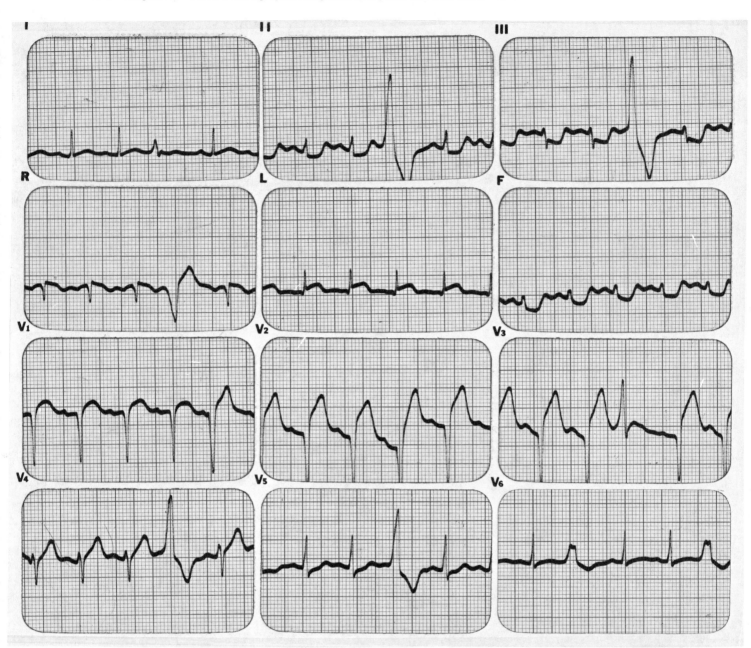

Figure 15.20. *Acute anteroseptal myocardial infarction.* The key findings are ST segment elevations in lead aVL and V1-V3, along with significant Q waves in V1-V3. Note that the ST segments are markedly depressed in leads II, III and aVF, reflecting *reciprocal* changes in these inferior leads. Frequent PVCs are also present.

Inferior Myocardial Infarction

Myocardial infarction involving the inferior wall of the left ventricle is characterized by an infarction pattern—deep Q waves, raised ST segments, and sharply inverted T waves—in *leads II, III and aVF* (Figure 15.21). Unlike anterior infarctions, the precordial leads do not demonstrate an infarction pattern, and are often normal. However, on some occasions in ST segment depression is noted in the precordial leads, reflecting a *reciprocal* change (in which the pre-cordial leads show a mirror image of the ST segment elevation found in leads II, III and aVF). Also, inferior infarctions may be accompanied by infarction of the lateral ventricular wall (an *inferolateral* myocardial infarction). In this circumstance, in addition to signs of an acute inferior infarction the outer precordial leads (V5 and V6) and leads I and aVL may reveal characteristic ST segment and T wave changes. Examples of an acute inferior and an acute inferolateral myocardial infarction are shown in Figures 15.22 and 15.23.

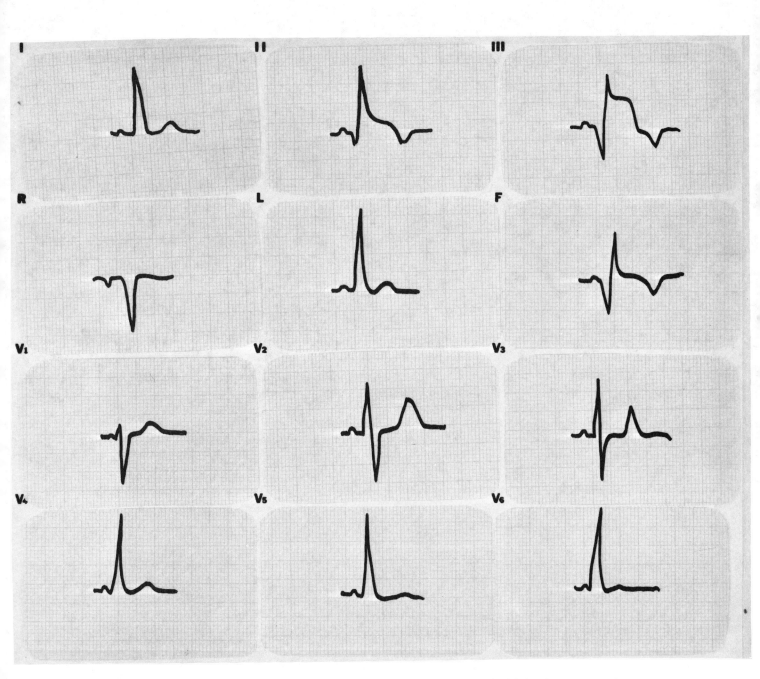

Figure 15.21. *Acute inferior infarction.* In this diagrammatic representation a typical infarction pattern—Q waves, elevated ST segments and inverted T waves—is noted in leads II, III and aVF.

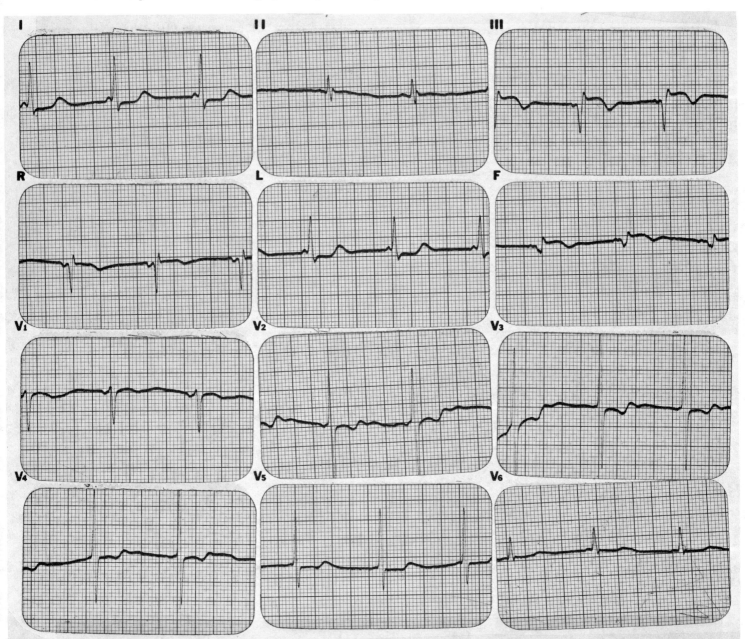

Figure 15.22. *Acute inferior infarction.* Note the typical Q waves and ST segment elevations in leads III and aVF. Reciprocal changes (ST segment depression) are seen in the anterior leads I, aVL.

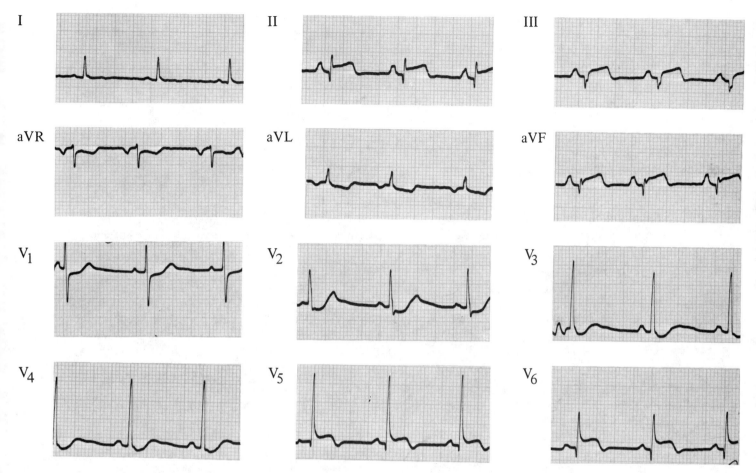

Figure 15.23. *Acute inferolateral myocardial infarction.* A characteristic infarction pattern is evident in the inferior leads (II, III, aVF) as well as in the lateral leads (V5 and V6).

STAGES OF
MYOCARDIAL INFARCTION

Besides identifying and localizing acute myocardial infarction, the ECG also provides valuable information about the stages of healing and the general age of an infarction. Clinically, myocardial infarction can be divided into three sequential phases: acute, recent, and old myocardial infarction. These phases are recognized by the ECG patterns that evolve at different time intervals after an attack.

The ECG pattern reflecting the *acute* stage of myocardial infarction consists of deep Q waves, elevated ST segments and inverted T wages, as described previously. After a few days the raised ST segments begin to return to the baseline and usually become normal within one to four weeks. The inverted T waves often show further deepening for several days, but then gradually resume a normal configuration. When the abnormalities of the ST segments and T waves finally disappear (or at least remain stable) the infarction may be classified as a *recent* myocardial infarction (in contrast to an acute myocardial infarction). Unlike the ST segments and T waves, the Q waves of acute myocardial infarction persist permanently and are the only diagnostic sign of an *old* myocardial infarction. (It is important to realize that small Q waves may be present normally in some leads; they do not indicate the presence of an old myocardial infarction.) Pathological Q waves are wide (more than 0.04 second) and deep (more than 4mm in depth). The ECG patterns of acute, recent, and old myocardial infarctions are shown diagramatically in Figure 15.24. Complete 12-lead ECGs of an old anterior and an old inferior myocardial infarction are presented in Figures 15.25 and 15.26.

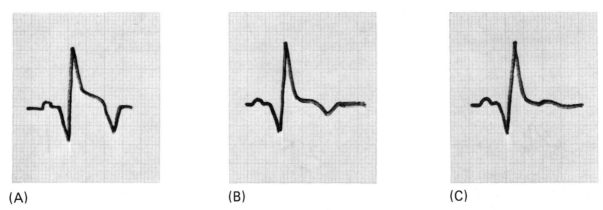

(A)   (B)   (C)

Figure 15.24.   Diagram illustrating ECG patterns of acute (A), recent (B), and old (C) myocardial infarction. Note the difference in the configuration of the ST segment and T wave in an acute infarction compared to an old infarction.

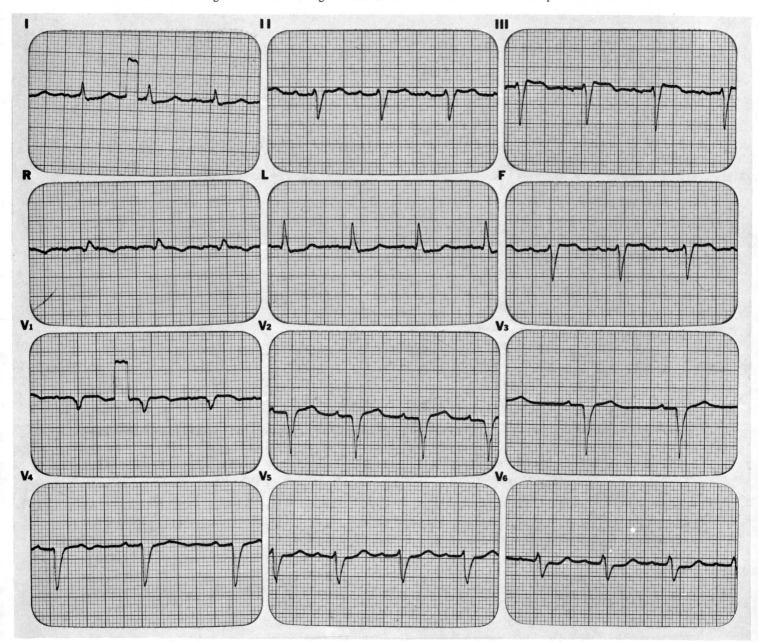

Figure 15.25.   *Old anterior myocardial infarction.* The Q waves in leads V1 through V4, without ST segment or T wave changes, indicate an old infarction.

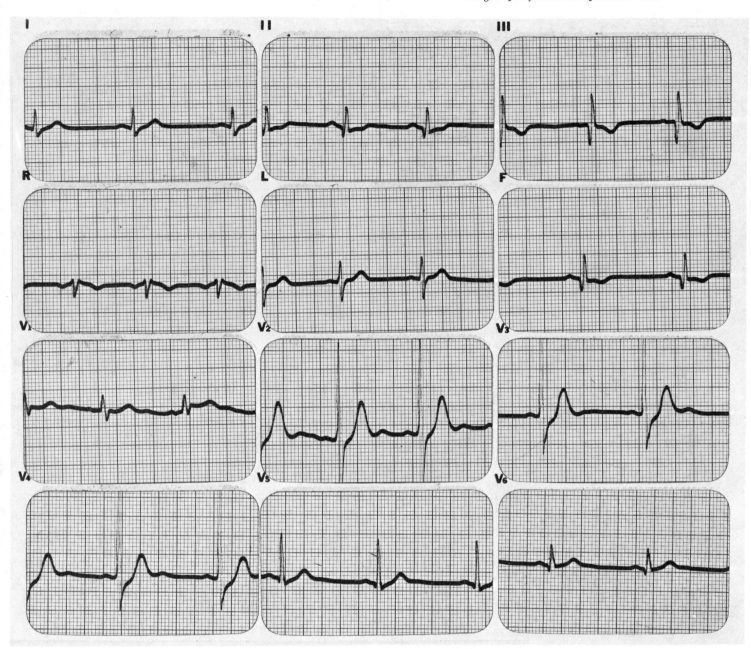

Figure 15.26. *Old inferior myocardial infarction.* The Q waves in leads II, III and aVF reflect a previous infarction of the inferior wall of the myocardium.

NONTRANSMURAL MYOCARDIAL INFARCTION

As noted in Chapter 1, infarctions that do not extend through-and-through the myocardium are called *nontransmural* infarctions. These infarctions are small and are associated with only patchy areas of necrosis. For this reason, nontransmural infarctions do *not* produce pathological Q waves, and the sole ECG evidence of myocardial infarction is elevated ST segments and, especially, symmetrical, deeply inverted T waves. The ST segment changes may be transient so that by the time an ECG is recorded, the only remaining abnormality is T wave inversion. In fact, nontransmural infarctions are sometimes called "T wave infarctions," indicating that the diagnosis rests on the T wave abnormalities alone. Since T waves may invert from dozens of causes other than myocardial ischemia and, as such, are a nonspecific ECG sign, it is essential to correlate this ECG evidence with the patient's history and enzyme studies before concluding that a nontransmural infarction has actually occurred. Acute nontransmural myocardial infarction may be detected electrocardiographically in the anterior and inferior wall of the left ventricle. An anterior nontransmural infarction, like an anterior transmural infarction, produces ST segment and T wave changes in leads I, aVL, and the precordial leads, as shown in Figure 15.27. An inferior nontransmural infarction is determined by leads II, III and aVF (Figure 15.28). Q waves never develop with nontransmural infarction and thus there is no definite way to identify an old nontransmural infarction.

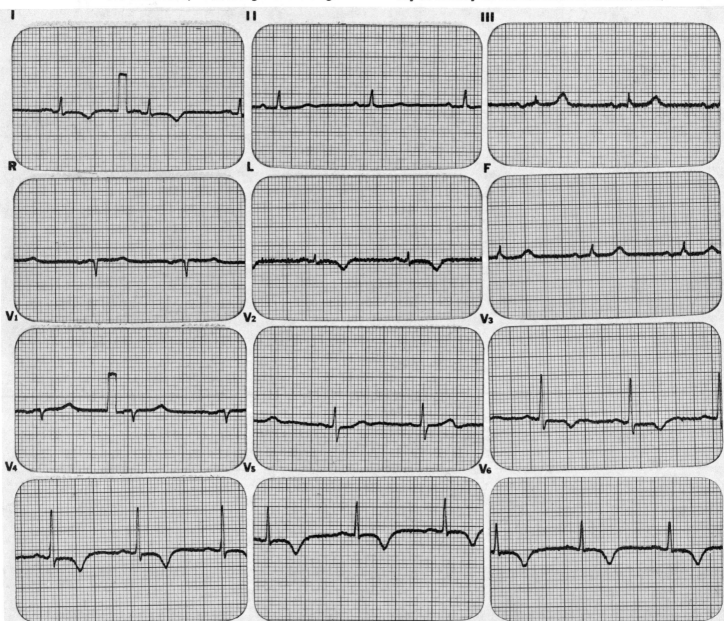

Figure 15.27. *Nontransmural anterior myocardial infarction.* The T waves are sharply inverted in leads I, aVL and V3-V6, but the absence of Q waves indicates that the infarction does not exceed through-and-through the myocardium.

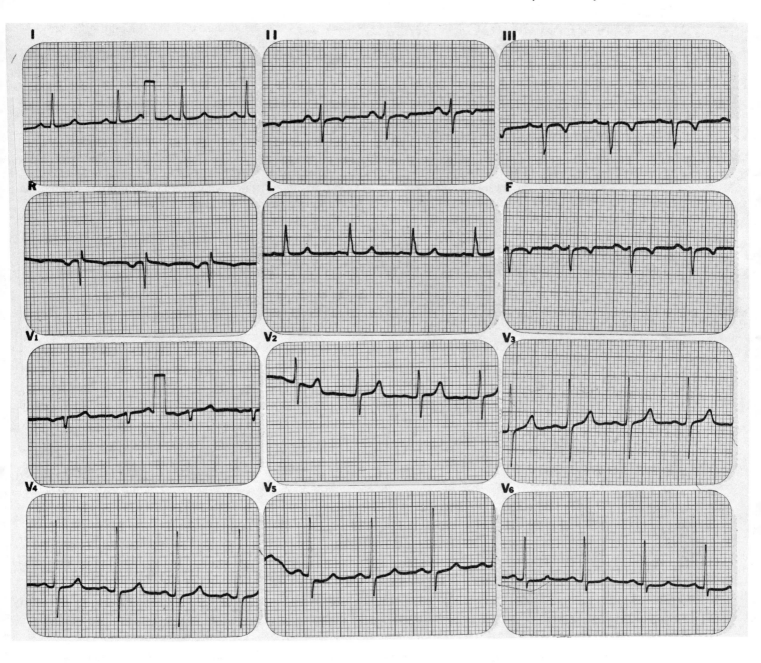

Figure 15.28. *Nontransmural inferior myocardial infarction.* T wave inversion is evident only in the inferior leads (II, III, aVF). Note the absence of Q waves.

TRANSIENT MYOCARDIAL ISCHEMIA (ANGINA PECTORIS)

Aside from its role in the diagnosis of myocardial infarction, electrocardiography is utilized extensively to detect or verify other manifestations of coronary heart disease (CHD), particularly *transient* myocardial ischemia.

Transient myocardial ischemia, the underlying cause of *angina pectoris,* can occur spontaneously or it may be induced by exercise (stress) testing to confirm the diagnosis of CHD. In either case transient myocardial ischemia is identified electrocardiographically by characteristic changes in the ST segments and, to a lesser degree, by changes in the T waves.

The most reliable ECG sign of transient myocardial ischemia is ST segment *depression.* The reason the ST segments show depression (rather than ST elevation, as expected with acute myocardial injury) is that the ischemic area of the myocardium associated with angina pectoris involves the *subendocardial* portion of the ventricles, as depicted in Figure 15.29. Note particularly that the chest electrodes do not face the subendocardium; they face away from this area. As discussed earlier in this chapter, a lead facing an injured area reveals ST segment elevation while a lead facing away from the injury will show depressed (or reciprocal) changes. Since the subendocardial area of ischemia faces away from the chest electrodes, the ST segments are depressed in these leads during an episode of angina pectoris. The depressed ST segments are typically horizontal or downsloping in shape (Figure 15.30), which distinguishes them from nonischemic causes of ST segment depression. An illustration of the ECG changes associated with angina pectoris is shown in Figure 15.31.

In addition to ST segment depression, myocardial ischemia also produces T wave changes. These T wave changes, however, are not as dependable or diagnostically significant as the ST segment changes just described (because many conditions other than myocardial ischemia can cause similar T wave abnormalities). Nevertheless, the development of *inverted* T waves which are sharply pointed and symmetrically shaped are frequently noted during myocardial ischemia (Figure 15.32).

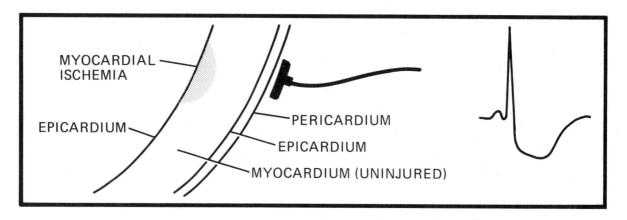

Figure 15.29. Illustration of *subendocardial* location of myocardial ischemia during angina pectoris. Note that the chest electrode faces away from the area of ischemia, causing downward depression of ST segment.

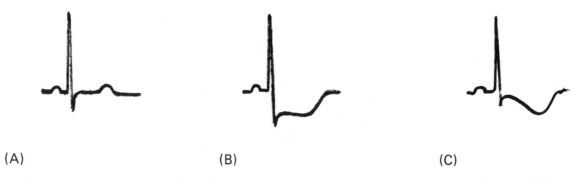

(A)   (B)   (C)

Figure 15.30. Diagrammatic illustrations comparing a) normal ST segment, b) horizontal depression of ST segment and c) downsloping of ST segment. Myocardial ischemia is manifested by either horizontal or downsloping ST segments.

BEFORE ANGINA   DURING ANGINA

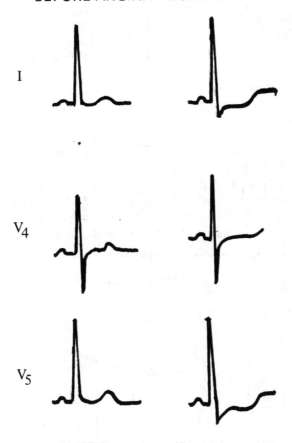

Figure 15.31.   Electrocardiographic changes (diagrammatic) associated with angina pectoris. Note that the ST segments are depressed during an angina episode, particularly in the three leads shown here.

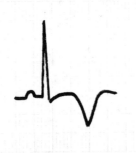

Figure 15.32. T wave changes of myocardial ischemia. Typically, the T waves are sharply pointed with symmetrical limbs.

VARIANT (PRINZMETAL'S) ANGINA

Variant angina pectoris (also called Prinzmetal's angina) is characterized by chest pain occurring at rest rather than with activity. Also unlike typical angina, variant angina is caused by coronary artery spasm, which diminishes blood flow through large- and medium-sized vessels. Because the coronary arteries lie on the epicardial surface of the ventricles, the effect of arterial spasm is to produce *subepicardial* ischemia (in contrast to subendocardial ischemia of typical angina). Subepicardial ischemia is manifested by ST segment *elevation* in the leads facing the injured surface (Figure 15.33). Thus there is a clear distinction electrocardiographically between typical stable angina, reflected by ST segment depression, and variant angina, reflected by ST segment elevation. Moreover, instead of diffuse ST segment depression seen with typical angina, the ECG during arterial spasm shows *localized* ST segment elevation in certain leads (depending on which artery is involved). This ECG pattern of localized ST segment elevation is very similar to the injury pattern of acute transmural myocardial infarction. However, with variant angina the ST segment elevation is only transient, resolving as soon as the arterial spasm abates (Figure 15.34). Indeed, ST segments that do not return to the baseline promptly after the chest pain stops usually indicate acute myocardial infarction.

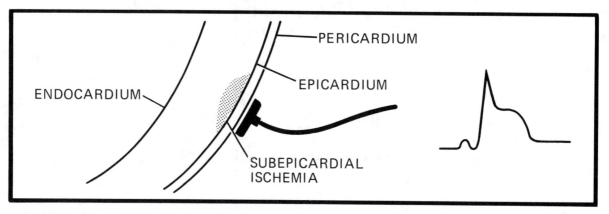

Figure 15.33. Subepicardial ischemia resulting from coronary artery spasm (variant angina). The ST segments are *elevated* in leads that face the injured area.

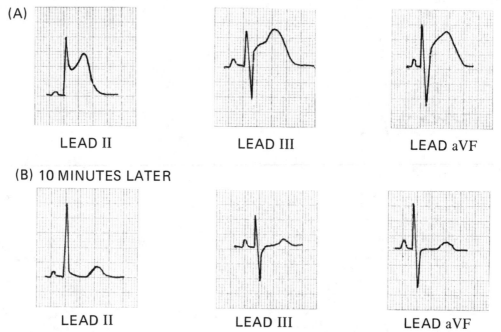

Figure 15.34. A. Transient myocardial ischemia during an episode of *variant angina pectoris*. Note elevated ST segments in leads II, III and aVF, indicating involvement of inferior wall of left ventricle probably from spasm of right coronary artery. B. 10 minutes later, after the pain has ended, the elevated ST segments have returned to the baseline. Coronary artery spasm may occur with normal vessels or in conjunction with coronary obstructive disease.

EXERCISE (STRESS) TESTING

The diagnosis of angina pectoris is usually established on the basis of the patient's history alone. On some occasions, however, the history is not clearcut and certain diagnostic studies must be performed to determine whether the chest pain is due in fact to angina pectoris. The most common test for this purpose is the exercise, or stress, test. The object of the procedure is to increase myocardial oxygen demands by exercising. If coronary flow is inadequate to meet these additional demands, an electrocardiogram recorded during (and immediately after) the exercise period will usually reveal signs of myocardial ischemia, as manifested by ST segment depression.

After the exercise (walking on a treadmill or riding a stationary bicycle) is completed, and oxygen supply and demand are again balanced, the ST segments return to the baseline. A stress test is interpreted primarily on the basis of the behavior of the ST segments during exercise; other criteria are of much less importance. A positive test is defined as horizontal or downsloping ST segment depression of more than 1 mm in depth. A typical example of a positive exercise test is shown in Figure 15.35.

It is important to realize that exercise testing is not an entirely reliable diagnostic method. In some instances, ST segment depression does not occur, despite significant coronary artery narrowing. Equally defeating is that the test sometimes appears positive, even though coronary disease is not present (a false positive result).

(A)

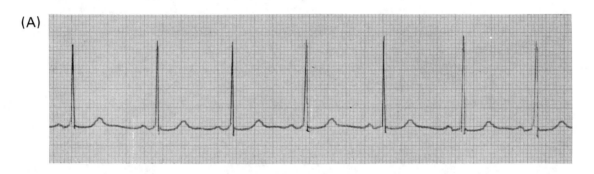

(B)

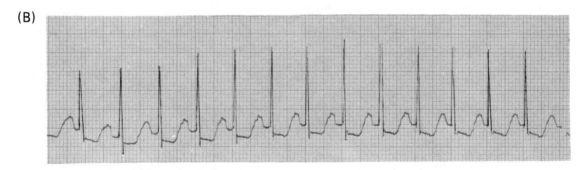

Figure 15.35. *Positive exercise (stress) test.* Strip A, recorded immediately *before* the exercise test was started, shows a heart rate of about 70/minute with normal ST segments. After 3 minutes of exercise (strip B), the heart rate increased to 150/minute. Note the downsloping ST segment depression, 2 mm in depth, that developed at this time, defining the test as positive.

16

Antiarrhythmic Drugs

It is apparent from the foregoing chapters that the successful management of arrhythmias depends not only on the recognition and diagnosis of the particular rhythm or conduction disturbance, but also on the selection and proper use of appropriate antiarrhymic therapy. The object of this chapter is to elucidate the actions and methods of administration of the main drugs used in treating arrhythmias associated with acute myocardial infarction. Before discussing the antiarrhythmic agents individually, it is worthwhile to consider the basic mechanisms by which this group of drugs affects the heart's electrical activity and controls arrhythmias.

MECHANISMS OF ANTIARRHYTHMIC ACTION

Antiarrhythmic drugs act by altering automaticity, excitability, or conductivity of cardiac cells. *Automaticity* refers to the ability of certain cells within the heart to initiate electrical impulses spontaneously. An increase or a decrease in automaticity (spontaneous firing) produces certain types of arrhythmias. For example, increased automaticity of pacemaker cells within the atria, AV junctional tissue, the His-Purkinje network, or the ventricles results in ectopic beats or tachyarrhythmias. In contrast, sinus bradycardia is due to decreased automaticity of the cells comprising the SA node. One of the fundamental actions of antiarrhythmic drugs is to restore normal automaticity. Many agents—including lidocaine, quinidine, procainamide, and beta-blockers—serve to

decrease spontaneous firing (particularly of ectopic rhythms), while other drugs such as atropine and isoproterenol are used to increase automaticity.

Excitability refers to the ability of cardiac cells to respond to stimulation. As noted, there is a critical (threshold) level at which the heart will respond completely or not at all to an electrical stimulus. If this threshold level for stimulation is reduced (because of low potassium levels, for example), the cells become more easily excitable and rapid-rate arrhythmias or repetitive firing may develop. On the other hand, if excitability is decreased (because of inadequate myocardial perfusion), a normal stimulus will not evoke a response (i.e., ventricular depolarization and contraction). The beneficial effects of antiarrhythmic drugs are often related to the control of excitability, either decreasing or increasing the responsiveness of myocardial cells.

Conductivity refers to the velocity at which impulses are transmitted through the specialized fibers of the conduction system. Certain arrhythmias are characterized by slow conduction velocities, and others by accelerated propagation of impulses. Among the antiarrhythmic drugs, atropine and isoproterenol increase the velocity of conduction, while digitalis, quinidine, and procainamide decrease conduction velocity.

CLASSIFICATION OF ANTIARRHYTHMIC DRUGS

Antiarrhythmic drugs exert their effect by altering automaticity, excitability, or conductivity of cardiac cells. Several different types of drugs possess these properties, but antiarrhythmic agents can be categorized broadly into four groups, on the basis of their electrophysiologic effects:

1. Drugs That Act Directly on Cardiac Cells

When a cardiac cell is stimulated by an impulse, the cell membrane immediately responds by allowing sodium ions to enter and potassium ions to leave. This exchange and flow of ions creates an electrical current (depolarization). During repolarization, potassium ions reenter the cell and sodium ions leave. The effect of the movement of ions across the cell membrane on the electrical behavior of the heart has been demonstrated in the animal laboratory by recording the electrical events that occur after stimulation of a single cardiac muscle fiber. The recording (which, in effect, represents an electrocardiogram taken from one cell) is called a *transmembrane action potential.* A typical transmembrane action potential tracing is shown in Figure 16.1.

After the cell membrane is stimulated (Figure 16.1, arrow) there is a sharp upstroke from the resting baseline (called phase 0), which represents depolarization of the cell. Unless the stimulus is strong enough to exceed the threshold level, the cell will not respond. After depolarization, repolarization occurs (phases 1, 2, and 3), and finally the potential return to the

baseline (phase 4). Critical to an understanding of antiarrhythmic drug action is the fact that the cell is insensitive (refractory) to another stimulus and cannot be reexcited until the repolarization curve has descended below the threshold level. In other words, if an impulse arrives at any time during the *effective refractory period,* the myocardium will not respond to the stimulus.

Antiarrhythmic drugs that act *directly* on cardiac cells produce a generalized depression of all cellular electrophysiologic activity. This means that antiarrhythmic agents of this class (of which quinidine is the prototype) reduce automaticity, diminish excitability, and slow conductivity. These effects are accompanied by changes in the transmembrane action potential. Of particular importance in this regard is the ability of these drugs to prolong the effective refractory period. (In principle, any drug that lengthens the effective refractory period should serve to suppress or terminate arrhythmias, since the myocardium cannot respond to stimulation while the refractory period is present.) Antiarrhythmic drugs of the direct-acting type currently available for use in the United States are:

Quinidine
Procainamide (Pronestyl)
Disopyramide phosphate (Norpace)
Lidocaine
Diphenylhydantoin (Dilantin)

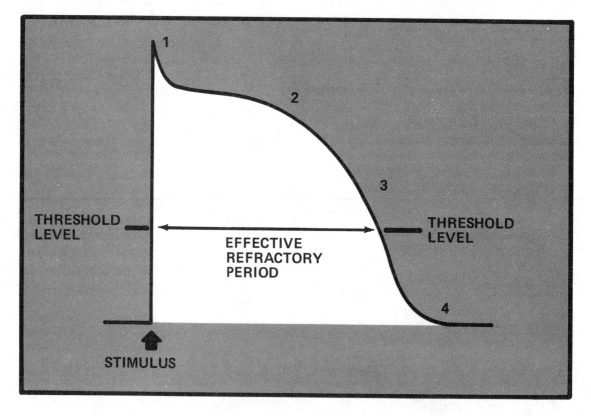

Figure 16.1

2. Drugs That Act Indirectly on Cardiac Cells

Drugs in this category control arrhythmias *indirectly* by either stimulating or blocking the cardiac effects of the autonomic nervous system. As mentioned previously, the sympathetic and parasympathetic nervous systems have antagonistic actions on the heart. Stimulation of sympathetic nerves results in an increase in the rate of impulse formation (heart rate) and an increase in conduction velocity. In addition, sympathetic stimulation causes an increase in the force of contraction of the atria and ventricles (positive inotropic effect). The effects of parasympathetic (vagus) stimulation are just the opposite—the inherent heart rate slows and the speed of conduction decreases. At the same time, the force of atrial contraction is diminished. (Ventricular contraction is not affected directly by parasympathetic stimulation because the ventricles do not contain vagal fibers.)

Drugs used to treat arrhythmias by influencing the autonomic nervous system's control of the heart include:

a. agents that *stimulate* sympathetic nervous system activity, e.g., epinephrine and isoproterenol (Isuprel);
b. agents that *block* sympathetic nervous system activity, e.g., propranolol (Inderal);
c. agents that *block* vagal activity, e.g., atropine.

3. Drugs With a Combined Direct and Indirect Action

A few agents have both direct and indirect actions on cardiac cells; for this reason they are considered as a separate class of antiarrhythmic drugs. At present, however, bretylium tosylate is the only drug in this unique group that is available for clinical use. The net effect of the combined actions of bretylium is an increase in the refractory period, along with a decrease in excitability, which inhibits cardiac cells from discharging spontaneously.

4. Calcium Blocking Agents

Although used primarily to treat angina pectoris by relieving coronary artery spasm, calcium blocking agents also possess impressive antiarrhythmic properties. These drugs act by blocking the entry of calcium through cell membranes, which affects various electrophysiologic mechanisms of the myocardium. The calcium blocking agent that has received the widest clinical application to date as an antiarrhythmic is verapamil (Calan, Isoptin). (Nifedipine and deltiazem, the two other calcium blockers now available, are less effective than verapamil in the treatment of arrhythmias.) The major effect of verapamil is on the AV node, where it slows conduction by increasing the refractory period. This action makes the drug especially useful in controlling (terminating) supraventricular tachycardias and in slowing the ventricular rate during atrial fibrillation.

Newer Antiarrhythmic Agents

Several new antiarrhythmic drugs are currently being studied here and abroad, and will soon be available for regular clinical use. In fact, many of these agents are already used widely in Europe but are still awaiting approval in the United States. Because some of these investigational drugs hold great promise and may replace or alter existing methods of antiarrhythmic therapy in the near future, a brief discussion of the following newer agents is included in this chapter: Amiodarone, Aprinidine, Encainide, Flecainide, Mexilitene, and Tocainide.

ANTIARRHYTHMIC DRUGS

Quinidine

Uses

1. To control or terminate atrial arrhythmias, particularly atrial fibrillation.
2. To suppress ventricular ectopic activity that has not responded to lidocaine or procainamide.
3. To prevent recurrent supraventricular tachycardia (prophylactic treatment).

Action

Quinidine acts directly at the cell membrane level and also inhibits vagal influences on the heart (vagolytic action).

The direct cellular action produces a decrease in spontaneous impulse formation (automaticity), a decrease in excitability (of atrial cells in particular), and a slowing of conduction (especially in the AV node). As with other antiarrhythmic drugs of its class, quinidine prolongs the effective refractory period. However, in achieving these desirable antiarrhythmic effects, quinidine depresses myocardial cells and thereby reduces the strength of myocardial contractility; this results in a reduction in stroke volume and cardiac output.

Because quinidine also has an inhibitory (blocking) effect on vagal impulses to the heart, the drug can cause the heart rate to increase and the conduction time to decrease. This vagolytic action may sometimes counteract the direct cellular effects.

Methods of Administration and Dosage

1. Although quinidine can be administered orally, intramuscularly, or intravenously, the oral route is by far the safest and is the method of choice (except perhaps in rare emergency situations).
2. When quinidine therapy is started, it is advantageous to begin treatment with a loading dose. This usually consists of 300 mg orally every 3 hours for 3 doses.
3. The oral dose thereafter (the maintenance dose) is 200-600 mg every 6 hours; the average dose is 400 mg every 6 hours. The daily dosage should not exceed 1.6 grams unless serum quinidine levels can be measured regularly (to identify toxic levels).
4. The customary prophylactic dose for preventing recurrence of arrhythmias is 200-300 mg every 6 hours.
5. The drug usually acts within 2-4 hours after oral administration, when peak blood level concentrations are reached.
6. Quinidine is available in long-acting form (Quinaglute).

Contraindications

1. Quinidine should *not* be given to patients who have evidence of a ventricular conduction disturbance (manifested by widened QRS complexes), nor should it be administered in the presence of advanced AV heart block.
2. Patients with known sensitivity or adverse reactions to quinidine should *not* be treated with this drug.
3. The drug should be used *cautiously* in patients with elevated BUN levels.

Side Effects

Cardiac Effects

1. Quinidine may cause atrioventricular and intraventricular heart block.
2. It may produce excessive depression of myocardial contractility, predisposing to, or exaggerating, heart failure.
3. In *toxic* doses, quinidine may lead to ventricular tachycardia or ventricular fibrillation (sudden death).

Systemic Effects

1. Gastrointestinal symptoms (nausea, vomiting and, especially, diarrhea) may occur.
2. Visual and auditory symptoms (blurred vision, tinnitus and deafness) may develop, often in conjunction with gastrointestinal symptoms.
3. Allergic reactions (fever, skin rashes, thrombocytopenic purpura and hemolytic anemia) are uncommon responses.

Nursing Implications

1. Careful electrocardiographic monitoring is essential to detect signs of cardiac toxicity. Progressive widening of the QRS complexes, the development of AV heart block, and major increases or decreases in the heart rate are of great significance and should be reported to the physician promptly.
2. Manifestations of systemic reactions always should be considered before the next dose is administered. Diarrhea, nausea, or vomiting is the most frequent side effect.
3. When there is reason to suspect quinidine toxicity, serum quinidine levels should be measured. A serum quinidine level greater than 8 mg/liter is in the toxic range (desired serum level is 5-7 mg/liter).

Procainamide

Uses

1. To suppress or terminate premature ventricular contractions or ventricular tachycardia.
2. To prevent recurrent ventricular arrhythmias.
3. To treat supraventricular tachyarrhythmias not controlled by quinidine (or when quinidine cannot be used because of hypersensitivity or side effects).

Actions

The electrophysiological effects of procainamide are very similar to those of quinidine. The drug (a myocardial depressant) decreases automaticity, excitability, conductivity, and myocardial contractility. In addition, procainamide inhibits vagal activity, but this action is usually not of sufficient magnitude to cause an increase in the heart rate.

Procainamide is now seldom used as a primary drug in the treatment of arrhythmias. It is less effective than lidocaine in terminating ventricular arrhythmias and less effective than quinidine in controlling supraventricular arrhythmias. The drug is employed most often to prevent the recurrence of ventricular arrhythmias.

Methods of Administration and Dosage

1. Procainamide can be given orally, intravenously, or intramuscularly. The parenteral routes are used to terminate or suppress arrhythmias, while oral administration is reserved mostly for prophylactic treatment.
2. When procainamide is used intravenously to terminate ventricular arrhythmias, 2 grams of the drug are diluted in 500 cc 5% dextrose in water and administered by continuous drip at a rate of 100 mg every 5 minutes (25 cc). (In this dilution each milliliter contains 4 mg of procainamide.) The total intravenous dosage should not exceed 1 gram in an hour (250 cc).
3. If the arrhythmia is successfully controlled, maintenance therapy is usually continued intravenously for the first 24 hours. In this circumstance the customary dosage is 2-4 mg of procainamide per minute (or a total of about 1 gram each 6 hours).
4. If for some reason an intravenous line has not been established (for example, while the patient is enroute to the hospital), procainamide may be injected intramuscularly. The usual intramuscular dose is 500 mg.
5. In less urgent situations the drug should be given orally. A loading dose of 1 gram procainamide produces effective blood levels in less than an hour (4-8 mg/liter). Because the action of the drug lasts only 3-4 hours, repeated doses of 500 mg are given every 4 hours. The total oral dosage in 24 hours should not be more than 3 grams.
6. When used for prophylactic purposes, the recommended oral dose is 250-500 mg every 4 hours.
7. Long-acting preparations of procainamide are now available. These sustained release drugs (Pronestyl-SR and Procan-SR) can be administered every 6 hours in doses of 500-1000 mg as maintenance therapy.

Contraindications

1. Procainamide should *not* be administered to patients with advanced atrioventricular heart block or intraventricular conduction defect (unless a demand pacemaker is functioning).
2. The drug is contraindicated in patients with known hypersensitivity to procaine and chemically related drugs.

Side Effects

Cardiac Effects

1. Procainamide may slow conduction velocity and produce atrioventricular or intraventricular heart block. Widening of the QRS complex by more than 50% of the pretreatment width, or the development of a prolonged P-R interval, is reason to discontinue the drug temporarily.
2. The drug may precipitate or potentiate heart failure because of its depressant action on myocardial contractility.
3. Occasionally procainamide may cause an acceleration of the heart rate (as a result of its vagolytic action) and induce ventricular tachyarrhythmias.

Systemic Effects

1. A fall in blood pressure is often observed after parenteral administration of the drug (rarely after oral administration). In most instances the drop in pressure is less than 15 mm Hg. However, in some patients procainamide produces serious hypotension. As a general rule, if the blood pressure falls more than 20 mm Hg, the drug should be discontinued.
2. Gastrointestinal symptoms develop in about 10% of patients. These side effects include anorexia, bitter taste, nausea, vomiting, abdominal pain, and diarrhea.
3. A syndrome resembling lupus erythematosus may develop during the course of prolonged procainamide therapy. This reaction usually consists of chills, fever, skin lesions, joint and muscle discomfort, and pleuritic pain.
4. In patients sensitive to procainamide, allergic reactions manifested by urticaria and chills and fever may be noted.
5. Agranulocytosis, leukopenia, and thrombocytopenia occur rarely after the administration of procainamide.

Nursing Implications

1. The nurse should examine the electrocardiogram (monitor strip) before each dose of procainamide is administered. Of particular importance is the development of intraventricular blocks (widening of the QRS complexes) or signs of atrioventricular block (particularly prolongation of the P-R interval). These findings may represent cardiotoxicity and, if present, should be brought to the attention of the physician. The drug should be withheld if the QRS complex widens more than 50% of its original

duration, or if first- or second-degree AV block is observed. Also of concern is a significant reduction or acceleration of the heart rate. Again, a rate change may reflect a toxic effect.

2. The blood pressure should be carefully recorded before the drug is administered initially, and then checked at regular intervals thereafter. A reduction in blood pressure of more than 15 mm Hg should be reported to the physician.

3. Because of its myocardial depressant action, procainamide may cause or worsen heart failure. Careful assessment of the patient's clinical condition is essential in detecting early signs of this complication.

4. The nurse should be aware of the diverse systemic side effects of procainamide. If there is any suspicion of drug-induced reactions, the physician should be notified before the next dose is given.

Disopyramide (Norpace)

Uses

1. To suppress premature ventricular contractions and ventricular tachycardia.
2. To terminate or prevent supraventricular tachycardias, including atrial tachycardia, atrial flutter, or atrial fibrillation.

Actions

The electrophysiologic effects of disopyramide are similar to quinidine: a decrease in automaticity, slowing of conduction, and prolongation of the effective refractory period. Disopyramide, however, also exerts an atropine-like (vagolytic) effect, which can paradoxically speed conduction through the AV node (thus increasing rather than decreasing the ventricular response to atrial flutter or atrial fibrillation).

Methods of Administration and Dosage

1. Disopyramide is administered orally. The customary dosage schedule is 300 mg initially (loading dose), followed by doses of 150 mg every 6 hours.
2. In patients with decreased renal function or signs of left ventricular failure, the loading dose is often omitted and the maintenance dose is usually reduced to 100 mg every 6 hours.
3. Effective blood levels following oral administration of the drug are seen within 2 hours, and persist (on an average) for about 6 hours.

Contraindications

1. The drug must be used cautiously in patients with clinical evidence of even mild heart failure because disopyramide reduces myocardial contractility significantly and, therefore, can worsen heart failure (as mentioned below).
2. Patients with renal or hepatic insufficiency are not good candidates for disopyramide therapy because the effects of the drug are not predictable.
3. Disopyramide should *not* be used in patients with previous symptoms of urinary retention or glaucoma; the drug, as the result of its atropine-like properties, can precipitate frank attacks on both of these conditions.

Side Effects

Cardiac Effects

1. The most serious cardiovascular side effect of disopyramide is its tendency to reduce myocardial contractility (negative inotropic effect) and, in turn, to produce congestive heart failure. Although other direct-acting drugs possess this hemodynamic property, none affects myocardial function to the marked degree of disopyramide.
2. Disopyramide is capable of *inducing* ventricular tachycardia in the presence of high drug blood levels.

Systemic Effects

1. Signs or symptoms of the drug's atropine (anticholinergic effect occur in at least one-third of all patients taking the drug. These reactions include dryness of the mouth, blurry vision, urinary hesitancy, and constipation.
2. More serious is the risk of precipitation of urinary retention or closed angle glaucoma.

Nursing Implications

1. Repeated evaluation of the patient is necessary to detect any signs of congestive heart failure developing as the result of the drug's powerful negative inotropic effect.
2. The possibility of drug-induced ventricular arrhythmias, including ventricular tachycardia, must always be considered. The drug should be discontinued immediately if this possibility exists.
3. Anticholinergic effects are to be anticipated in a high percentage of patients receiving disopyramide. These symptoms are sufficiently disabling in 10-15% of patients to require discontinuance of the drug.

4. Urinary retention, particularly in elderly men with prostatic disease and attacks of glaucoma (both caused by drug therapy) must be recognized and treated promptly.

Lidocaine

Uses

1. To terminate premature ventricular contractions and ventricular tachycardia.
2. To suppress ventricular ectopic activity prophylactically and to prevent recurrent ventricular arrhythmias.

Actions

Lidocaine controls ventricular arrhythmias by depressing automaticity in the His-Purkinje network and by raising the excitability threshold of the ventricles. (The drug has little or no effect on the atria and therefore is not particularly useful in treating atrial tachyarrhythmia.)

Unlike quinidine and procainamide, lidocaine in customary doses does not affect conduction velocity; consequently, it does not produce atrioventricular or intraventricular conduction disturbances. (In higher dosages conduction may be depressed.)

In usual doses lidocaine has only a minimal effect on myocardial contractility and peripheral vascular resistance. Therefore, cardiac output and systemic blood pressure are not ordinarily decreased during drug administration.

The drug penetrates cardiac tissues very rapidly, and its onset of action occurs within 60 seconds following an intravenous bolus dose. Lidocaine is successful in abolishing ventricular arrhythmias in more than 75% of cases.

Methods of Administration and Dosage

1. Lidocaine is administered intravenously, except in rare circumstances when an intramuscular route must be used.
2. For the initial treatment of ventricular arrhythmias, an intravenous bolus injection of lidocaine is given. The dosage is 50-100 mg (or 1 mg/kg of the patient's body weight). Effective blood levels are achieved at once. If the ventricular arrhythmia is not controlled with this injection, the same dose may be repeated every 5 minutes until the arrhythmia is terminated, or until a total dosage of 300 mg has been administered during a 1 hour period.
3. Because the effect of the bolus dose lasts no more than 15 minutes, it is necessary to start a continuous infusion of lidocaine to maintain effective blood levels and prevent the recurrence of ventricular ectopic activity. This infusion is prepared by diluting 3000 mg 2% lidocaine in 500 cc 5% dextrose solution. This dilution provides a solution containing 6 mg lidocaine per milliliter. The infusion is administered at a rate of 1-4 mg/minute (10-40 microdrops/minute), depending on the clinical response. Although maintenance doses of lidocaine can be continued for several days, if necessary, it is desirable to discontinue therapy as soon as the cardiac rhythm appears to be stable in order to maintain toxic effects.
4. When an intravenous route is not immediately feasible, lidocaine may be administered intramuscularly. The intramuscular dose is 200 mg and may be repeated every 5-10 minutes. However, intravenous administration is always preferable.

Contraindications

1. Lidocaine should *not* be used in the presence of complete heart block since the drug may suppress or abolish the ventricular focus that is maintaining the heartbeat. The same principle applies wherever sinus node activity is depressed (e.g., sinoatrial block or marked sinus bradycardia), or when there is evidence of advanced atrioventricular or intraventricular block.
2. Because lidocaine is metabolized primarily in the liver, the drug must be administered with great caution, if at all, in patients with severe liver disease or congestive failure. In these conditions lidocaine may accumulate in the blood and produce toxic levels.
3. Although lidocaine does not depress myocardial function in usual doses, large doses may reduce myocardial contractility, especially when the heart is severely damaged. For this reason the drug may be hazardous in patients with cardiogenic shock or pulmonary edema.
4. Patients with known hypersensitivity to local anesthetics should *not* receive the drug.

Side Effects

Cardiac Effects

The toxic effects of lidocaine on the heart have been described previously.

Systemic Effects

1. The most serious side effects of lidocaine involve the central nervous system. Of particular importance is the occurrence of convulsions (grand mal seizures), which result most often when large doses of the drug are administered for prolonged periods.
2. Other common central nervous system manifestations of lidocaine toxicity are drowsiness, paresthesias, difficulty in hearing, and muscle twitching. Patients also may become acutely disturbed, agitated, or disoriented when lidocaine is administered on a continuous basis.
3. Nausea and vomiting are less common side effects than those involving the central nervous system, but are by no means rare.

Nursing Implications

1. The maintenance dosage of lidocaine must be adjusted according to the clinical response. A microdrip technique should be used for accurate titration. As a general rule the rate of infusion should not exceed 4 mg lidocaine per minute.
2. The nurse should be aware of the total dosage of lidocaine that has been administered in a given period (e.g., total mg in 8 hours).
3. Because of the high incidence of side effects involving the central nervous system, the nurse must seek manifestations of such reactions at frequent intervals. In the event of seizures, the drug should be discontinued. If the convulsions persist, the physician may choose to administer a short-acting barbiturate. Less obvious central nervous system reactions (especially drowsiness or behavioral changes) can be recognized only by thoughtful repeated assessment of the patient's clinical state. The latter effects often can be controlled by reducing the rate of infusion.
4. Although lidocaine is a relatively safe drug and does not usually cause heart block or depression of myocardial function, the possibility of these cardiac side effects must be kept in mind. Widening of the QRS complexes, prolongation of the P-R interval, a change in rate or rhythm, the development of hypotension, or left ventricular failure should be brought to the physician's attention at once.

Diphenylhydantoin (Dilantin)

Uses

1. To terminate digitalis-induced tachyarrhythmias.
2. To control ventricular ectopic beats when lidocaine and procainamide have been ineffective.
3. To prevent or treat supraventricular tachyarrhythmias, but only as a secondary choice to quinidine or other agents.

Actions

Dilantin, well known for its antiepileptic action, also has antiarrhythmic properties. These electrophysiologic actions are unlike those of other antiarrhythmic agents, and the drug is unique in this sense. The main effect of Dilantin is to accelerate conduction velocity through the atria (by increasing the rate of depolarization). As a result, the greatest use of the drug is in combating depressed AV conduction resulting from digitalis or other drug toxicity. In effect, diphenylhydantoin (DPH) reduces automaticity without decreasing conduction through the heart.

Clinically, Dilantin does not affect the QRS complex, but may shorten the P-R interval.

Methods of Administration and Dosage

1. When used in emergency situations, Dilantin is administered intravenously. In less critical circumstances or when used as maintenance therapy, oral dosages are employed.
2. The initial intravenous dose is 125-250 mg; this amount is injected *slowly* over a period of 3-5 minutes (about 50 mg/minute). The drug usually acts within 15 seconds, and its maximal effect is evident at 5 minutes. If not successful in controlling the arrhythmia, the same dose may be repeated every 15 minutes, if necessary; however, the total dosage should not exceed 750 mg in 1 hour.
3. The drug should *not* be given by continuous intravenous infusion because a precipitate forms within most intravenous solutions.
4. Oral administration consists initially of 200 mg, followed by 100 mg every 6 hours.
5. Following termination of the arrhythmia, Dilantin may be continued for maintenance purposes in dosages of 100 mg 3 times a day.

Contraindications

1. Because Dilantin decreases automatic firing of the SA node and ectopic pacemakers, the drug probably should *not* be used in patients with marked sinus bradycardia or sinus arrest. Similarly, the drug should be avoided in patients with complete heart block, in whom depression of the ventricular focus may lead to ventricular standstill.

2. Hypersensitivity to diphenylhydantoin, although rare, is a specific contraindication to the use of the drug in treating arrhythmias.

Side Effects

Cardiac Effects

1. Depression of automaticity may lead to excessive slow heart rates.
2. Atrioventricular heart block may develop during the course of Dilantin therapy; however, AV conduction is only rarely affected.

Systemic Effects

1. When administered intravenously, Dilantin may cause hypotension, particularly if the rate of injection is too rapid.
2. Drowsiness, ataxia, dizziness, incoordination, and nystagmus are central nervous system side effects. (It is believed that, if these findings are allowed to persist, they may become permanent.)
3. Nausea, vomiting, pruritus, urticaria, and skin rashes may occur; these effects are probably allergic manifestations of the drug.
4. Gingival hypertrophy is commonly observed in patients on long-term treatment with Dilantin. This effect, however, is seldom observed during acute therapy for arrhythmias.

Nursing Implications

1. Dilantin should *not* be given as a bolus injection intravenously. Rather, the drug should be injected slowly, at a rate of 50 mg/minute.
2. Continuous observation of the monitor is essential during intravenous administration, particularly since the drug may begin to act within seconds. Blood pressure monitoring during the postinjection period also is available.
3. Complaints of drowsiness, nervousness, and depression should alert the nurse to the possibility that these behavioral changes are toxic manifestations of the drug.
4. When the drug is given orally, it is good practice to have the patient drink at least a half glass of water to minimize gastric upset.

Epinephrine

Uses

1. To restore the cardiac rhythm after cardiac arrest (especially ventricular asystole).

2. To increase conduction and lessen the degree of heart block. (Isoproterenol, discussed next, is a more effective drug for this purpose.)

Actions

Epinephrine acts by stimulating sympathetic nervous system receptors in the heart. The drug causes an increase in heart rate and in the strength of myocardial contraction. It also stimulates pacemaker cells, which explains its use after cardiac arrest. In addition, when used in large doses, epinephrine elevates the blood pressure and peripheral resistance.

Methods of Administration and Dosage

1. The drug may be given subcutaneously, intravenously, or as an intracardiac injection. The customary subcutaneous dose is 0.1 to 0.5 mg.
2. A direct intravenous dose is usually 0.25 to 0.5 mg. When administered as an intravenous infusion, the flow rate generally is 2-8 μg per minute, adjusted according to the response.
3. In resuscitation attempts after cardiac arrest, epinephrine may be injected directly into the heart by way of a long needle inserted through the rib cage (intracardiac injection). In this circumstance, 5 or 10 cc of a 1:10,000 epinephrine solution is used.

Contraindications

1. Special caution must be exercised when epinephrine is given to patients with angina or myocardial infarction because the drug augments myocardial ischemia.
2. In general, the drug should be reserved for emergency situations such as the treatment of ventricular asystole. Cerebrovascular accidents have occurred after intravenous use of epinephrine.
3. Although epinephrine can be used to treat advanced heart block, it is a far more dangerous drug than isoproterenol for this purpose.

Side Effects

Cardiac Effects

1. Ventricular arrhythmias, including ventricular tachycardia and ventricular fibrillation, may develop during the administration of epinephrine.

2. Epinephrine may precipitate angina and intensify myocardial ischemia, as the result of the increased myocardial oxygen demands it creates.
3. A substantial rise in blood pressure and a marked increase in the heart rate occur with large doses of epinephrine.

Systemic Effects

1. Throbbing headaches and tremors are common systemic side effects.
2. Anxiety, sweating, and a sensation of warmth often occur after the administration of epinephrine.

Nursing Implications

1. Ventricular ectopic beats can be expected to develop in most patients treated with epinephrine. Continuous surveillance of the electrocardiogram during (and after) drug administration is therefore important, particularly because of the risk of precipitating ventricular tachycardia or ventricular fibrillation during this period.
2. Epinephrine increases the heart rate, blood pressure, and the oxygen demands of the myocardium. Therefore, the possibilities of drug-induced angina or symptoms of additional myocardial ischemia must be considered.
3. Systemic side effects (especially headaches, anxiety, and sweating) develop in a high percentage of patients receiving epinephrine. The nurse should explain to the patient that these side effects are related to treatment, and are only temporary in nature.
4. Repeated measurements of the blood pressure and heart rate are essential to monitor the effects of increased sympathetic nervous system stimulation.

Isoproterenol (Isuprel)

Uses

1. To accelerate the heart rate in advanced heart block (especially complete heart block) until a temporary pacemaker can be inserted.
2. To control Stokes-Adams attacks due to marked bradycardia.
3. To treat symptomatic bradyarrhythmias that do not respond to atropine (or when atropine cannot be used).

Actions

The effect of isoproterenol is very similar to that of epinephrine. The drug is a sympathetic nervous system stimulant.

Isoproterenol increases automatic firing of both supraventricular and ventricular pacemakers, and produces an increase in the heart rate. In addition, the drug improves AV conduction. (Other than these antiarrhythmic properties, isoproterenol causes a marked increase in the force of myocardial contractility.)

Methods of Administration and Dosage

1. Isoproterenol can be given in any of the following ways: subcutaneously, intramuscularly, intravenously (directly or by continuous infusion), or sublingually. In addition, an intracardiac injection may be used in the emergency treatment of ventricular standstill. The route of administration depends on the arrhythmia being treated and urgency of the clinical situation, but the most common method of administration is by continuous intravenous infusion.
2. An intravenous infusion of isoproterenol is prepared by diluting 1 mg isoproterenol in 250 ml 5% dextrose in water (in this dilution, each milliliter contains 4 μg). Microdrip administration and the use of "piggyback" technique are essential. The infusion rate initially is 2-4 μg per minute. If this dosage is ineffective in maintaining the heart rate at 60/minute or more, the infusion rate may be increased to 6-10 μg/minute.
3. When used to treat ventricular standstill or severe Stokes-Adams attacks, the customary intracardiac or direct intravenous dosage is 0.02 or 0.04 mg; however, 0.1 mg may sometimes be necessary.
4. The customary subcutaneous or intramucular dosage is 0.1-0.4 mg isoproterenol every 2-4 hours as required.
5. Sublingual administration (the least common method of administration in a CCU) consists of 10-20 mg every 3 hours. The action begins within 15-30 minutes.

Contraindications

Isoproterenol increases the heart's oxygen consumption and therefore must be used cautiously in patients with signs of coronary ischemia. For this reason, the drug is reserved for *emergency* use until a temporary pacemaker can be inserted.

Side Effects

Cardiac Effects

1. The most serious effect of isoproterenol is that it may provoke ventricular tachycardia or ventri-

cular fibrillation! This complication stems from the drug's ability to increase automatic firing of ectopic ventricular foci.

2. Angina may develop during isoproterenol therapy, reflecting the increased oxygen demand created by the drug.

Systemic Effects

1. Sweating, flushing of the skin, and a feeling of weakness are perhaps the most common side effects.
2. Nervousness, excitement, tremors, headaches, and dizziness also occur frequently.
3. Hypotension may develop because of the vasodilating effect of the drug on skeletal and mesenteric vessels.

Nursing Implications

1. During the course of continuous intravenous administration of isoproterenol, the nurse should remain near the patient at all times. The threat of ventricular tachycardia or ventricular fibrillation is ever present, even when small doses are used.
2. In the event premature ventricular contractions develop with increasing frequency, the rate of infusion should be reduced. A syringe filled with lidocaine should be available at the bedside.
3. Monitoring blood pressure and vital signs is essential.
4. Since most patients treated with isoproterenol are likely candidates for temporary pacemaker insertion, preparations should be made for this procedure.

Propranolol (Inderal)*

Uses

1. To control supraventricular tachyarrhythmias associated with rapid ventricular rates.
2. To terminate tachyarrhythmias due to digitalis toxicity.
3. To suppress ventricular ectopic beats not controlled by other antiarrhythmic drugs.

---

*Propranolol is just one of several beta-blocking agents now in use. However, it was the first drug of this class available and served as a prototype for the newer agents. Because clinical experience with propranolol (for antiarrhythmic purposes) is far more extensive than with the other drugs, and because it would be impractical to discuss each of the other beta-blockers separately, the following discussion is limited to propranolol, a typical beta-blocking agent.

Actions

The primary effect of propranolol is to reduce sympathetic stimulation of the heart. This is accomplished by blocking beta receptor cells in the heart, thus inhibiting the secretion of catecholamines (norepinephrine) at the receptor sites.

Propranolol also has a direct action on the electrophysiological properties of cardiac tissue. Specifically, the drug decreases automatically in the SA node, atria, the AV junctional, and the His-Purkinje system. Furthermore, propranolol slows electrical conduction through the atria and bundle of His.

At the same time, propranolol seriously decreases the strength of ventricular contraction and in turn reduces cardiac output.

Methods of Administration and Dosage

1. When used in the emergency treatment of arrhythmias, propranolol is given intravenously. The drug is injected slowly at a rate of 1-2 mg/minute. If necessary, the same dose may be repeated after 5 minutes. Further intravenous doses are not advisable for at least 4 hours. Following intravenous administration, the drug acts within minutes, and the effect persists for at least 3 hours.
2. In noncritical situations (e.g., to suppress premature ventricular contractions), propranolol is administered orally in doses of 10-30 mg every 4-6 hours.

Contraindications

1. Because propranolol decreases the heart rate and prolongs AV conduction time, it should *not* be used in patients with marked sinus bradycardia, sinus arrest (or block), or second- or third-degree heart block.
2. As the result of its adverse effect on myocardial contractility, propranolol is extremely dangerous in the presence of heart failure or cardiogenic shock. The reduction in cardiac output induced by the drug can only exaggerate or intensify the pumping failure of the heart.
3. Propranolol should *not* be given to patients with a known history of bronchial asthma or bronchospasm because the blocking of beta receptors in the lung may produce severe airway resistance.

Side Effects

Cardiac Effects

1. Excessive slowing of the heart rate may develop, even after small doses of propranolol. This

bradycardia may be accompanied by syncope, hypotension, and angina pectoris.
2. In patients with acute myocardial infarction, propranolol may precipitate heart failure or cardiogenic shock.
3. The drug may decrease atrioventricular conduction sufficiently to cause complete heart block, particularly in patients with pre-existing conduction disorders.

Systemic Effects

1. Gastrointestinal symptoms (including nausea, vomiting or constipation) may occur.
2. Weakness, fatigue, and lassitude are common side effects.
3. Confusion, insomnia, hallucinations, and mental depression are sometimes observed.
4. Allergic reactions including skin rashes, fever, and paresthesias of the hands are rare toxic manifestations.

Nursing Implications

1. Intravenous propranolol should be injected slowly (1 mg/minute) and not as a bolus.
2. Continuous observation of the monitor is essential during and following intravenous administration of the drug. Particular attention must be given to the heart rate. If severe bradycardia (a rate less than 50/minute) develops, the physician may order 1 mg atropine intravenously to combat this complication.
3. The possibility of second- and third-degree AV block developing in patients receiving propranolol should be considered.
4. The nurse should examine the patient at regular intervals for signs or symptoms of heart failure or hypotension. Any evidence of this untoward effect should be reported promptly to the physician.
5. If patients develop wheezing or other signs of bronchospasm, discontinue the drug and notify the physician.
6. Behavioral changes, particularly lassitude and depression, resulting from propranolol treatment should be considered in the nursing assessment of the patient.

Atropine

Uses

1. To accelerate the heart rate in sinus bradycardia, sinoatrial arrest, and slow junctional rhythms caused by parasympathetic (vagal) overactivity.
2. To increase the rate of conduction through the AV node in first- and second-degree AV block.

Actions

1. Atropine inhibits parasympathetic (vagal) activity on the SA node (and AV junctional area) and permits the sympathetic nervous system to gain control of the heart rate.
2. The increase in conduction velocity occurring after the administration of atropine is also related to vagal blockade. (Conduction disturbances due to organic damage to the SA or AV nodes are not benefited by atropine.)
3. Atropine may produce an increase in blood pressure and cardiac output. This effect is particularly apparent in patients with bradycardia and hypotension.

Methods of Administration and Dosage

1. Although atropine can be given subcutaneously and intramuscularly, intravenous administration is preferable in the treatment of arrhythmias. The initial intravenous dose may range from 0.3 to 1 mg; the average dose is 0.5 mg. The drug is injected as a bolus. The onset of action is rapid, usually within 1-3 minutes.
2. If the heart rate does not increase to a satisfactory level with this initial dose, a similar dosage may be given in 5 minutes.
3. The drug is usually active for 4 hours, at which time an additional dose may be required. The cumulative dosage, however, should not exceed 4 mg.
4. When used intramuscularly, a 2 mg dose of atropine is generally used.

Contraindications

1. Patients with known glaucoma should *not* receive atropine because of the risk of increasing intraocular pressure to dangerous levels.
2. Because atropine has an antispasmodic effect and decreases urinary bladder tone, caution must be exercised in using the drug in patients with symptoms of urinary obstruction. The danger of causing urinary retention is particularly high in men with prostatic hypertrophy.

Side Effects

Cardiac Effects

1. The heart rate response to atropine is not wholly predictable, and certain patients may develop

excessively rapid heart rates after receiving only small amounts of atropine.

2. The drug can produce atrioventricular dissociation because the atrial rate may be accelerated more than the ventricular rate.
3. Ventricular tachycardia and ventricular fibrillation have been reported following the administration of atropine; however, this arrhythmic complication is rare.
4. A *decrease* in the heart rate may occasionally develop before the rate increases. This paradoxical effect usually develops if atropine is injected too slowly or if the dosage is too small (less than 0.3 mg).

Systemic Effects

1. Atropine inhibits glandular secretions and, therefore, produces dryness of the mouth and diminished sweating.
2. Dilation of the pupils and blurred vision are common side effects. As noted, atropine may cause an exacerbation of glaucoma.
3. Atropine sometimes has a stimulating effect on the central nervous system and causes euphoria, excitability, and mental confusion.

Nursing Implications

1. For a period of at least 5 minutes after atropine is administered intravenously, the monitor should be observed continuously to determine the effect of the drug on the heart rate. The possibility of inducing an overly rapid rate must be considered. Also, paradoxical rate slowing may be noted immediately after the injection.

2. The duration of action, as manifested by the maintenance of an adequate heart rate, should be carefully observed. If bradycardia returns within a short time, temporary pacing may be required.

3. The nurse should ask the patient if he or she has a known history of glaucoma or difficulty in voiding. (Normally the physician would have determined these facts prior to ordering atropine, but for safety's sake, it is a wise practice to recheck this possibility.)

4. Because a dry mouth and blurred vision are common side effects of atropine, the nurse should advise the patient that these symptoms may occur, but are only temporary.

5. If the patient does not void for several hours after receiving atropine, suspect urinary retention and notify the physician.

Digitalis (Digoxin)*

Uses

1. To control atrial fibrillation associated with a rapid ventricular rate.
2. To terminate other rapid-rate supraventricular arrhythmias, particularly paroxysmal atrial tachycardia.

Actions

Digoxin exerts multiple and diverse effects on the electrophysical properties of the heart. Its main action is to increase the strength of myocardial contraction, but this effect is unrelated to its antiarrhythmic activity. Fundamentally, the drug controls arrhythmias by increasing vagal activity and slowing the rate of conduction in the AV node and in the bundle of His.

Methods of Administration and Dosage

1. Digoxin may be given intravenously or orally, depending on the urgency of the clinical condition.
2. In patients with rapid ventricular rates due to supraventricular arrhythmias, it is customary to administer 0.5 mg digoxin intravenously as an initial dose. Slowing of the ventricular rate begins within 15 minutes, and a maximum effect is usually reached within 1 hour. Depending on the heart rate response, an additional dose of 0.25 mg digoxin can be given within 3 hours if necessary; however, if the ventricular rate is adequately controlled by the initial dose, the second injection can be administered at 6 hours. Further doses of 0.25 mg or 0.125 mg digoxin may be given at 12 and 18 hours after the first injection. The total intravenous dose of digoxin in patients with acute myocardial infarction should not exceed 1.2 mg in 24 hours.
3. Oral administration of digoxin produces an effect within 2-6 hours and can be used in less critical situations. The oral dosage consists of 0.5 mg initially, followed by 0.25 mg every 6 hours for 2 additional doses, or until a satisfactory rate control is achieved. Subsequent doses of 0.125 mg or 0.25 mg digoxin may be given at

---

*This discussion considers digoxin only as an antiarrhythmic agent. (The use of digoxin in the treatment of heart failure has been discussed previously.) Although digoxin is but one of several cardiac glycosides used in the management of arrhythmias, it is by far the most popular digitalis preparation. Other agents, such as digitalis leaf, digitoxin, deslanoside, and ouabain, are not discussed here.

6-hour intervals if needed until a total dose of 1.5 mg is reached.
4. After a supraventricular tachyarrhythmia is terminated (or controlled) by digoxin, oral doses of 0.125 mg or 0.25 mg digoxin are administered once a day for maintenance purposes.

Contraindications

1. Digoxin should *not* be used to treat any arrhythmia that may in itself be a manifestation of digitalis toxicity (e.g., junctional tachycardia).
2. Because digoxin decreases conduction through the AV node, it should be administered with great caution in patients with ECG evidence of first- or second-degree AV block.
3. The presence of frequent premature ventricular contractions may be a relative contraindication to the use of digoxin because the drug tends to increase automaticity and to stimulate ectopic pacemakers; this action may precipitate ventricular tachycardia.
4. Acidosis, alkalosis, hypokalemia, and other electrolyte disturbances are known to increase sensitivity to digoxin. Thus the risk of inducing digitalis toxicity in patients with these conditions must always be weighed before selecting digitalis as an antiarrhythmic agent.
5. The combined use of digoxin and quinidine can produce elevated serum digoxin levels, leading to digitalis toxicity.

Side Effects

Cardiac Effects

1. In toxic doses, digitalis may induce practically any type of rhythm disturbance. Premature ventricular contractions (particularly in the form of bigeminy), nonparoxysmal junctional tachycardia, and paroxysmal atrial tachycardia with block are the most frequent digitalis-induced arrhythmias.
2. Digitalis toxicity also may produce second-degree heart block and, less frequently, sinus arrest.

Systemic Effects

1. Gastrointestinal symptoms include anorexia, nausea, and vomiting.
2. Central nervous system manifestations of digoxin overdosages are mental depression, confusion, and lassitude.
3. Visual complaints, although mentioned frequently in textbooks, are not especially common. Abnormal color perception and blurred vision are sometimes noted.

Nursing Implications

1. It is important for the nurse to ascertain precisely which digitalis preparation is to be administered. The dosages of the various drugs in the digitalis group are distinctly different. For example, the oral maintenance dose of digitalis (leaf) is 100 mg, the maintenance dose of digoxin is 0.25 mg, and the maintenance dose of digitoxin is 0.1 mg. Administering the wrong digitalis preparation may have fatal consequences.
2. There is only a narrow margin between a therapeutic and a toxic dose. Consequently it is essential to constantly seek signs suggesting digitalis toxicity.
3. If ECG or systemic signs of digitalis toxicity are noted or suspected, the nurse should withhold the next dose of digoxin until the physician has been consulted.
4. If the heart rate decreases to below 60/minute, the physician should be advised before further doses of the drug are given.
5. Because hypokalemia is a common cause of digitalis toxicity, the nurse should be aware of the serum potassium level before administering digoxin. This caution is particularly important in patients being treated concomitantly with diuretic therapy.

Bretylium Tosylate (Bretylol)

Uses

1. To control ventricular fibrillation that persists or recurs, despite conventional treatment, including electrical defibrillation and lidocaine.
2. To suppress or terminate recurrent or refractory ventricular tachycardia that fails to respond to adequate doses of lidocaine, procainamide, or other first-line antiarrhythmic drugs.

Actions

The exact mechanism of action of bretylium is still uncertain, but a combination of direct and indirect effects on myocardial cells is probably involved; the indirect effect (involving the autonomic nervous system) is more important. The key action of bretylium is to block sympathetic nervous system discharge at the nerve endings of the heart. However, before this beneficial action occurs, the drug may cause a release of stored catecholamines, which, unfortunately, can produce ventricular arrhythmias during the initial stages of therapy. In any case, the drug has a unique antifibrillatory effect: it is capable of restoring sinus rhythm in patients with ventricular fibrillation when other treatment measures have failed. Also, the drug differs from most other antiarrhythmic agents in that it does not reduce myocardial contractility in achieving its antiarrhythmic effect.

Methods of Administration and Dosage

1. In unconscious patients with ventricular fibrillation (or sustained ventricular tachycardia), undiluted bretylium is administered intravenously in a dosage of 5 mg/kg, as a bolus injection.
2. If ventricular fibrillation persists after the initial injection, resuscitation procedures must be continued, and another rapid intravenous injection given, in a dosage of 10 mg/kg. This larger dosage can be repeated every 15-30 minutes, if necessary, until a total dosage of 30 mg has been administered. Defibrillation should be attempted before and after each injection.
3. For conscious patients with recurrent ventricular arrhythmias, bretylium is administered in diluted form (e.g., 500 mg bretylium in 50 cc dextrose solution) over a period of 10 minutes, at a dosage of 5-10 mg bretylium/kg.
4. Maintenance therapy to prevent repeated episodes of life-threatening ventricular arrhythmias involves either a constant intravenous infusion of a diluted solution of bretylium (given at a dosage of 1-2 mg/minute) or intermittent intravenous infusions (5-10 mg/kg at 6-hour intervals).
5. Bretylium also may be administered intramuscularly. The customary dosage is 5-10 mg/kg. It can be repeated in 1-2 hours if the arrhythmia has not been suppressed.

Contraindications

1. There are no specific contraindications to bretylium in the treatment of ventricular fibrillation or other life-threatening ventricular arrhythmias.
2. The drug should *not* be used, however, as a first-line antiarrhythmic agent; it is reserved only to treat life-threatening ventricular arrhythmias that cannot be controlled with standard therapy.

Side Effects

Cardiac Effects

1. By far the most common adverse effect of bretylium is significant *hypotension*, often accompanied by lightheadedness, fainting, and vertigo. At least 50% of patients develop postural hypotension, which results from the blocking action of the drug on the nerve endings of the sympathetic nervous system (described as a "chemical sympathectomy").
2. The sudden release of stored catecholamines shortly after the drug is administered may produce transient *hypertension* and an increase in the frequency of ventricular ectopic activity. Also, the initial release of norepinephrine can precipitate digitalis toxicity; therefore, the concomitant use of digitalis and bretylium is potentially dangerous.
3. Bretylium potentiates the pressor effects of drugs like dopamine and Levophed; therefore, the dosages of these agents must be reduced when bretylium is used.

Systemic Effects

Nausea and vomiting are relatively common, particularly when the drug is given intravenously. These gastrointestinal symptoms, however, can usually be diminished by slowing the rate of the intravenous infusion.

Nursing Implications

1. Hypotension should be anticipated whenever bretylium is used. The patient should be kept in a supine position until a tolerance develops to the hypotensive effect of the drug, and the blood pressure stabilizes.
2. If the systolic blood pressure falls below 80 mm Hg (with the patient in a supine position), an intravenous infusion of dopamine or norepinephrine may be used to raise the pressure and control the hypotension. Careful monitoring of the blood pressure is mandatory during and after the administration of bretylium.
3. The possibility of hypertension or additional ventricular arrhythmias developing during the early stages of bretylium therapy must be kept in mind. Remember, too, that the hypertension is transient and will be followed by hypotension.
4. Because bretylium may be administered in several different ways according to clinical circumstances (diluted or undiluted, as a bolus injection or as an intravenous infusion, and intramuscularly), it is essential to verify the physician's order regarding the exact manner in which the drug is to be given.

Verapamil (Calan, Isoptin)*

Uses

1. To terminate episodes of paroxysmal atrial tachycardia (and other supraventricular tachycardias).
2. To slow the ventricular rate in atrial flutter and especially in atrial fibrillation.

Actions

As an antiarrhythmic agent, verapamil blocks the entry of calcium into cardiac cells. The main effect of this blockade is a slowing of conduction across the AV node. This particular effect explains the effectiveness of the drug in treating rapid atrial arrhythmias, but its ineffectiveness in treating ventricular arrhythmias. In addition, verapamil slows the sinus node and thereby reduces the heart rate. The drug causes only a mild reduction in cardiac contractility; however, cardiac performance can be diminished greatly under certain circumstances (see Contraindications).

Methods of Administration and Dosage

1. When used to terminate paroxysmal atrial tachycardia (or other supraventricular tachycardias), verapamil is administered intravenously in a dosage of 5-15 mg over 1-2 minutes. The drug acts very rapidly (usually within 1-5 minutes) and is successful in converting at least 80% of supraventricular tachycardias to sinus rhythm.
2. When used to slow the ventricular response to chronic atrial fibrillation, the drug is given orally in doses of 80 mg or 120 mg q.i.d.

Contraindications

1. Verapamil should *not* be used in patients with existing AV nodal conduction disorders. The slowing effect of the drug on conduction across the AV node may result in advanced heart block.
2. This agent is also contraindicated in the presence of sinus node disease, manifested by brady-

cardia. Verapamil slows sinus node discharge and, in this circumstance, can lower the heart rate to dangerous levels. Patients with sinus and AV nodal disorders can develop asystole during verapamil therapy.
3. Although verapamil does not usually reduce cardiac performance significantly, the drug should be used with great caution in patients with a past or present history of congestive heart failure. Of particular importance in this regard is that an overdose of verapamil may cause a marked decrease in cardiac contractility, leading to severe heart failure.
4. In general, the drug should *not* be used together with beta-blockers since the combination of drugs may precipitate congestive heart failure. At least 24 hours should elapse after discontinuation of beta-blocker therapy before calcium blocking agents are started.

Side Effects

Cardiac Effects

1. Verapamil may cause high-grade AV heart block or asystole, particularly in the presence of existing conduction disorders. However, the drug's slowing effect on the AV node is sufficient in itself to induce serious heart block.
2. Bradycardia is a frequent side effect, resulting from the inhibitory effect of the drug on the SA node. Moreover, sinus node slowing may be potentiated when verapamil is used in conjunction with other bradycardic drugs (e.g., digitalis and beta-blocking agents).
3. Hypotension develops occasionally; it is seldom severe.

Systemic Effects

1. The most common side effects of verapamil (and other calcium blockers) are nausea and constipation. The constipation can be very severe, sometimes necessitating discontinuation of the drug. On many occasions, however, adverse gastrointestinal effects abate after a few days.
2. Vertigo and headache are uncommon complaints during verapamil therapy. These central nervous system effects are usually mild and seldom are cause to discontinue the drug.

Nursing Implications

1. The heart rate should be monitored carefully during verapamil therapy to detect bradycardia from sinus node slowing.

---

*Verapamil is one of three types of calcium blocking agents now approved for clinical use. It has been evaluated more extensively than the two other drugs in this class (nifedipine and deltiazem), particularly as an antiarrhythmic agent. Since nifedipine has minimal antiarrhythmic activity and deltiazem resembles verapamil (as an antiarrhythmic), the following discussion concerns only verapamil, the prototype drug. As calcium blockers become better defined and their modes of action better understood, several new agents will probably be developed in the future.

2. Prolongation of the P-R interval, usually the first sign of decreased conduction across the AV node, can be detected only by frequent measurements of the ECG.
3. The possibility of the development of advanced AV heart block must always be considered in patients receiving verapamil.
4. Because the verapamil may potentiate other drugs being used concomitantly, it is important for the CCU team to review the patient's medications regularly. Drugs such as beta-blockers (Inderal), digitalis, disopyramide (Norpace), and other antiarrhythmic agents are potential sources of trouble.
5. Gastrointestinal side effects, especially constipation, must be evaluated carefully because decisions about the discontinuation of therapy may depend on the severity of these symptoms.

Potassium*

Uses

1. To abolish digitalis-induced tachyarrhythmias (e.g., paroxysmal atrial tachycardia with block or junctional tachycardia).
2. To suppress premature ventricular contractions that may be caused by a deficiency of potassium in myocardial cells.

Actions

The basic effect of potassium is to decrease the threshold of excitability and to increase intraventricular conduction. These actions are related to alterations in the exchange of sodium and potassium across the myocardial cellular membrane.

Methods of Administration and Dosage

1. In patients with acute myocardial infarction in whom arrhythmia control must be achieved promptly, potassium is often administered intravenously. In less critical situations the drug is given orally.
2. For intravenous use, 40 mEq potassium chloride is diluted in 500 ml 5% dextrose solution and the infusion is administered by slow drip during a 2- to 3-hour period. *Potassium should never be injected directly into a vein without being diluted.*
3. Oral dosage consists of a total 40-80 mEq potassium per day. This amount is divided into two, three, or four doses, depending on the concentration of potassium in the particular preparation being used. Oral potassium preparations should be given after meals with a full glass of water to minimize the saline laxative effect and gastrointestinal irritation.
4. The ultimate amount of potassium required to combat digitalis-induced arrhythmias is not constant; it depends on the severity of digitalis toxicity and the response to therapy.

Contraindications

1. Because of the threat of producing *hyperkalemia,* potassium should *not* be given to patients with evidence of renal insufficiency or failure (e.g., oliguria, elevated BUN) who are unable to excrete potassium loads.
2. A high serum potassium level is a definite contraindication for the use of potassium therapy. (Potassium should never be administered until the serum potassium level has been determined.)
3. Elevating the serum potassium level may increase atrioventricular block in patients with normal serum potassium levels. For this reason, potassium should *not* be used in the presence of second-degree or complete heart block unless the serum potassium level is markedly low to begin with.

Side Effects

Cardiac Effects

Although the initial effect of potassium is to decrease excitability and increase intraventricular conduction, these desirable effects may be reversed with prolonged infusion of potassium. Ultimately, conduction slows and excitability diminishes so that bradycardia or heart block may develop.

Systemic Effects

1. Nausea, vomiting, diarrhea, and abdominal discomfort may occur with the use of oral potassium.
2. Overdosage of potassium may lead to toxicity. Common manifestations of potassium intoxication are weakness, a feeling of heaviness of the extremities, listlessness, mental confusion, and a fall in blood pressure.

---

*Although not a true antiarrhythmic agent (in the sense of the drugs described in previous pages), potassium is nevertheless used frequently to treat digitalis-induced arrhythmias and ventricular arrhythmias. It is included in this section in light of its important role in the overall management of arrhythmias.

3. With intravenous administration, patients may experience pain or a burning sensation at the infusion site and along the venous pathway.

Nursing Implications

1. Potassium must *never* be injected directly into an intravenous line; the drug should always be diluted in at least 500 cc of fluid and administered by slow drip. The flow rate should not be greater than 20 mEq/hour. If the patient experiences pain at the intravenous site, the rate of infusion must be decreased.
2. Any change in heart rate, rhythm, or the duration of the QRS complexes occurring during potassium administration should be reported immediately to the physician.
3. The nurse should consider the possibility that continuous potassium infusion may produce hyperkalemia and therefore should observe the patient for signs of toxicity. In addition, the ECG should be examined carefully. Findings such as a narrowed peaked T wave, shortened QR interval, prolonged P-R interval, and diminished P waves may reflect hyperkalemia.
4. Oral potassium preparations should be given with a full glass of water (for reasons explained previously).
5. Serum potassium levels should be monitored regularly in all patients receiving potassium. The normal serum potassium level is 3.8-5.1 mEq. If the laboratory reports a serum level in excess of 5.1 mEq, the physician should be notified.

NEW ANTIARRHYTHMIC DRUGS

Amiodarone

Amiodarone, an investigational drug at present, has been used successfully to treat both supraventricular and ventricular arrhythmias. Also, it appears that this new agent is effective in preventing recurrent ventricular fibrillation and improving the long-term prognosis after resuscitation from sudden death.

The drug's actions are not fully understood at this stage, but it seems to antagonize the effects of sympathetic nervous system activity (although it is not a beta-blocking agent). In small doses it has very little effect on myocardial contractility.

Amiodarone can be administered intravenously and orally. The oral dose is usually 1200-2000 mg daily for 2-4 weeks, and then 200-800 mg daily as maintenance therapy. The intravenous dose is 5-10 mg/kg. The full antiarrhythmic effect of the drug may not be apparent for several days or weeks. However,

once effective, the drug has a remarkably prolonged effect, even after maintenance dosage is stopped. Indeed, the drug's antiarrhythmic effect may persist for 30-45 days after cessation of therapy, making it an ideal agent for long-term use against ventricular fibrillation and sudden death.

The main disadvantage of the drug is that it may slow the heart rate greatly and produce advanced AV block. The noncardiac side effects of amiodarone are of interest because of their uniqueness. For example, the drug causes the development of yellow-brown microdeposits on the cornea. The deposits generally impair vision and disappear after therapy is stopped. Among other reported side effects, probably more serious than the corneal deposits, are pulmonary fibrosis and infiltrates.

Despite these side effects, some believe that amiodarone has many attributes of an ideal antiarrhythmic agent, most particularly its very long duration of action, along with its minimal effect on myocardial contractility.

Aprinidine

Aprinidine is an investigational antiarrhythmic agent with demonstrated effectiveness in the treatment of ventricular arrhythmias and (to a lesser extent) supraventricular arrhythmias. Studies have shown that the drug is capable of controlling even the most serious ventricular arrhythmias, such as recurrent ventricular tachycardia and ventricular fibrillation.

The drug acts directly on cardiac cells and, therefore, its basic electrophysiologic properties resemble those of other direct-acting drugs, such as quinidine and procainamide. Aprinidine can be administered orally or parenterally. The drug is well absorbed from the gastrointestinal tract; its antiarrhythmic effect is evident within 2 hours. The usual oral dose is 100-150 mg per day in 2 or 3 doses.

Adverse systemic effects are very common with aprinidine therapy, and the toxic : therapeutic ratio is extremely narrow. Neurologic side effects, the most frequent complications, include tremor, ataxia, double vision, and nervousness. Jaundice and agranulocytosis also have been reported. Although the neurologic side effects are related to serum drug concentrations and perhaps can be controlled by dose reduction, the high incidence of these adverse effects may well limit the clinical use of aprinidine.

Encainide

This new antiarrhythmic agent appears to be very effective in the long-term suppression of ventricular ectopic beats. One of encainide's most attractive features is its prolonged antiarrhythmic effect, which may last for 12 hours or more during chronic oral therapy. This sustained action is related to two metabolites produced by the drug, which accumulate in the body and exert potent antiarrhythmic activity on their own.

The antiarrhythmic effect of encainide is associated with prolongation of the P-R interval and widening of the QRS complexes, indicating that the drug slows conduction significantly. This cardiac side effect can have serious consequences (e.g., the development of heart block), and for this reason encainide probably should be discontinued if the duration of the QRS complexes increases more than 30-40%. Other side effects include blurred vision, dizziness, and worsening of congestive heart failure. The side effects seem to be dose-related, and can be reduced by decreasing the dosage.

Flecainide

Flecainide, a relatively new antiarrhythmic drug, is structurally different than any other antiarrhythmic agent. The drug is reported to be highly effective against ventricular arrhythmias (both acute and chronic), as well as supraventricular tachycardias.

The drug is administered orally, and effective blood levels are achieved within 2-4 hours. The antiarrhythmic action is prolonged (about 16 hours), probably because the metabolites of the drug are excreted slowly. The recommended oral dose is only 200 mg twice daily. Intravenous administration is used less often; the IV dosage is 1-2 mg/kg, over a 5- to 10-minute period.

Flecainide is predominantly a direct-acting drug, but other effects are also being evaluated. The drug has no significant effect on heart rate or blood pressure. It does, however, slow conduction and prolongs the P-R and QRS intervals. In addition, flecainide reduces myocardial contractility (negative inotropic effect), but this undesirable action seems to be mild.

The attraction of the drug is its wide range of antiarrhythmic activity, its prolonged effect, and its relative safety. Nevertheless, the drug is contraindicated in patients with second- or third-degree AV heart block, because of the risk of inducing complete heart block or asystole. It is also withheld in the presence of advanced heart failure or cardiogenic shock.

Mexilitene

Like lidocaine, this drug is a local anesthetic agent that is effective in controlling ventricular arrhythmias. Its electrophysiologic properties closely resemble those of lidocaine, but unlike lidocaine, mexilitene can be administered orally. In this broad sense, the drug can be considered an oral form of lidocaine.

Mexilitene is highly effective in suppressing both acute and chronic premature ventricular contractions (and refractory ventricular tachycardia). The drug is absorbed rapidly after oral ingestion; however, when used in conjunction with analgesic agents or narcotics, which slow gastric emptying, absorption can be delayed significantly. The usual oral dose is 200-300 mg every 6 hours. Mexilitene can also be administered intravenously.

The main problem with mexilitene is its high incidence of side effects. Especially distressing are nausea and vomiting, which often necessitate the use of cimetidine (Tagamet) and antacids. Even more important are central nervous system side effects. including tremors, nystagmus, dizziness, ataxia, and confusion. The high frequency of adverse effects has tended to limit the use of mexilitene as a single antiarrhythmic agent and, therefore, attempts have been made to combine the drug in small doses (that do not produce toxicity) with other agents, such as propranolol. Combination therapy of this type may reduce or eliminate serious side effects, while retaining mexilitene's effective antiarrhythmic action. In any case, mexilitene appears to be a very useful oral agent for suppression of chronic PVCs (e.g., after acute myocardial infarction), but its toxic effects may be defeating.

Tocainide

Unlike lidocaine, which must be administered intravenously (or intramuscularly), tocainide is one of several new drugs resembling lidocaine that can be taken orally.

Tocainide is rapidly and almost completely absorbed within 60 minutes after oral administration, and its antiarrhythmic action is almost identical to that of lidocaine. It is used primarily to suppress ventricular ectopic beats and recurrent ventricular tachycardia, particularly if refractory to customary antiarrhythmic agents. In emergency situations, the drug also can be administered intravenously. However, the main advantage of the drug (in contrast to lidocaine) is that it can be used prophylactically on a long-term basis. The daily maintenance dose of tocainide has ranged from 400-1000 mg every 8 hours by mouth. The intravenous dosage is 0.5 mg/kg.

The drug is generally well tolerated and is considered a safe method of treatment. Gastrointestinal side effects, usually nausea and vomiting, are relatively common, but most often are mild and transient. Neurologic side effects have also been reported, but these are much less severe than those occurring with lidocaine. The drug can produce dizziness, vertigo, tremor, and nervousness; however, these neurologic side effects seem to be dose-related.

Appendix

EXERCISES IN THE
INTERPRETATION OF ARRHYTHMIAS

The 30 electrocardiograms presented in this section are meant to provide the reader with additional experience in interpreting arrhythmias. These exercises should not be considered a formal examination since, indeed, some of the arrhythmias were not discussed in detail in the text.

In interpreting these arrhythmias it is important to recognize that more than one arrhythmia may be present in the same rhythm strip. Therefore, do not jump to a conclusion about the interpretation of an arrhythmia. A particular abnormality may seem so obvious that it obscures other disorders. This problem can be avoided by always adhering to the basic 5-step format for interpreting arrhythmias used throughout this book. Remember that the use of an orderly process underlies successful ECG interpretation. Never make snap decisions.

Also to be considered in interpreting these (or any other) arrhythmias is the fact that many arrhythmic disorders cannot be identified specifically from a single monitoring lead. In order to reach a firm diagnosis, multiple ECG leads may be required. For this reason, whenever there is uncertainty about a particular finding (e.g., are P waves present or absent?), it is a sensible practice to simply state that more than one diagnostic possibility exists: the arrthythmia may be *either* sinus tachycardia *or* atrial tachycardia, for example.

The authors' interpretation of the 30 arrhythmias, along with pertinent comments about the diagnosis process, are found on the back of each page.

ECG 1

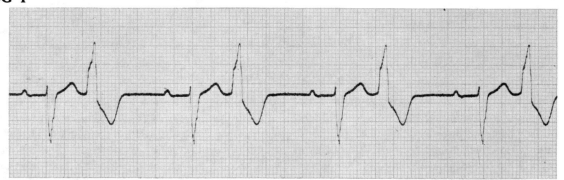

Interpretation:

_____
_____
_____
_____

ECG 2

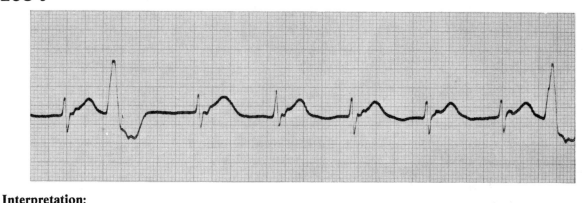

Interpretation:

_____
_____
_____
_____

ECG 3

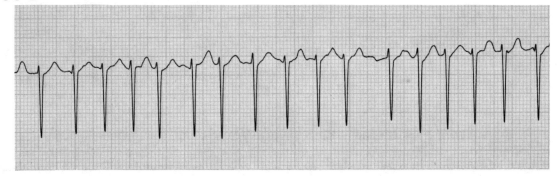

Interpretation:

_____
_____
_____
_____

ECG #1

Ventricular Bigeminy

First-Degree AV Heart Block
Intraventricular Conduction Defect

This ECG shows a disorder of impulse formation in conjunction with two disorders of conduction. The impulse formation disorder is manifested by PVCs occurring every other beat (ventricular bigeminy). The conduction disorders are a first-degree AV block (P-R interval of 0.28 second) and an intraventricular conduction defect (QRS is widened to nearly 0.12 second). The combination of a first-degree block and an intraventricular conduction defect reflects widespread involvement of the conduction system—a fact that must be taken into account when selecting an antiarrhythmic drug to control the PVCs.

ECG #2

Atrial Fibrillation with a Rapid Ventricular Response

The *irregular* ventricular rhythm and the absence of P waves clearly signify atrial fibrillation. The very rapid ventricular rate (180/minute) indicates that a high number of atrial impulses pass through the AV node to the ventricles. This rapid ventricular response can be slowed greatly with digitalis (or verapamil), which increases the extent of AV block. Atrial fibrillation with a fast ventricular rate is a hemodynamically inefficient rhythm and may lead to or precipitate heart failure.

ECG #3

Accelerated Junctional Rhythm
Premature Ventricular Contractions

Other than two PVCs, the remaining beats in this recording originate in the AV junction, as evidenced by P waves occurring *after* the QRS complexes. These junctional beats occur at a rate of 75/minute, which is faster than the inherent rate of an AV junctional pacemaker (40-60/minute); therefore the arrhythmia is designated an *accelerated junctional rhythm.*

ECG 4

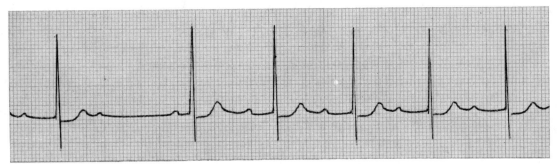

Interpretation:

_____

_____

_____

_____

ECG 5

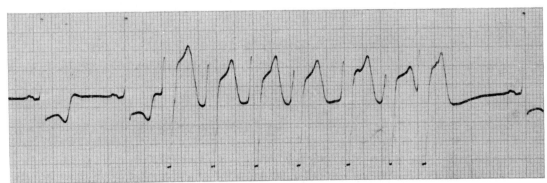

Interpretation:

_____

_____

_____

_____

ECG 6

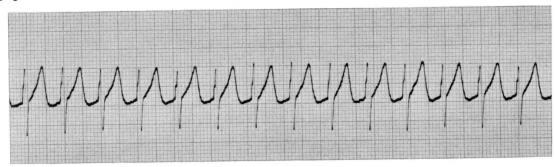

Interpretation:

_____

_____

_____

_____

ECG #4

Second-Degree Heart Block (Wenckebach-type)

The most characteristic feature of Wenckebach-type second-degree AV heart block is progressive lengthening of the P-R interval until a P wave is finally blocked. This sequence is demonstrated in the accompanying ECG, which shows the end of one Wenckebach period and the beginning of another. Note that the longest P-R interval (0.40 second) occurs immediately before the blocked beat (which ends one Wenckebach cycle). The shortest P-R interval (0.20 second) occurs immediately after the blocked beat, with the start of the next Wenckebach cycle.

ECG #5

Ventricular Tachycardia

After two sinus beats, seven consecutive premature ventricular contractions occur at a rate greater than 100/minute. Any run of three or more consecutive PVCs at a fast rate represents *ventricular tachycardia.* Although the episode shown here stopped spontaneously, as is often the case with ventricular tachycardia, lidocaine therapy was utilized subsequently to prevent further recurrences of this serious arrhythmia.

ECG #6

Supraventricular Tachycardia

From a single monitor lead recording, it is difficult to classify this arrhythmia in any more specific terms than "supraventricular tachycardia." The normal duration of the QRS complexes indicates that the tachycardia (140/minute) originated in either the atria or the junctional tissue (supraventricular) but not in the ventricles. Because of the inability to identify P waves specifically in this tracing, it cannot be determined if the arrhythmia is paroxysmal atrial tachycardia, paroxysmal junctional tachycardia, or atrial flutter with 2:1 block. Only by using additional leads can a definite interpretation be made.

ECG 7

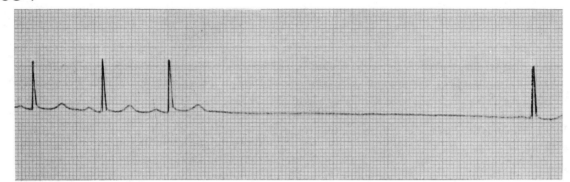

Interpretation:

_____

_____

_____

_____

ECG 8

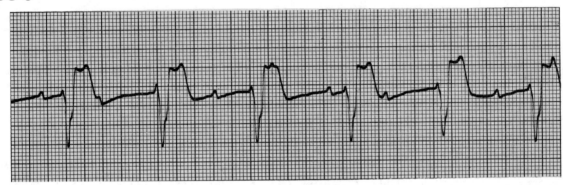

Interpretation:

_____

_____

_____

_____

ECG 9

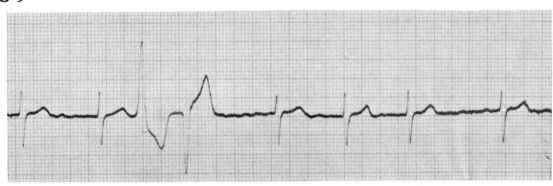

Interpretation:

_____

_____

_____

_____

ECG #7

Sinoatrial (SA) Arrest (or Block)

After two normal sinus beats, all electrical activity ceases for about 4 seconds (20 large boxes) before the next beat appears. The absence of P waves and QRS complexes during this period indicates that the SA node failed to initiate impulses (SA arrest) or that the impulses were blocked within the node (SA block). Prolonged episodes of asystole, as shown in this example, may result from ischemic injury to the SA node or from chronic disease of the SA node (sick sinus syndrome). In either case the temporary absence of a heartbeat for 4 seconds can produce syncope.

ECG #8

Complete (Third-Degree) Heart Block with Accelerated Idioventricular Rhythm

The P waves and QRS complexes bear no relationship, indicating that the atria and ventricles are beating independently of each other. The atrial rate is 100/minute while the ventricular rate is 60/minute. Since none of the atrial impulses is conducted to the ventricles, the disorder can be classified as a complete (third-degree) AV heart block. That the QRS complexes are wide (more than 0.12 second) suggests that the block is below the AV junctional area (subjunctional block) and that the ventricles are activated by a focus in the ventricles. In this circumstance the ventricular rate would be expected to be only 30-40/minute (the inherent rate of a ventricular pacemaker), but here the rate is 60/minute. This faster-than-anticipated ventricular rate probably reflects an accelerated idioventricular rhythm.

ECG #9

Premature Ventricular Contractions (PVCs) Occurring as a Couplet
Atrial Fibrillation

The underlying rhythm is atrial fibrillation, as evidenced by the absence of P waves and an irregular ventricular response. In this setting, two PVCs occur consecutively as a couplet (or pair). Couplets are a dangerous form of ventricular ectopic activity, often warning of ventricular tachycardia or ventricular fibrillation. The development of PVCs in patients with atrial fibrillation being treated with digitalis may be an indication of digitalis toxicity.

ECG 10

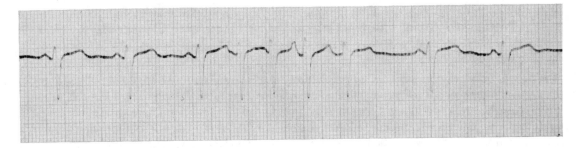

Interpretation:

_____
_____
_____
_____

ECG 11

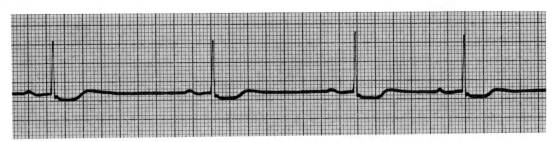

Interpretation:

_____
_____
_____
_____

ECG 12

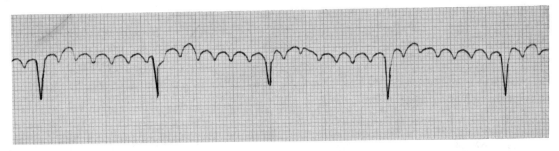

Interpretation:

_____
_____
_____
_____

ECG #10

Premature Atrial Contractions (PACs) Occurring Consecutively as a Short Run of Atrial Tachycardia

The fourth beat in this rhythm strip occurs prematurely and is associated with an abnormally shaped P wave (partially hidden in the preceding T wave). The configuration of the QRS complex is the same as normal sinus beats. From these facts we know the beat originates in the atria and that it is a premature atrial contraction (PAC). This atrial ectopic beat triggers 3 consecutive PACs (a total of 4 PACs) at a rate of about 150/minute, after which sinus rhythm returns. This brief burst of 4 consecutive PACs represents a very short run of paroxysmal atrial tachycardia. Brief runs of this type are the most common form of atrial tachycardia.

ECG #11

Sinus Bradycardia

Sinus Arrhythmia

First-Degree AV Heart Block

The average heart rate is about 40/minute. Since each QRS complex is preceded by a normal P wave, this slow rate arrhythmia is sinus bradycardia. However, the rhythm is distinctly irregular—a finding not normally anticipated with sinus bradycardia. The uneven rhythm is the result of sinus arrhythmia and is related to vagal changes during respiration. Sinus bradycardia and sinus arrhythmia often occur together because both arrhythmias are expressions of increased vagal activity. In addition, a first-degree AV block is also evident in this example (P-R interval 0.28 second). First-degree block may also be a manifestation of increased vagal tone. In other words, the combination of sinus bradycardia, sinus arrhythmia (disorders of impulse formation) and first-degree AV block (disorder of conduction) may all reflect vagal effects on the heart.

ECG #12

Atrial Flutter with Advanced AV Block

The typical sawtooth flutter waves (occurring at a rate of about 300/minute) identify this arrhythmia immediately as atrial flutter. The unusual feature of the ECG is the slow ventricular rate (about 50/minute). Most often atrial flutter is associated with a ventricular rate of 140-160/minute (atrial flutter with 2:1 block) or 70-80/minute (atrial flutter with 4:1 AV block). In this example, however, the extent of AV block is more advanced, with 6 flutter waves between each QRS complex (6:1 AV block). This indicates that the AV node is either injured or that the advanced block is due to drug therapy (e.g., digitalis). The administration of any drug that may increase AV block is clearly dangerous in this circumstance, and should be avoided.

ECG 13

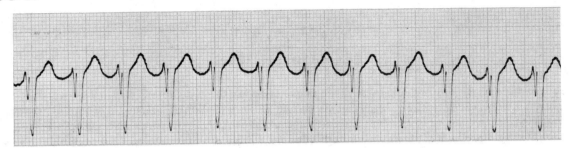

Interpretation:

_____

_____

_____

_____

ECG 14

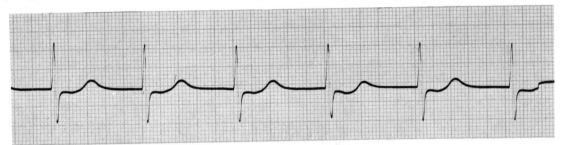

Interpretation:

_____

_____

_____

_____

ECG 15

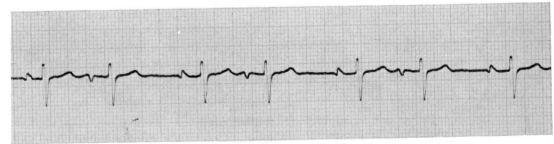

Interpretation:

_____

_____

_____

_____

ECG #13

Sinus Tachycardia

Bundle Branch Block

The lead from which this recording was made does not demonstrate definite P waves; however it does not exclude their presence. Therefore we cannot be certain if the arrhythmia is sinus tachycardia, an atrial or junctional rhythm or, even, a ventricular tachycardia (especially in light of the wide, distorted QRS complexes). Recognizing the importance of identifying this arrhythmia precisely, the nurse changed electrode positions, after which a normal P wave became clearly visible before each QRS complex (see ECG below). On this basis, the interpretation of the arrhythmia is sinus tachycardia. In addition to this disturbance in impulse formation (sinus tachycardia), there is evidence of an unrelated disturbance of conduction. The wide, distorted QRS complexes (0.16 second in duration) reflect a bundle branch block.

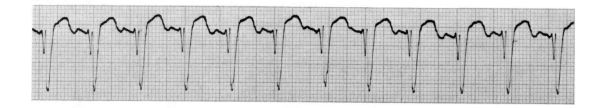

ECG #14

Junctional Rhythm

The ECG reveals a heart rate of about 60/minute, with a regular rhythm. No P waves are evident, indicating that the arrhythmia did not originate in the SA node or the atria. Since the QRS complexes are normal, it can be reasoned that impulses arise in the junctional area, and that the arrhythmia is a *junctional rhythm*. That a junctional pacemaker has assumed command means that the SA node must be discharging at a rate *slower* than the inherent rate of junctional tissue (40-60/minute). In this sense, a junctional rhythm is an escape rhythm.

ECG #15

Atrial Bigeminy

First-Degree AV Block

Every other beat is a premature atrial contraction (PAC) and, therefore, this arrhythmia is described as *atrial bigeminy*. Note that in this example the beats that arise in the atria are characterized by inverted P waves (in contrast to the upright P waves of the sinus beats). The P-R intervals of the sinus beats and the atrial ectopic beats are prolonged beyond 0.20 second, reflecting a delay in passage of all impulses through the AV node (first-degree AV block).

ECG 16

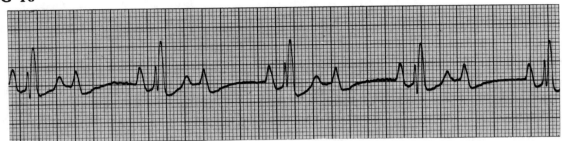

Interpretation:

_____

_____

_____

_____

ECG 17

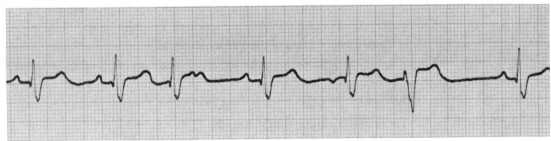

Interpretation:

_____

_____

_____

_____

ECG 18

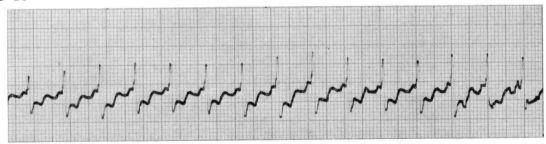

Interpretation:

_____

_____

_____

_____

ECG #16

Second-Degree AV Heart Block (Mobitz II Type)

There are two (tall) P waves between QRS complexes. Thus the atrial rate is twice the ventricular rate—a 2:1 heart block. This second-degree heart block is classified as a Mobitz II type because the P-R intervals are *constant* (unlike Wenckebach-type second-degree AV block, in which the P-R intervals lengthen progressively before a beat is dropped). The QRS complexes are very wide because Mobitz II blocks occur *below* the AV node.

ECG #17

Premature Atrial Contraction (PAC)
Premature Junctional Contraction (PJC)
Premature Ventricular Contraction (PVC)
Intraventricular Conduction Disorder

This tracing demonstrates three different types of ectopic beats: atrial, junctional, and ventricular. The third beat on this strip is a PJC, with the P wave occurring after the QRS complex. The fifth beat is a PAC, as evidenced by the abnormal (inverted) P wave. The following beat (the sixth on the strip) is a PVC. In addition to these ectopic beats, the QRS complex is widened (0.12 second), reflecting an intraventricular conduction defect.

ECG #18

Atrial Flutter with 2:1 Block

As a general rule, any supraventricular arrhythmia with a regular rhythm and a heart rate between 140-160/minute should be regarded as atrial flutter with 2:1 block, until proven otherwise. The heart rate in this example is 150/minute, and the rhythm is regular. Two P waves (which are initially inverted) occur between QRS complexes, creating the "sawtooth" appearance that characterizes atrial flutter. The diagnosis of atrial flutter with 2:1 block can easily be missed, unless its characteristic heart rate (140-160/minute) arouses suspicion of the problem.

ECG 19

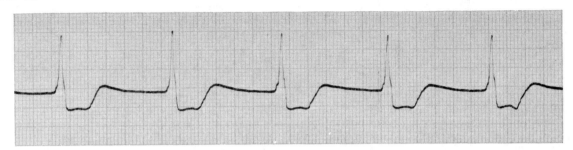

Interpretation:

_____

_____

_____

_____

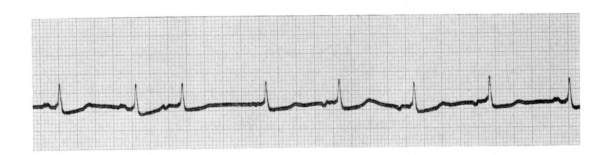

Interpretation:

_____

_____

_____

_____

ECG 21

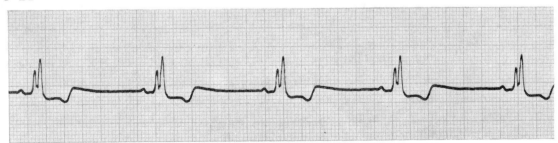

Interpretation:

_____

_____

_____

_____

ECG #19

Idioventricular Rhythm
Atrial Standstill

All of the beats in this rhythm strip originate in the ventricles, as revealed by the wide, bizarre QRS complexes and the absence of P waves before the QRS complexes. Although these ventricular ectopic beats occur consecutively, they do *not* represent ventricular tachycardia, since their rate is only 50/minute. The reason that the ventricles have taken over as pacemaker is that the atria have stopped initiating impulses (atrial standstill) and the junctional tissues have not come to rescue the heartbeat. In general, the complete absence of impulses from higher centers (atria and AV junctional area) usually indicates severe ischemia of these tissues, and is a manifestation of *downward displacement of the pacemaker* (before death occurs).

ECG #20

Wandering Pacemaker
Premature Atrial Contraction

The main diagnostic feature of a wandering pacemaker is a changing configuration of the P waves, indicating that the pacemaker is shifting between the SA node and an adjacent site in the atria or AV nodal area. In this particular example, the pacemaker moves temporarily from the SA node to the atria (the beats with the inverted P waves) after the occurrence of a premature atrial contraction. The last beat in the rhythm strip shows the return of a sinus pacemaker (upright P wave).

ECG #21

Bundle Branch Block
Sinus Bradycardia

The QRS complexes are wide (more than 0.12 second) and distorted. Since each complex is preceded by a normal P wave (and constant P-R interval), we know that these beats originate in the SA node and that the abnormal ventricular complexes are due to an intraventricular conduction defect (bundle branch block). The heart rate is only 45/minute, reflecting slow impulse formation (sinus bradycardia), which is unrelated to the bundle branch block.

ECG 22

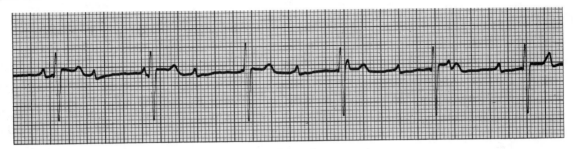

Interpretation:

_____

_____

_____

_____

ECG 23

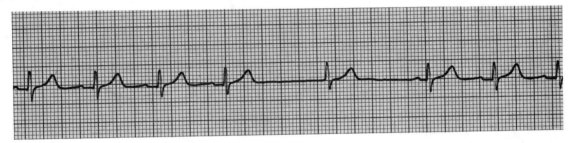

Interpretation:

_____

_____

_____

_____

ECG 24

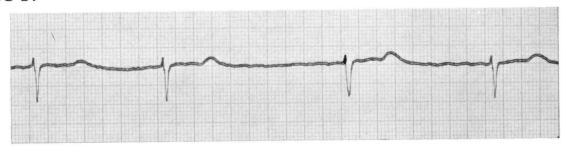

Interpretation:

_____

_____

_____

_____

ECG #22

Complete Heart Block with Narrow QRS Complexes (Junctional Pacemaker)

The diagnosis of complete heart block is based on the fact that the atria and ventricles are beating independently of each other and that no atrial impulses are conducted to the ventricles. The atria, activated by the SA node, are beating on their own at a rate of 100/minute. The ventricles are stimulated independently by a pacemaker in the AV junctional area, as evidenced by the ventricular rate of 60/minute along with narrow QRS complexes (with a ventricular pacemaker the anticipated heart rate would be less than 40/minute and the QRS complexes would be abnormally wide).

When the atria and ventricles beat independently, as in complete heart block, the condition is described by the broad term *atrioventricular (AV) dissociation.* However, AV dissociation is not synonymous with complete heart block since it may also occur with several other arrhythmias.

ECG #23

Junctional Escape Beat

After 4 normal sinus beats the SA node fails to discharge on impulse on schedule (probably as a result of sinus arrest or sinus arrhythmia). This causes a pause in the rhythm which finally ends when the AV junction "escapes" from SA control and produces a junctional escape beat. Unlike premature junctional contractions (PJCs) which occur before the next anticipated sinus beat, junctional escape beats occur only when sinus beats are delayed or absent. Thus, a junctional escape beat can be considered a protective mechanism to preserve the heartbeat when the SA node defaults.

ECG #24

Atrial Fibrillation with Advanced Atrioventricular (AV) Block

The rhythm is atrial fibrillation, as evident from the irregular R-R intervals and the absence of P waves. The very slow ventricular response reflects advanced block in the AV node, and may be due to drugs (especially digitalis) or AV nodal disease. In either case, atrial fibrillation with a ventricular rate of less than 50/minute results in serious hemodynamic consequences.

ECG 25

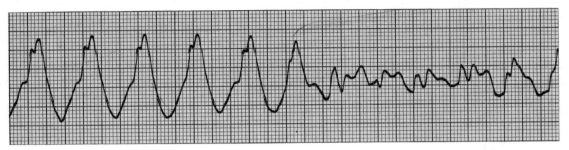

Interpretation:

_____

_____

_____

_____

ECG 26

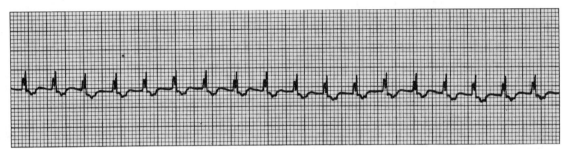

Interpretation:

_____

_____

_____

_____

ECG 27

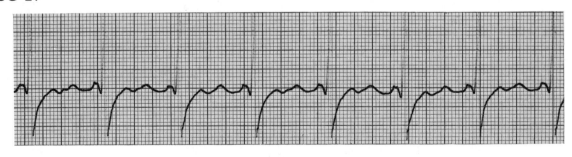

Interpretation:

_____

_____

_____

_____

ECG #25

Ventricular Tachycardia Deteriorating into Ventricular Fibrillation

The first 6 complexes in this strip represent a series of consecutive premature ventricular contractions in the form of *ventricular tachycardia.* Suddenly, the rhythm deteriorates into *ventricular fibrillation.* The onset of ventricular fibrillation after extremely widened, bizarre QRS complexes of the type demonstrated here, is often seen as a terminal event in patients dying of pump failure (secondary ventricular fibrillation).

ECG #26

Junctional Tachycardia

The key features of this ECG example are a very rapid ventricular rate (about 180/minute), with inverted P waves that *follow* the QRS complexes. The position of the P waves indicates that the arrhythmia originates in the AV nodal area (rather than the atria). The low amplitude of the complexes, as recorded in this particular monitoring lead, is disadvantageous, and makes interpretation more difficult.

ECG #27

Normal Sinus Rhythm with Prominent U Waves
Intraventricular Conduction Defect

At first glance this arrhythmia seems to resemble atrial flutter with 3:1 block. However, more careful inspection makes it evident that the three waves between each QRS complex are different in configuration and, more significicantly, are not regularly spaced (as they would be with atrial flutter). The wave between the T wave and P wave is called a U wave. It is frequently associated with low serum potassium levels. Also noted in this recording is abnormal widening of the QRS complexes (greater than 0.12 second), which reflects an intraventricular conduction defect.

ECG 28

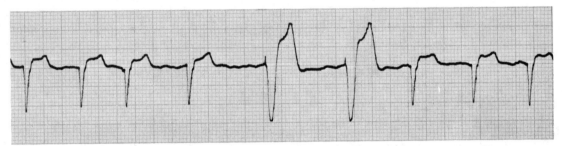

Interpretation:

_____

_____

_____

_____

ECG 29

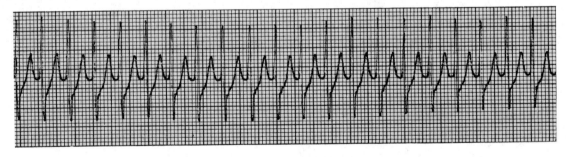

Interpretation:

_____

_____

_____

_____

ECG 30

Interpretation:

_____

_____

_____

_____

ECG #28

Ventricular Standstill
Atrial Standstill

After two isolated ventricular complexes, ventricular activity stops completely (ventricular standstill or asystole). That no P waves are visible before or after the onset of ventricular standstill suggests that atrial activity has ceased (atrial standstill) even before the terminal event. The cessation of atrial activity with the subsequent development of ventricular standstill usually indicates that death is due to *downward displacement of the pacemaker.*

ECG #29

Normally Functioning Demand Pacemaker
Atrial Fibrillation

The diagnosis of atrial fibrillation is readily apparent from the grossly irregular rhythm and the absence of P waves. After 4 atrial beats are conducted to the ventricles, the AV node blocks the next impulses, causing the ventricular rate to fall to 68/minute (22 small boxes). The pacemaker (which had been inserted because of periods of a slow ventricular rate) correctly senses this pause and discharges an impulse to stimulate the ventricles directly. A second pacing impulse is delivered when the advanced AV block persists. Atrial fibrillation with a faster ventricular rate then returns on its own after the 2 paced beats. The pacemaker functioned normally in this case: it sensed the pause created by the advanced block, and discharged impulses on demand. Also, the pacing impulses produced ventricular capture.

ECG #30

Atrial Tachycardia

The heart rate is 210/minute. It is evident that this tachycardia originated *above* the ventricles (supraventricular) since the QRS complexes are normal (0.08 second). Although it is agreed that this is a supraventricular tachycardia (SVT), how do we know the arrhythmia is atrial tachycardia (rather than junctional tachycardia or other SVT)? The key to the diagnosis is the unusual configuration of the T waves, which are sharp and peaked as the result of superimposed P waves.

Index